The Palgrave Lacan Series

Jacques Lacan is one of the most important and influential thinkers of the 20th century. The reach of this influence continues to grow as we settle into the 21st century, the resonance of Lacan's thought arguably only beginning now to be properly felt, both in terms of its application to clinical matters and in its application to a range of human activities and interests. The Palgrave Lacan Series is a book series for the best new writing in the Lacanian field, giving voice to the leading writers of a new generation of Lacanian thought. The series will comprise original monographs and thematic, multi-authored collections. The books in the series will explore aspects of Lacan's theory from new perspectives and with original insights. There will be books focused on particular areas of or issues in clinical work. There will be books focused on applying Lacanian theory to areas and issues beyond the clinic, to matters of society, politics, the arts and culture. Each book, whatever its particular concern, will work to expand our understanding of Lacan's theory and its value in the 21st century.

Max Maher

Symptom Invented

Lacan and the History of Marxism

palgrave
macmillan

Max Maher
De Montfort University
Leicester, UK

ISSN 2946-4196 ISSN 2946-420X (electronic)
The Palgrave Lacan Series
ISBN 978-3-032-12266-7 ISBN 978-3-032-12267-4 (eBook)
https://doi.org/10.1007/978-3-032-12267-4

Cover credit: Artefact

This Palgrave Macmillan imprint is published by the registered company Springer Nature Switzerland AG
The registered company address is: Gewerbestrasse 11, 6330 Cham, Switzerland

Acknowledgements

This book is based on my doctoral thesis, which I completed at the University of Essex in 2022. Many thanks to my doctoral supervisor Matt ffytche, for patient guidance and support throughout my studies at Essex. I am also very grateful to the Department of Psychosocial and Psychoanalytic Studies and the CHASE Doctoral Training Partnership, for generously funding my research. Thanks and salutations also to Ralph Hawkins, Tom Kügler, Neil Pattison, Véronique Voruz, the New Lacanian School, and everyone who has been part of the Psychoanalysis Society at Essex, for education, companionship, and everything else.

Competing Interests The author has no competing interests to declare that are relevant to the content of this manuscript.

Contents

1

Introduction

This book is about Lacan's place in the history of Marxist thought. It attempts to offer a more subtle, more complex, and more extensive account of Lacan's relationship with Marx than those that currently exist. The book reunites Lacan with a number of figures in and adjacent to French Marxism, with whom he is not usually understood to have been in dialogue, and it also adds nuance to existing accounts of the relationships he had with some of his better-known interlocutors. It reads these figures—including Jean Wahl, Jean Hyppolite, Alexandre Koyré, Alexandre Kojève, Lev Vygotsky, Georges Politzer, Henri Wallon, Louis Althusser, and others—in the context of a history of Marxist thought, and as participants in a moment of profound intellectual change, disruption, and anxiety. Dramatic shifts in the history of Marxism took place during the years this book focuses on. It reads each of these figures as contributors to a movement that did not leave Marx unchanged, and that put significant pressure on both his theories and their political implications. The book begins to narrate the history of a seismic shift in reading Marx, and it locates an apex of this shift in Lacan's work.

Lacan has recently come to be viewed, by many of his readers, as something of a true heir of Marxism. In a reading that has become increasingly

M. Maher, *Symptom Invented*, The Palgrave Lacan Series,
https://doi.org/10.1007/978-3-032-12267-4_1

dominant since Althusser's writings of the 1960s, Lacan has been hailed by a set of influential scholars as the messenger of a reformation of psychoanalysis, which is supposed to have restored the ways, as enigmatic as they are fundamental, in which Freud's project is in agreement with Marx's. Readings of this kind tend to make good use of the claims Lacan makes, in the late 1960s and early 1970s (when he starts to play up to, and take the wheel of, Althusser's application of his theories) that there exists a 'homology' between psychoanalysis and Marx's critique of political economy, and that Marx 'invented' the logic of the Freudian symptom. In light of these claims, Samo Tomšič, for example, is able to formulate that '[t]he place of the proletarian and the place of the subject of the unconscious is the same', and that 'psychoanalysis, as far as it consists in modifying the subjective relation to *jouissance*, should be considered in logical continuity with Marx's project of a critique of political economy'.[1] Tomšič's work is an extreme example of an attempt to unite Lacan and Marx. There are many other readers of Lacan—whose work is, for the most part, not published in English—who take the approach of putting forward a series of ways Lacan can be used to fine-tune or adapt something in Marx, to maximise the revolutionary potential of Marx's theories; pressing towards what David Pavón-Cuéllar calls a 'Lacanian Marxism'.[2] By this reading, Lacan can be used to complete something in Marx, because there is something inherently but unintentionally Marxist about his work.

But what of Lacan's other clearly articulated, and theoretically significant, points of divergence from Marx? Offsetting his supposed fidelity to Marx are the other well-known, enigmatic comments in which Lacan is fiercely critical of him: that he turned surplus *jouissance* into calculable surplus value, for example, or that communism is reliant on a misguided

[1] Samo Tomšič, 'Homology: Marx and Lacan', in *Journal of the Jan van Eyck Circle for Lacanian Ideology Critique*, 5 (2012), pp. 98–112 (pp. 110–111).

[2] David Pavón-Cuéllar, 'Lacanianizing Marxism: The Effects of Lacan in Readings of Marx and Marxist Thinkers', *Critique*, 6, no. 1 (May 2019), 262–289. For examples of this approach, see Pietro Bianchi, 'The Discourse and the Capitalist. Lacan, Marx, and the Question of the Surplus', *Filosofski vestnik*, 31, no. 2 (2010), 123–137; Ceren Özselçuk and Yahya M. Madra, 'Enjoyment as an Economic Factor: Reading Marx with Lacan', *Subjectivity*, 3 (2010), 323–347; and Roger A. Salerno, 'Imagining Marx Imagining Lacan', *Critical Sociology*, 44, no. 2 (2018), 259–266.

fantasy that social cohesion is possible.[3] Comments like these are the reason why, for others, Lacan can appear equally clearly as being opposed to Marxism. Eli Zaretsky, for instance, in *Secrets of the Soul* (2005), frames, if briskly, how the New Left 'paved the way' for Lacan, whose 'return to Freud' then amounted to a 'waning' of its movement and the 'end of its hopes for a Marx/Freud synthesis'.[4] For this historian—one of the few who situate Lacan against the French New Left—Lacan can only be seen as having betrayed the ambitions of Freudo-Marxism, in favour of a clinic of narcissistic liberalism. This was the classic position of the Marxists who publicly criticised Lacan in the 1960s, particularly during the attempted revolution of 1968. Typical of this is the abuse he receives during a lecture at Vincennes in 1969, from students who accuse him of academic obscurantism and liberal political inaction.[5] Lacanian psychoanalysis clearly does problematise, as Pavón-Cuéllar observes, the basic Marxist psychological theory of 'reflection', that understands consciousness as a direct image of conditions in the external world, putting in question whether Lacan's theory of subjectivity is at all compatible with a Marxist understanding of subjectivity.[6] The more recent turn to emphasising a theoretical continuity between Lacan and Marx has been made partly in rejection of this contrasting position, which has been voiced by many others that Lacanianism amounts to a deflation or bathos of the Marxist tradition.[7]

Lacan's relation to Marx is in need of rigorous clarification. Neither a straightforward cleaving of Lacan to a Marxist project, nor a positioning of his work as an apolitical ossification of Marxism, is able to register the

[3] See Jacques Lacan, *Seminar XVII: The Other Side of Psychoanalysis*, trans. by R. Grigg (London: Norton, 1991), pp. 107–108.

[4] Eli Zaretsky, *Secrets of the Soul: A Social and Cultural History of Psychoanalysis* (London: Three Rivers Press, 2005), p. 320.

[5] Lacan, 'Appendix A. Analyticon', in *Seminar XVII*, pp. 197–213.

[6] Pavón-Cuéllar, 'Lacanianizing Marxism'. For the 'reflection' theory, see Vladimir Lenin, *Materialism and Empirio-Criticism* (1908) (Peking: Foreign Languages Press, 1972).

[7] For other proponents of this view, see Michèle Barrett, 'Althusser's Marx, Althusser's Lacan', in *The Althusserian Legacy*, ed. by E. Ann Kaplan and Michael Sprinkler (London: Verso, 1993), pp. 169–182; David Macey, 'Althusser and Lacan', in *Althusser: A Critical Reader*, ed. by Gregory Elliott (Oxford: Blackwell, 1994), pp. 142–158; and Joe Valente, 'Lacan's Marxism, Marxism's Lacan (from Žižek to Althusser)', in *The Cambridge Companion to Lacan*, ed. by Jean-Michel Rabaté (Cambridge: Cambridge University Press, 2010), pp. 153–172.

complexities and subversions that were—as is made clear by a serious reading of his work—put in play by him. Both of the approaches summarised above reduce Lacan and Marx to inert, monadic objects, who were not already, at the time when Lacan was working, thoroughly and inextricably intertwined. To read Lacan as a theoretical appendage of, or a supplement to Marx's theories, is to affix Lacan to Marx as if the two came from separate worlds, and were not already part of the same history. On the other hand, to read Lacan as the enemy of Marx abstracts him both from the serious engagements he makes with Marx, and from the whole set of themes and questions that he takes, and often significantly develops, from the Marxists working around him. A relationship between Lacan and Marx does not need to be improvised by contemporary scholars in the way that it has been so far. Their relationship simply needs to be articulated, by thorough, sustained work on the history of their connections. This book begins to demonstrate the extent of this historical entwinement.

There is a history of Marxism that goes unacknowledged by the literature summarised above. The following chapters read Lacan as a *part* of the history of Marxism. They argue that an elision of the historical context of Lacan's relationship with Marx has resulted in a portrayal of their relationship as something straightforward, simple, and unequivocal. The reason why Lacan looks like a miraculous missing piece of Marxist theory to many contemporary scholars, and as a defacer of Marx to others, is, this book argues, because his theories converged onto so many of the points of crisis encountered in the work of his Marxist contemporaries. Lacan was part of a specific historical movement of readers of Marx, which had its own themes, its own trajectory, and its own key problems. His unique responses to these can only be understood by restoring this history as a context for his work.

Lacan the French Marxist

In the fourth lesson of *Seminar XVI: From an Other to the other* (1968–69), Lacan recalls reading *Capital* for the first time, in 1921, as a young medical student.[8] This first reading of the book took place, he reminisces, on the Paris Metro on the way to work. The 20-year-old Lacan's copy of *Capital*—which is 'falling apart' as he gives the seminar in 1968—was already, when he first read it in 1921, an object representing a precarious history of Marxist thought in France. Lacan's copy of the book would have been the translation *Le Capital*, which was worked on by Marx himself, and which had been published in serial form between 1872 and 1875. This was, as Kevin Anderson asserts, in an article on this "unknown" version of the text, 'no mere translation'; it contained 'greatly expanded' versions of the two pivotal sections on accumulation and fetishism of commodities, and remains 'to this day the standard text of the work' in French.[9]

Whilst the French benefitted in this respect from a version of *Capital* that Marx himself claimed to possess 'a scientific value independent of the original', which 'should be consulted even by a reader familiar with German', aside from this volume, the only writings of Marx that existed in French before 1914 were *The Communist Manifesto* and the political histories.[10] In general, Marxism had a relatively slow incorporation into French intellectual life. There was no Communist Party in the country until 1920, and a definitively French voice in Marxism would only appear after the First World War.[11] Due in part to reticence by the dominant Durkheimian circle of sociologists and anthropologists to engage almost at all with Marxists, the French academy initially resisted assuming

[8] Lacan, Lesson of 4 December 1968, 'IV. Facts and What is Said', in *Seminar XVI: From an Other to the other*, ed. by Jacques-Alain Miller, trans. by Bruce Fink (London: Polity, 2024), pp. 48–61, (p. 49).

[9] Kevin Anderson, 'The "Unknown" Marx's *Capital*, Volume I: The French Edition of 1872–75, 100 Years Later', *Review of Radical Political Economics*, 15, no. 4 (1983), 71–80 (pp. 71–3).

[10] Karl Marx, *Capital: A Critique of Political Economy, Volume 1* (1867), trans. by Ben Fowkes (London: Penguin, 1976), p. 105.

[11] See Arthur Hirsh, *The French New Left: An Intellectual History from Sartre to Gorz* (Boston: South End Press, 1981), p. 8.

responsibility for, or advocating Marxism.[12] French Marxism then went through a famously prolific expansion during the inter-war period, stimulated in part by the social inequality made visible by the First World War and Wall Street Crash. It was in this context that, in 1920, in the wake of the 1917 October Revolution, the French Socialist Party became the French Communist Party. Intellectually, this began an era characterised by a return to reading Marx as a philosopher in France, and the proliferation there of new connections between Marxist theory, science, and everyday life.[13]

During the 1920s and 1930s, translations of Marx and Engels, and secondary writings on dialectical materialism, began to trickle into France from Eastern Europe. But this period also saw the emergence of an indigenous French Marxist theory with its own concerns, which, often explicitly rejecting the materialist dogma of the USSR, tended to return to the philosophical basis and context of Marx's work. Towards the end of the 1920s (alongside, incidentally, a decline in the CFP's working-class membership), three significant groups of intellectuals began to associate themselves with the Party, and to explore themes and questions that would be crucial in the following decades, in writing that was published in a host of new journals centred on Marxist thought.[14] The first of these were the writers and artists of the Surrealist movement. Founded by Andre Breton, and including Louis Aragon, Paul Eluard, and Tristan Tzara, they were committed to the fermentation of revolution through their provocative art, and their theories were explicitly, if eccentrically, dialectical. The

[12] See Pradeep Bandyopadhyay, 'The Many Faces of French Marxism', *Science & Society*, 36, no. 2 (Summer, 1972), 129–157 (p. 134). Bandyopadhyay notes Durkheim's own later reading and assessment of Marxist thought, and cites his reviews of historical materialism, mainly Labriola's, in his *Sociologie et l'Action Sociale* (Paris, 1969). As Bandyopadhyay describes, the hard divisions between disciplines in French universities enabled Marx's decisively interdisciplinary writings to be cloven up and deposited into economic, historical, and anthropological pigeon-holes, and thus made it possible for the Durkheimians to overlook them; even so, French economists still had no interest in the theories of *Capital*, committed as they were to Böhm-Bawerk's and Pareto's theories of marginal analysis, nor did historians pay serious attention to his work.

[13] For accounts of early French Marxism, see Bandyopadhyay, 'The Many Faces of French Marxism'; Hirsh, *The French New Left.*; Tony Judt, *Marxism and the French Left: Studies on Labour and Politics in France, 1830–1981* (Oxford: Oxford University Press, 1985); Kelly, *Modern French Marxism* (London: Wiley-Blackwell, 1982); Paul McGarr, Alex Callinicos & John Rees, *Marxism and the Great French Revolution* (London: International Socialism, 1989).

[14] Bandyopadhyay, 'The Many Faces of French Marxism', p. 135.

second of these new groups was a small association of philosophers who produced work, between 1929 and 1934, facilitating a more assured grasp of Marxist theory. The group centred around the *Philosophies* journal, whose contributors included Henri Lefebvre, Georges Friedmann, Georges Politzer, Pierre Morhange, and Paul Nizan, who sought to challenge the dominant French traditions of Cartesian rationalism and Bergsonian vitalism.[15] A third group, this one comprised of scientists, centred on another journal, *La Pensée, revue du rationalisme moderne*, and included physicists Paul Langevin and Frédéric Joliot-Curie, biologist Marcel Prenant, and the psychologist Henri Wallon. Both of these latter groups—in stark contrast to the Surrealists—sought to cast Marxism as the apotheosis of positivism, and to ally dialectical materialism with the natural sciences: Marx's theories, Politzer claimed, amounted to 'no more than the scientific understanding of the universe', and were the heir of Diderot's eighteenth-century materialism.[16]

There was a sense amongst French Marxist intellectuals at this time—one that was clearly influenced by the reformations being carried out in all areas of human life in the early, pre-Stalinist years of the Soviet Union—that Marxism could be the basis for a revived, alternative canon of intellectual life and culture across all areas. This was reflected in the scope of the three groups described above: Marxist exhibitions on the frontiers of philosophy, science, and art. There was, however, a crisis clearly underlying this era of French Marxism, in the tension between this spirit of liberation and innovation, on the one hand, and the Stalinist orthodoxy that dominated the Communist Party, on the other.[17] Stalin's interpretation of Marx and Lenin was taken by many European communists to be authoritative, and was for the most part open to no debate in Communist Parties. His reading of dialectical materialism, or 'diamat', as

[15] Mark Poster, *Existential Marxism in Postwar France: From Sartre to Althusser* (Princeton: Princeton University Press, 1975), p. 36.

[16] Georges Politzer, *Principes élémentaires de philosophie* (1935–1936) (Paris: Éditions sociales, 1970), p. 21. See Poster, *Existential Marxism in Postwar France*, p. 37.

[17] The oppressive intellectual atmosphere created by the Communist Party under Stalin is widely documented. See Poster, *Existential Marxism in Postwar France*, pp. 36–42 for an exemplary account. Bandyopadhyay argues well for the overlooked innovations made by intellectuals affiliated with the Party, though her account weighs heavily on the developments made by the group normally associated with Althusser and with structuralist thought in the 1960s.

it was labelled, was a reduced form of Marx and Engels's theories, that presented them as a completed dogma to be accepted by intellectuals, with no room for development.[18] This bolus of Marxist theory divided it, in summary, into dialectical materialism—which, as Mark Poster comments, was a 'phrase never used by Marx'—and historical materialism.[19] According to Stalin, the dialectic was the metaphysical abstraction of objective reality, the 'secondary [...] reflection of matter' in the mind, and materialism referred to the 'primary' material exterior. Historical materialism amounted essentially, in his account, to an economic theory, which presented the superstructure as entirely, mechanically dependent on the material base, without any level of autonomy.[20] Diamat was imposed by the Party as a script that its intellectuals could only rehearse and re-rehearse, making them actors in the drama of the Cold War conflict between Sovietism and capitalism; Marxism, in the guise enforced by the Communist Party under Stalin, had been metabolised, and put purely into the service of defending Sovietism. An appropriately scandalous symbol of this state of decadence was the support, in the utilitarian interest of preserving a stable Europe, that Stalin gave to Charles de Gaulle after WWII. French communist intellectuals were left with a dilemma: kowtow to the Stalinist distortions, or risk being lumped with American anti-communists.

A backlash against this deadlock came partly in the form of a return to Marx's texts, and partly by the sudden emergence of a new tradition of Marxist thought in Europe of the early 1920s. The publication of György Lukács' *History and Class Consciousness* in 1923 began the intellectual movement usually known as Western Marxism (emphasising its distinction from the 'Eastern', Soviet interpretation). Lukács's work salvaged a latent humanist, subjectivist, and undogmatic Marxism from the Stalinist dogma, which reduced the disillusionment and sense of stagnation it had

[18] Mark Poster, *Existential Marxism in Postwar France: From Sartre to Althusser* (Princeton: Princeton University Press, 1975), p. 39.

[19] See Joseph Stalin, 'Dialectical and Historical Materialism', in *Leninism: Selected Writings* (New York, 1942), pp. 406–433.

[20] Reducing man, as this does, to a robotic *homo economicus*, would be a decisive point of contention by the existentialist movement. See Poster, *Existential Marxism in Postwar France*, p. 40.

produced, and reinvigorated hopes of emancipation in socialist thought.[21] One hallmark of this new tradition was the close attention it paid to the relationship between Marx and Hegel, particularly as it existed in Marx's early work. In France, this drama between Marx and Hegel both expressed, and acted as the stage on which the reservations of French intellectuals to Soviet dogma could be played out. The narrative of Marx's departure from and correction of Hegel had already become a commonplace in Marxist writings prior to the 1930s: Marx and Engels themselves had made it clear in key works exactly what use they understood Marx to have made of Hegel, in the 'Afterword' to *Capital* (1867), for example, or the beginning of *Anti-Dühring* (1877).[22] Influential works by Lenin and Georgi Plekhanov translated into French in the late 1920s had also paid due service to the Hegelian origins of dialectical materialism, but Hegel manifests in them as a figure in the background, rather than a presently active force for enabling the comprehension of Marxist theory. The 1930s saw much greater attention being paid in France to Marx's intellectual origins in Hegel. These early years of the 1930s also saw a famously significant upsurge in French Hegelianism itself: Alexandre Koyré called for a revival in French Hegel studies in 1930, Alexandre Kojève began his Seminar on Hegel at the Ecole Normale Supérieure in 1933, and Jean Hyppolite began to write about and translate Hegel in 1935. Auguste Cornu's *Karl Marx, l'homme et l'oeuvre* (1934), an intellectual biography of Marx's early life, sought, in this context, to 'expose the formations' of Marx's thought by tracing its early development. The biography definitively places the intellectual development of the young Marx as having

[21] See Martin Jay, *Marxism and Totality: The Adventures of a Concept from Lúkaks to Habermas* (Berkeley: University of California Press, 1984), p. 2. Following Lúkacs were the equally influential figures of Antonio Gramsci, Karl Korsch, and Ernst Bloch. Martin Jay further expands the remit of Western Marxism to include the Frankfurt School, Marcuse, and even Habermas. Decisively with regards to psychoanalysis, some of these later Western Marxists were open to supplementing Marx with psychological theories, and used Freud to think about alienation as a psychic phenomenon; others drew on Gestalt psychology or the work of Jean Piaget.

[22] See Karl Marx, 'Afterword to the Second German Edition' (1873), in *Capital: A Critique of Political Economy*, trans. by Samuel Moore and Edward Aveling (London: Lawrence and Wishart, 1974), pp. 12–22 (p. 19). 'The mystification which dialectic suffers in Hegel's hands, by no means prevents him from being the first to present its general form of working in a comprehensive and conscious manner. With him it is standing on its head. It must be turned right side up again, if you would discover the rational kernel within the mystical shell.'

been 'dominated by the thought of Hegel', and as 'situated in the setting of the evolution of the Left Hegelians'.[23] Cornu's biography provided the connection between Hegel and Marx on a historical level that Kojève was offering at the same time on an epic, almost prophetic one. *L'homme et l'œuvre* also made a direct challenge, from the new historical angle of biography, to any diminishment of the role Hegel had played in Marx's development, and signalled the arrival of a definitively French Marxism alongside, and intertwined with, the self-consciously French Hegelianism developing simultaneously.

Broadly speaking, the proponents of the French Marxist movement were acknowledging that political progress was not just a case of necessary resourcefulness—of sensitivity to their material, historical conditions, or awareness of the tools at their disposal. It was becoming clear at this time—most explicitly with regards to Hegel—that there was a much more pressing need for Marxists to come to terms, and better collaborate, with their own historical inheritance, and with their own context in the history of philosophy. Revolution—for the likes of Henri Lefebvre and Norbert Guterman, in their Leninist interpretation of Marx, or following the incremental acceptance of Hegel aided by philosophers such as René Maublanc—would, it increasingly seemed, be dependent on subtlety of interpretation and intellectual shrewdness, not least because of serious contradictions and aporias in Marx which had been made clear to his students of this era.[24]

Accounts of the history of French Marxism do not give Lacan a significant position. On the one hand, historical studies of the French New Left—and its development out of the anguished conflict between Hegelio-Marxist phenomenology, and the vanguards of a Communist Party dominated by the Stalinist Second Internationale—tend, overlooking that Lacan's earliest work had a basis in phenomenological psychology, to reduce him to a representative of structuralism, mouthing his

[23] Auguste Cornu, *Karl Marx, l'homme et l'œvure: De l'hégélianisme au matérialisme historique (1818–1845)* (Paris: Librairie Félix Alcan, 1934), p. 394.

[24] See Norbert Guterman and Henri Lefebvre, *La Conscience mystifiée* (Paris: Gallimard, 1936); and René Maublanc, 'Hegel et Marx', in *A la lumière du Marxisme* (Paris: Editions Sociales Internationales, 1935), pp. 189–232.

name off a list including, invariably, Althusser, Barthes, and Foucault.[25] On the other hand, studies that attempt a more sensitive, comprehensive immersion of Lacan in the context of philosophy contemporary to him, whilst usually covering useful ground, do so with a lack of precision that risks eliding Lacan's deliberate ambivalence towards philosophy, and tend to overlook the potential incompatibility between philosophy and psychoanalysis.[26] This is especially surprising considering that Lacan's reading of Marx is entirely in keeping with the dedication to purity, precision, and idol-smashing that characterised readings of Marx from this era. The confusions created by the *1832 Manuscripts*, or by the question of Marx's general relationship with Hegel, or by the major questions posed to and by Stalinism, meant that Marx could definitively not, for Lacan's contemporaries, be viewed as a static endpoint to an unveiling of truth that had been completed in the late nineteenth century. All serious readers of Marx from Lacan's era had to offer a stance on where Marx could be positioned with respect to the idealism epitomised by Hegel, and on how the contradictions and transitions in Marx's own oeuvre could be reckoned with. Their writings also make it clear just how many potential answers there were to this question.[27] Lacan is not usually thought of as one of those weighing into these debates—but his interventions, as the following chapters will show, contribute to them with just as much sophistication and relevance as any of his contemporaries.

Rather than understanding Lacan as either Marxist or anti-Marxist, then, this book instead presents him as a part of an intellectual

[25] In addition to the histories of French Marxism referenced above, the following give Lacan either surprisingly little attention, or none at all: Nathan Coombs, *History and Event: From Marxism to Contemporary French Theory* (Edinburgh: Edinburgh University Press, 2015); Kelly, *Modern French Marxism*; William S. Lewis, *Louis Althusser and the Traditions of French Marxism* (Lanham: Lexington Books, 2005); Poster, *Existential Marxism in Postwar France: From Sartre to Althusser*.

[26] See, for example Phillippe van Haute, 'Psychanalyse et existentialisme: A propos de la théorie lacanienne de la subjectivité' *Man and World: An International Philosophical Review* (October 1990), 453–472; Daniel C. Knudsen, Jillian M. Rickly, Elizabeth S. Vidon, 'The Fantasy of Authenticity: Touring with Lacan', *Annals of Tourism Research*, 58 (May 2016), 33–45; Louis A. Sass, 'Lacan: The Mind of the Modernist', *Continental Philosophy Review*, 48, no. 4 (December 2015), 409–443.

[27] See, for example, Maurice Godelier, *Rationalité et Irrationalité en Economie* (Paris: Éd. Maspéro, 1966); Lucio Colletti, *Il Marxismo e Hegel* (Laterza, 1969); Trần Đức Thảo, 'Le "noyau rationnel" dans la dialectique hégélienne', in *La Pensée* (Jan-Feb 1965), 4–5; and Kelly, *Modern French Marxism*, for a historical summary of these different approaches.

movement that was making it increasingly unclear, firstly, what it would mean to be 'Marxist'; secondly, whether it was possible to be Marxist; and thirdly, whether carrying the effort of Marxism to fruition would mean sacrificing something of Marx. The book also reads Lacan's work in the context of a set of serious questions that were being asked about how to think about history, and specifically how to think about Marx's position in history. Lacan's contemporaries were concerned with the extent to which 'Marx' could be understood as the name for a profound shift that happened historically—or even the name for a profound shift in the nature of what history *is*—and they were attempting to formulate exactly what this shift amounted to. When Lacan's reading of Marx is approached in this way, it can be understood as having crystallised something acutely about the concerns of his generation's readers of Marx, and as having done so in ways that often took their own questions to a limit.

The Argument

This book will restore to Lacan some dimensions of the conceptual and sociological detail of French Marxism, and of traditions of thought closely associated with it, which preceded and were contemporary to his work. The four chapters of the book will carry out detailed historical studies of three fields—French Hegelianism, dialectical materialist psychology, and structuralist theories of history—with a focus on how conceptual impasses that were encountered in these areas formed the basis for Lacan's own theories. The book will show how central concerns in these fields are given a new designation in Lacan's reading of Marx.

The following two chapters of the book discuss two intellectual movements in philosophy and science that presented pressing questions for French Marxist thought in the early twentieth century. Chapter 2 is about French Hegelianism. As described above, the question of the relationship between Hegel and Marx was of obsessive concern in mid-century France, but the way Hegel was read in this context was the result of a protracted and turbulent drama of his reception there. The history of French Hegelianism is usually made to pivot around a 'Hegel renaissance' supposed to have occurred the 1930s—and Lacan's own reading of Hegel is also routinely reduced to two of its main players, Kojève and Hyppolite. This chapter gives an account of Hegel's French reception that sees it as a less straightforward narrative. It was, the chapter illustrates, a drama of confusion and misrecognition that created a set of pressing questions for French readers of Hegel. The chapter pays close attention to one particular theme of French Hegel studies from the early decades of the century, which is not usually associated with Lacan: the conflict that was first articulated by Kierkegaard, between existence and concept, which centred in France on readings of the figure of the 'unhappy consciousness' from Hegel's *Phenomenology of Spirit* (1807). Lacan distils a theoretical schema from Hegel that is crucial to the way he later approaches Marx. This, the chapter argues, was a response to questions first raised by the French readers of Hegel that it discusses.

Both French Marxists and French Hegelians encountered a problem in the early twentieth century, in a conflict they identified in these philosophers' oeuvres, between dialectical logic, on the one hand, and the ephemera of subjective existence on the other. Chapter 3 describes how this same problem was addressed in a different field, by the movement, begun in the Soviet Union, and continued in France, that sought to give the spiritualistic, introspective science of psychology a dialectical materialist revival. As a consequence of this theoretical experiment, the chapter illustrates, psychology came to act as a screen for the most significant pressure-points of the relationship between idealism and materialism. The unconscious repeatedly appeared as an equivocal concept for the psychologists who were attempting to produce this new psychology. It seemed, for several of them, to hold great materialist potential, yet also to bear witness to the idealist sins committed by Freud. This chapter makes detailed discussion of three materialist psychologists from Russia and France who made significant but ambivalent use of Freud: Lev Vygotsky, Georges Politzer, and Henri Wallon. The chapter then performs a close reading of Lacan's responses to the materialist psychological movement. It shows how Lacan sought to rewrite instabilities he identifies at the conceptual foundation of materialist psychology, in his own theory of the instance of the signifier in the unconscious. Lacan, the chapter illustrates, also thereby apprehends flaws that he considers to exist at the conceptual basis of materialism itself.

Following the discussions of these early twentieth century intellectual movements, the final two chapters of the book discuss two specific readings of Marx made in the 1960s and early 1970s—that of Louis Althusser, and Lacan's own. These chapters focus on the attention given by both Althusser and Lacan to Marx's position in the history of science. As summarised in Chap. 3, one of the main questions facing materialist psychology was how this science could view its subjects independently of any spiritual, subjective excess, whilst also giving an adequate model for phenomena that were usually located on this extra-material level. Chapter 4 picks up this theme by outlining how an equivalent problem was encountered by Althusser, when he attempted, in his rendition of Bachelard's 'epistemological break', to theorise the role played by Marx's subjective personhood in the shift he takes Marx to have brought about in the history of science. Althusser's work of the 1960s attempted to solve this problem by adopting from Spinoza a logic of the 'symptom'. The chapter describes how Althusser expanded this 'symptomatic' reading of Marx into a model for the movement of the history of science in general. It identifies the problems that resulted from his attempt to make this expansion. The conceptual errors Lacan finds at the foundation of materialist psychology recur, the chapter argues, in Althusser's theory of the history of science. As a result, despite Althusser's attempt to ascribe a pivotal position to psychoanalysis in the history of science, Lacan's own understanding of this history should be viewed in stark contrast to Althusser's own.

The final chapter discusses in detail the extended use of Marx made by Lacan in the late 1960s and early 1970s. It gives particular attention to the positions he attributes, in these years, to Marx and to psychoanalysis in the history of science. In 1968, in *Seminar XVI: From an Other to the other* (1968–69), Lacan announces that a 'homology' exists between his and Marx's theories—that they have a continuous logic—and he develops a theory of the signifier and *jouissance* that redeploys the theory of value laid out in Marx's critique of political economy. Though it usually goes without comment, Lacan also makes another impressive claim at this point. Marx, he argues, does not represent an antidote to capitalism, but, when his theories are understood by way of Lacan's theory of discourse, they can be seen to have actually played an unwitting, central role in the operation of capitalist logic. Marx, he claims in *Seminar XVII: The Other Side of Psychoanalysis* (1969–70), 'founded capitalism'.[28] Lacan gives Marx a fundamentally paradoxical status. This, the chapter illustrates, is a key element of what Lacan also demonstrates about psychoanalysis at this point. Tying together questions encountered in the fields discussed in previous chapters, Lacan gives psychoanalysis a historical position that would make it the inheritor of the paradox that Marx introduced into science. For Lacan, psychoanalysis is able to decipher something new about the natures of capitalism and science as a result. However, it also attributes to Marx a new degree of responsibility for their operations.

The aim of this study is not just to provide some much-needed historical context to Lacan's reading of Marx. It also seeks to demonstrate that using Lacan as a tool to modify Marx, or casting him as a nemesis of Marxism, makes no sense when either this context, or his texts, are taken seriously. It took Lacan time to articulate a position with respect to Marx, because this position is more subtle than the parties demanding his allegiance usually understand it to be. One clear obstacle to achieving this more precise reading of Lacan is that many of his texts, particularly his later ones, have not yet been published, and even fewer have been translated into English. This book builds up a historical account of the context in which Lacan responded to Marx. It uses this as a background to read some of Lacan's texts that have received less attention in English—the untranslated seminars of the mid-60s: *Seminar IX: Identification* (1961–62); *Seminar XII: Crucial Problems for Psychoanalysis* (1964–65); *Seminar XV: The Psychoanalytic Act* (1967–68); and Lacan's famous, but untranslated radio interview 'Radiophonie' (1970). What this study makes clear is the way in which these texts express and respond to impasses that already existed in Marxist thought. The contemporary fascination with Lacan as a political thinker, or as someone who enabled a new way of approaching politics, can then be re-evaluated without an oversimplification of his position.

[28] See Lacan, Lesson of 11 March 1970, 'VII. Oedipus and Moses and the Father of the Horde', in *Seminar XVII*, pp. 102–117 (pp. 107–108).

2

How to Repeat Hegel: Lacan and the French Hegelians

As the Introduction to this book summarised, the relationship between Marx and Hegel became an object of intense fascination and anxiety amongst French communists in the 1930s, to the extent that reading Marx with Hegel became a distinguishing feature of French Marxism. Lacan's own thinking about Marx is also intimately bound up with his thinking about Hegel. From the mid-1960s onwards, Lacan claims that Marx is responsible for the logic of the Freudian symptom.[1] This amounts to his own rearticulation of how Marx made the break from Hegel that was the subject of such controversy, and of so many different renditions, by mid-century French Marxist philosophers. The significance of Hegel's status in Lacan's work is a commonplace in virtually all literature about Lacan, and certainly in writing that documents his early influences.[2] The story is well known: amidst the vogue for reading Hegel in France of the 1930s, Lacan attended the seminars of Alexandre Kojève, butted heads

[1] See Lacan, 'On the Subject Who Is Finally In Question' (1966), in *Écrits*, trans. by Bruce Fink (London: Norton, 2006), pp. 189–196 (p. 194).

[2] See Juan Pablo Lucchelli and Todd McGowan, 'The Early Lacan: Five Unpublished Letters from Jacques Lacan to Alexandre Kojève', *American Imago* 73, no. 3 (Fall 2016), 325–341; David Macey, *Lacan in Contexts* (London: Verso, 1988); and Caroline Williams, 'Philosophy and Psychoanalysis: Lacan, Kojève and Hyppolite on the Concept of the Subject', *Parallax* 3, no. 1 (1997), 41–53.

M. Maher, *Symptom Invented*, The Palgrave Lacan Series,
https://doi.org/10.1007/978-3-032-12267-4_2

with the Existentialists, and hosted Jean Hyppolite in his own seminars—his early work is marked by enthusiastic Kojèvian Hegelianism, but this was put under greater pressure as he developed his theories further. One aim of this chapter is to find a different beginning to Lacan's relationship with Hegel, by extending its scope much further back, to Hegel's earliest reception in France. If the beginning of Hegel's role for Lacan is usually located in his attendance of Kojève's seminar in the 1930s, this chapter will locate this origin far earlier, in the historical background of the passion for Hegel that appeared in French intellectual life in this decade.

At the other end of the historical trajectory of the relationship between Lacan and Hegel is the work of Slavoj Žižek, and a moment where what is at stake is whether Lacan can be flattened into Hegel. In a project begun in *The Sublime Object of Ideology* (1989), and continuing into contemporary work, Žižek reads Hegel for the ways he strategically undermines attempts to outstrip his own thinking, so that all of Lacan's rejections of Hegel can be read as commentaries on the subtleties of Hegel's own thought. This chapter will argue that such a strategy of positing wilful slavery to Hegel has a history that goes back to the earliest years of Hegel's reception in France. This history does not surface in Žižek's work, but it conditions it inescapably. The reading of Hegel that Žižek weaponises is the product, the chapter will demonstrate, of a set of questions about Hegel that existed from the early phases of his reception in France.

The first part of this chapter summarises the history of the French reception of Hegel, with particular attention to its dramas of confusion and controversy, and for the assortment of very different ways that Hegel was represented in France before his resurgence of popularity there in the 1930s. It deliberately resists characterising these as 'misrepresentations' of Hegel. As the chapter will describe, the most astute and committed of Hegel's readers realised that reading Hegel amounted not to filtering off these misrepresentations to attain a pure version of Hegel, but to involving oneself, as a reader, in a drama *of* competing misrepresentations. French readers of Hegel discovered, the chapter shows, a conflict between fractional moments of a philosophy, each of which threatened to eclipse the others. The chapter then pays close attention to one particular theme of French Hegel studies from the early decades of the twentieth century:

the conflict between 'existence' and concept, which was played out in readings of the figure of the 'unhappy consciousness' from Hegel's *Phenomenology of Spirit* (1807). Lacan, the chapter will argue, revises Freud's theory of transference to capture the consequences of the flux that, as acknowledged by the French Hegelians, exists at the heart of Hegel.

The chapter positions Žižek as one of the characters who participated in the (long-) twentieth-century historical romance of French Hegelianism that it describes. It argues that Žižek's attempt to give a post-Lacanian reading of Hegel unintentionally produces a pre-Lacanian one, because it does not pay attention to the detail of the readings of Hegel that were made by Lacan's contemporaries. Žižek does not, as a result, communicate the particular ways in which Lacan responded to and modified the concerns of these readers of Hegel. The chapter seeks to restore this context to Lacan's Hegel, in order to articulate his particular strategy of reading the philosopher—a strategy which, as later chapters will develop, forms a vital component of the reading of Marx that he carries out in the late 1960s and early 1970s.

The Reception of Hegel in France

> [T]he Philosopher is the man who changes, essentially; and who changes consciously, who wants to change, who wants to become and to be other than he is, and wants all this solely because he does not know that he is satisfied by what he is. [...] If the Wise Man serves as the model for himself and for others (which means: for Philosophers, that is, for those who tend toward the ideal realized by the Wise Man), the Philosopher is, so to speak, a negative model: he reveals his existence only in order to show that one must not be like him, to show that man wants to be not Philosopher, but Wise Man. Hence the Philosopher changes because he *knows* what he ought *not* to be and what he *ought* to become. In other words, he realizes a progress in his changes.[3]

[3] Alexandre Kojève, 'Philosophy and Wisdom: Complete Text of the First Two Lectures of the Academic Year 1938–1939', in *Introduction to the Reading of Hegel*, trans. by James H. Nichols, Jr. (London: Cornell University Press, 1980), pp. 75–99 (p. 87).

> We must learn at every moment to dispense with this subject who is supposed to know. We cannot at any moment have recourse to it, this is excluded [...] the fact is that this subject of ours [...] we could not approach any closer than is done in this exemplary dream which is entirely articulated around the sentence: "he did not know that he had died".[4]

The first of the passages above is the concluding flourish of a lecture given in 1938 at the École Normale Supérieure, by Alexandre Kojève. It came towards the end of a seven-year Seminar, started in 1933, in which Kojève gave an extended, detailed commentary on Hegel's *Phenomenology of Spirit* (1807). He would begin each session of the Seminar by translating several lines of the original text into French, 'emphasizing certain words', as Raymond Aron recalls, before speaking for the remainder of the lecture 'with no notes, without ever stumbling over a word, in an impeccable French accent', made 'original and fascinating as well' by his Slavic intonation.[5] Giving a thorough exposition of a handful of lines each lecture, Kojève read through the *Phenomenology* in this way, passage by passage, from beginning to end. Like all the richest interpretations of Hegel made in France in these decades, Kojève's intent focus on a single text in no way diminishes the novelty of his concerns. Kojève is known equally well for making Hegel's dialectic of master and slave the formal principle that drives the dialectical narrative of the *Phenomenology* as he is for the realism that he gives to his rendition of Hegel's 'End of History'. The effusion of political peace and human contentment that this eschatological moment is supposed to bring is, as Kojève describes above, signalled by the replacement of philosophy's search for truth by the serene self-consciousness of Wisdom. At this point, as Kojève presents it, philosophy is to undergo an almost sacrificial disappearance.

Kojève's lectures had a decisive impact on French intellectual life. His regular audience included such headlining names in art and philosophy

---

[4] Lacan, Lesson of 22 November 1961, in *Seminar IX: Identification* (1961–1962), unpublished. Available in an unofficial English translation by Cormac Gallagher at <http://www.lacaninireland.com/web/wp-content/uploads/2010/06/Seminar-IX-Amended-Iby-MCL-7.NOV_.20111.pdf>, p. 13.

[5] Raymond Aron, *Mémoires: Cinquante Ans de réflexion politique* (Paris: Julliard, 1938), pp. 94–100. Cited in Denis Hollier ed., *The College of Sociology, 1937–39* (University of Minnesota Press, 1988), p. 86.

as George Bataille, Raymond Aron, André Breton, Maurice Merleau-Ponty, and of course, Jacques Lacan.[6] In addition to the dazzling content of his Seminar, Kojève's very presence in the institutional platform he had been given exerted a magnetic influence on his audience.[7] Kojève was a Russian emigré, and nephew of the abstract artist Wassily Kandinsky. He had completed his PhD in Berlin under Karl Jaspers, and since the 1920s had been friends with the French philosopher and historian of philosophy Alexandre Koyré, who he had met in Heidelberg.[8] When Koyré left Paris in January 1934 to teach in Cairo, he had enlisted Kojève to continue his course on Hegel at the École Pratique des Hautes Études.[9] Not only in his performative charisma and his celebrity, but also in his Russianness, and his sympathies with Stalinism, would Kojève—formerly Alexander Kojevnikoff—have been 'rather disconcerting to proper French university professors', John Heckman imagines, invoking figures such as 'the then influential Leon Brunschvicg'.[10] As Simone de Beauvoir reflects with regret in a memoir, Brunschvicg had 'systematically ignored Hegel and Marx' in his work and teaching.[11] Brunschvicg represents for Heckman, as he did for de Beauvoir, a traditional academic philosophy which was resistant to a radical spirit of innovation represented by Hegel. Kojève's provocative glamour made him an electrifying representative both of the neglected philosopher, and of a new generation of intellectuals in a process of a spirited break with the old.

This neglect had been addressed by Koyré two years before the start of Kojève's Seminar, in a presentation at the first Hegel Congress in La Haye

[6] For a full list of participants in Kojève's seminar, see Michael S. Roth, 'Appendix', in *Knowing and History: Appropriations of Hegel in Twentieth-Century France* (Cornell University Press, 1988), pp. 225–227.

[7] See Aron, *Mémoires*, pp. 94–100.

[8] Michael S. Roth, *Knowing and History*, p. 95.

[9] Roth, *Knowing and History*, p. 95, n. 3.

[10] John Heckman, 'Introduction', in Jean Hyppolite (1946), *Genesis and Structure of Hegel's Phenomenology of Spirit*, trans. Samuel Cherniak and John Heckman (Illinois, Northwestern University Press, 1974), pp. xv–xli (p. xxiii).

[11] Simone de Beauvoir (1958), *Memoirs of a Dutiful Daughter*, trans. by J. Kirkup (New York: Harper, 1959), p. 243. The specific text that 'systematically ignored Hegel and Marx', and that reduces Marx to 'one of the obscurest reactionary thinkers' is 'a big book' by Léon Brunschvicg 'on "the progress of consciousness in the Occident"', presumably *Le progrès de la conscience dans la philosophie occidentale* (Paris: Alcan, 1927).

in 1930. His 'Rapport sur l'état des études hégéliennes en France' ('Report on the State of Hegel Studies in France') began with an apology that this summary would appear 'very thin and very poor in comparison' to his German, English, and Italian colleagues, whose nations enjoyed a rich tradition of work on Hegel.[12] The article also summarises the approaches of the three main voices in French Hegelianism at the time. Firstly, Emile Meyerson, who enabled a vital rehabilitation of the infamous *Naturphilosophie*, a prevailing headache to even the most loyal of Hegelians, in his *De l'explication dans les sciences* (1922).[13] Secondly, Victor Basch, who not only made a happy emphasis on the importance of comprehending Hegel's work as a whole, rather than an isolated sketch of one corner of his work, but who also rescues Hegel, in his *Les doctrines politiques des philosophes classiques de l'Allemagne* (1927), from the allegations of totalitarianism and amorality which had so often beleaguered the French understanding of his politics. By contrast, Basch's Hegel is a teacher of morals and of liberty, his ethics amounting 'not [to] a morality of duty but to one of Being'.[14] Koyré turns, finally, to Jean Wahl, whose focus, anticipated by Emile Bréhier and Lucien Herr, on the unhappy consciousness of Hegel's *Phenomenology*, makes the young Hegel's Romanticism, mysticism, and Christianity the key to his entire system, and its 'life and blood'; the abstract formulas of the concept being, in this reading, only their 'pale and distant expressions'.[15] Though Koyré adds in passing his own course on Hegel at the École, and Charles Andler's teaching at the Collége de France, he considers Meyerson, Basch, and Wahl to represent the 'three roads leading to Hegel' in France, and optimistically regards their heretofore success as a sign of Hegel studies to come.

Even a short summary of the main points in Koyré's article shows its history of French Hegelianism to be broad and complex. In this respect, its disparity with many other accounts of this narrative is stark. Koyré's report is an important document in challenging the notion, regularly

[12] Alexandre Koyré (1930), 'Rapport sur l'état des études hégéliennes en France', in *Études d'histoire de la pensée philosophique* (Paris: A. Colin, 1961), p. 205. All citations from the article will be given in my English translation.

[13] Koyré, 'Rapport', p. 215.

[14] Koyré, 'Rapport', pp. 220, 222.

[15] Koyré, 'Rapport', p. 222.

invoked by more recent, oversimplified accounts of this reception history, of a French 'Hegel renaissance': the vignette of a 'sudden prominence of Hegel' after the Second World War signifying 'a break with traditions of thought', which, while attempting to account for a true phenomenon, is cartoonish after reading Koyré's rich, sensitive 1930 text.[16] And only a serious confusion could describe Koyré's report, as Mark Poster does in his history of French Existentialism, as a straightforward lamentation of 'utter absence of interest in Hegel'.[17] This neglects entirely Koyré's overall tone of hopeful optimism for contemporary French Hegelianism, and attentive respect for its antecedents.

Koyré concludes his 'Rapport' by voicing his hope for Andler to release a book which would be 'for Hegel, what the books of [Victor] Delbos and of Xavier Léon have been for Kant and for Fichte'.[18] In retrospect, this hope was misplaced: there was to be no single text to mark a clean entry-point for Hegel into French culture, nor a single delegate who would deliver it. It is a desire similar to Koyré's which has both misled so many with regards to this reception history, and motivated attempts to find some watershed or point of origin in Kojéve's 1933–40 Seminar, or Hyppolite's translated *La Phénomenologie de l'esprit* (1939), or Wahl's *Le Malheur de la conscience dans la philosophie de Hegel* (1929), or to generate conglomerates from them to serve this narrative function. The prejudice is unintentionally disclosed by Poster: before an 'abrupt turn to Hegel in the 1940s', he describes, '[o]nly "offbeat" intellectuals like André Breton's surrealists and a circle of young Marxists in the 1920s paid tribute to the German dialectician'.[19] If the tributes of these less savoury parties manifested the presence of Hegel in France, then they should not be glossed over. These unregistered, subtle undercurrents of Hegelianism which Poster brushes aside had been precisely the kind acknowledged by Koyré as the missing piece of this historical puzzle. Yet their 'offbeatness' is pronounced by Poster as being sufficient to justify their historical repression. Against this pursuit of a clean and simple narrative, the unclean, 'offbeat'

[16] Mark Poster, *Existential Marxism in Postwar France: From Sartre to Althusser* (Princeton: Princeton University Press, 1975), p. 3.

[17] Poster, *Existential Marxism*, p. 3

[18] Koyré, 'Rapport', pp. 226–27.

[19] Poster, *Existential Marxism*, pp. 3–4.

Hegel who existed in glimpses and caricatures beyond the institution of French academia was not separable from the Hegel who was read and, frequently, misunderstood by philosophers in France. Even more conservative readers of Hegel could not quarantine themselves from the awkwardness of this history, and the myth of Hegel fashioned by it. The version of Hegel formed from a texture of caricature and rumour created the negative space into which the mirage of the 'Hegel renaissance' was projected.

The Hegel of Surrealism

Hegel was equally, perhaps more, popular beyond traditional academic circles. The 'Hegel renaissance' inspired not only philosophy, but also an abundance of theological, mystical thought. This work almost always drew on the revolutionary theories of the Surrealists, a key component of which was, and had been since the movement's foundation in the 1920s, Hegelian dialectics. André Breton, the founder of the Surrealist movement, had been reading Hegel as early as 1924, the year he wrote the first 'Manifesto of Surrealism'—five years before Wahl would publish *Le Malheur de la conscience* (1929), and three years before even Basch's *Les doctrines politiques* (1927). Hegel's texts had already become orthodox for Breton by this point: Henri Lefebvre, the Marxist philosopher and early affiliate of the Surrealist movement, recalls, meeting Breton that year, how '[h]e showed me a book on his table, Véra's translation of Hegel's *Logic*, a very bad translation, and said something disdainfully of the sort: "You haven't even read this?"'.[20] The founder of Surrealism might be described as an unsung hero, if a Quixotic one, of this entire reception history. Breton envisaged the Hegelian dialectic as the process by which a plane of unconscious reality could be brought together with everyday, conscious life, imagining 'the future resolution of these two states, dream

[20] Henri Lefebvre, *Les temps des méprises* (Paris: Stock 1975), p. 49.

and reality, which are seemingly so contradictory, into a kind of absolute reality, a *surreality,* if one may so speak'.[21]

A loose appropriation of Hegel's dialectical mechanism informed this theory of revolutionary process. Breton later makes a more explicit engagement with Hegel in his 'Second Manifesto' of 1930. Invoking Hegel to belittle the objections cast against the Surrealist's extension of poetic innovation to political struggle, Breton refers to the distinction made in Hegel's *Elements of the Philosophy of Right* (1820) between the 'formal conviction' of morality and the 'true conviction' which 'occurs initially only in social life'.[22] But the 'Second Manifesto' also proclaims Breton's intention to take Hegel, not only beyond idealism, but even beyond philosophy. The Surrealists, Breton adds compellingly, 'also intend to place ourselves at a point of departure such that for us philosophy is "outclassed"'—in part by dialectical materialism, but also by the surreality to which their movement was dedicated.[23]

Despite the moments of doe-eyed commitment to Hegel espoused above, the Surrealists' Hegelianism was realised at best erratically. The Surrealists, as Martin Jay comments, certainly rejected Hegel's 'rationalist logocentrism';[24] and, where the Hegelian dialectic eventually overcomes contradictions in a final synthesis, Surrealism advocates the continuous preservation of dissonance, to reveal 'a new whole'.[25] Worse is the

---

[21] André Breton, 'Manifesto of Surrealism' (1924), in *Manifestoes of Surrealism,* trans. by Richard Seaver and Helen R. Lane (University of Michigan Press, 1969), pp. 1–48 (p. 14).

[22] Breton, 'Second Manifesto of Surrealism' (1930), in *Manifestoes of Surrealism,* pp. 117–194 (p. 138).

[23] After the reservations voiced in the 'Second Manifesto', Breton returned to Hegelian aesthetics a year later as the basis for that of Surrealism, in a lecture on the 'Surrealist Situation of the Object' (1935). His praise for Hegel in the lecture is unguarded: Hegel had, says Breton, not only already 'attacked all the problems that on the plane of poetry and art may today be considered to be the most difficult', but 'with unparalled lucidity he solved them for the most part', so that only an obstinate ignorance and 'lack of knowledge' could lead to 'anxiety or pretexts for endless controversy' over these already-defeated problems. See Breton, 'Surrealist Situation of the Object' (1935), in *Manifestoes of Surrealism,* pp. 255–278 (p. 258). The principal achievement of Hegel's philosophical machine was, Breton says here, '*dialectically* reconciling these two terms—perception and representation—that are so violently contradictory for the adult man', allowing the Surrealists to 'thro[w] a bridge over the abyss that separated them' (p. 278).

[24] Martin Jay, *Marxism and Totality: The Adventures of a Concept from Lukáks to Habermas* (Berkeley: University of California Press, 1984), p. 286.

[25] Jay, *Marxism and Totality*, pp. 286–287.

diagnosis of Ferdinand Alquié, who not only 'do[es] not believe Breton's project is the same as Hegel's', but who also suspects that 'the confusion of the two projects—partly responsible for the obstinacy of Surrealists in declaring themselves partisans of the Marxist dialectic—has done the greatest disservice for Surrealism'.[26] Alquié emphasises the disjunction between, on the one hand, Hegel's preference of 'History to the individual', 'discursive language to intuitive evidence' and 'universal verity to personal certitude', and on the other, Breton's affirmation of the 'rights of the individual man', along with the value placed by Surrealism on errancy and singularity.[27]

The fact that Surrealism slipped questionably far from Hegelian philosophy of any real rigour is a useful indicator of Hegel's part in French intellectual life at this point. That Hegel could be taken up and assimilated by a community of thought as chimerical, disorderly, and revolutionary as the Surrealist movement is a further indication of the place of unstable, forbidden object that his work had come, since the nineteenth century, to occupy in France. Breton's wielding of Hegel like a weapon or battle standard also bears witness to a common association of the philosopher's name with power, intrigue, and countercultural vogue. Though Alquié might resist it, his very frustration indicates that Hegel had already been assimilated to intellectual currents beyond those of traditional philosophy. Despite Alquié's critique, the Surrealists have a place reserved in every account of French Hegelianism, many of which address them with far less dismissiveness than Poster.[28] Their appropriation was no more dubious than any other French reading of Hegel—indeed, than Alquié's own. It was certainly more promising for French Hegelianism than the

---

[26] Ferdinand Alquié, *The Philosophy of Surrealism*, trans. by Bernard Waldrop (University of Michigan Press, 1965), p. 34.

[27] Alquié, *The Philosophy of Surrealism*, p. 35. Though Alquié acknowledges the genuine attraction posed to Breton by a Hegelian collapse of metaphysics into subjectivity, he attributes Breton's 'seduc[tion]' by the dialectic as, not only a mere means 'to explain his own poetic demands', but chiefly as a rebellious 'reaction of the young Breton against the anti-Hegelian sarcasms of his philosophy professor, the positivist Andre Cresson' (p 37).

[28] Their Hegelianism is summarised in Roth's Knowing and History as a fundamentally political utilisation of the philosopher that complimented their Marxism; two chapters of Baugh's *French Hegel: From Surrealism to Postmodernism* are dedicated to Breton and Bataille; and the chapter of Martin Jay's *Marxism and Totality* on the reception of Hegelian Marxism in France is focused on the Surrealists.

contemptuous Hegelian phantoms, like the despotic anti-liberal who Basch dispelled as a fake, whose gradual banishment Koyré documents in his report.

There was a series of compelling writers in France of the 1930s and 1940s, working outside of the academy, who combined an often fiercely political interest in Hegel and Marx with research into mysticism and the esoteric. Several of these writers, including George Bataille, came together in 1937 in a self-titled 'College of Sociology', to conduct research and discussion of 'Sacred Sociology': their name for the study of 'all manifestations of social existence where the active presence of the sacred is clear'.[29] Joining Bataille as a founding member of the group was Roger Caillois, whose esoteric and wide-ranging work began with two essays on insects published in the 1930s, which speculated on the unconscious significance of the praying mantis, and on the origins of morphological mimicry.[30] Lacan would famously make reference to this in his 1949 article on 'The Mirror Stage as Formative of the *I* Function as Revealed in Psychoanalytic Experience', where he recalls how Caillois, 'young and fresh from his break with the sociology school', conducted valuable research into the 'derealising effect of an obsession with space' in living organisms.[31]

Caillois's 'Introduction' to the College's foundation gives a vibrant description of the unstable mood amongst intellectuals of the time[32] and prescribes the alternative field of investigation opened by the College as a response to these 'present circumstances'. He refers by this to a twenty-year inter-war period, which had, he reflects, 'seen as extensive an intellectual turmoil as one could imagine. Nothing durable, nothing solid, no basis: Everything crumbles already and loses its edges, while time so far has taken only one step'.[33] These decades had also seen

[29] Roger Caillois et al., 'Note on the Foundation of a College of Sociology' (1937), in Hollier ed., *The College of Sociology*, pp. 3–5 (p. 5).

[30] The College's other founding members were the physicist Georges Ambrosino; the artist and translator of Walter Benjamin, Pierre Klossowski; the sociologist Jules Monnerot; and Pierre Libra (Hollier, *The College of Sociology*, p. 5).

[31] Lacan, 'The Mirror Stage as Formative of the *I* Function as Revealed in Psychoanalytic Experience', in *Écrits* (London: Norton, 2006), pp. 75–81 (p. 77).

[32] Caillois, 'Introduction' (1938), in Hollier ed., *The College of Sociology*, pp. 9–11 (p. 9).

[33] Caillois, 'Introduction', p. 9.

> an extraordinary, almost inconceivable, fermentation: yesterday's problems posed again each day with many others that are new, extreme, disconcerting, indefatigably invented by tremendously active minds that are no less tremendously incapable of patience or continuity—in a word, a production that literally floods the market, and is out of proportion to needs and even to the capacity for consumption.

One result of this intellectual cacophony and 'inadequacy' identified by Caillois is that 'an entire side of modern collective life, its most serious aspect, its deep strata, eludes the intellect'.[34] Caillois's frustrated analysis of a culture hopelessly ignorant of its own 'most serious' underside echoes Breton's vision of a psychic revolution through the ecstatic release of repressed imaginative forces. But Caillois's version is baffled rather than agitating; his portrait of a culture in transition, fermenting in its own anxious expectancy, and eagerly attentive to any spark of guidance which might illuminate its way to escape from this disorientation into the future, should be seen as the background for the gravitation towards Hegel by French intellectuals of the time. Some form of 'Renaissance', whether Hegel's or anyone else's, was a myth keenly suited to the instability of this moment in France. The explosion of Hegel's popularity and fashionableness, still misunderstood by many historians as having been triggered by one or two individual members of the philosophical establishment, was made possible by galvanising a set of anxieties held by a new generation of intellectuals.

Caillois recalled in 1970 how he once tried to 'obtain the assistance' of Kojève for the College of Sociology.[35] Caillois's admiring description of the 'principal exegete of Hegel in France', who 'exerted an absolutely extraordinary influence on our generation', reiterates the magnetism his celebrity exerted over this generation which, Caillois felt, was in such pressing need of direction.[36] But Kojève was not as sympathetic towards the College's project as Caillois would have liked. After listening to their request for assistance, he 'dismissed the idea'. In his eyes, Caillois reflects,

[34] Caillois, 'Introduction', p. 10.

[35] Caillois, Interview with Gilles Lapouge, in *La Quinzaine littéraire* (June 1970). Cited in Hollier, *The College of Sociology*, p. 86.

[36] Caillois, in Hollier, *The College of Sociology*, p. 86

'we were putting ourselves in the position of a conjurer who wanted his magic tricks to make him believe in magic'.[37]

This metaphor apprehends much about the relationship between the central representative of Hegel in France, the esoteric school which accorded such importance to Hegelian philosophy, and the background of French Hegelianism against which it was set. It depicts the College of Sociology as being, from the point of view of a philosopher—even one as disruptive as Kojève—sincere to the point of absurd naivety. Kojève had envisaged the *Phenomenology*'s dialectic as actualised in a contemporary world lingering on a century after the End of History. Even he maintained, however, as Caillois's metaphor depicts him, a degree of cynicism with regards to this rich and strange world that Hegel's work had, according to him, conjured up. The College of Sociology renounced even this trace of cynicism. What they wanted from Hegel was a transformation of reality by the collapse of the divine, sacred, and mystical into the profane. This desire was a direct product of Hegel's ambivalent, anti-establishment integration into French culture.

Despite Kojève's scepticism, he did eventually give a lecture at the College, in December 1937. This lecture, says Caillois,

> left us all flabbergasted, both because of Kojève's intellectual power and because of his conclusion. You will remember that Hegel speaks of the man on horseback, who marks the closure of History and of Philosophy. For Hegel this man was Napoleon. Well! That was the day Kojève informed us that Hegel had seen right but that he was off by a century. The man of the end of History was not Napoleon but Stalin.[38]

Kojève would later renege on this particular interpretation of Hegel. But the drama of revisionism and retraction this plays out says as much about the status of Hegel in 1930s France as does Kojève's combination of reservation towards and participation in the College's activities. At stake in Kojève's altering location of the End of History is the position taken by the subject in relation to both History and philosophy. One

---

[37] Caillois, in Hollier, *The College of Sociology*, p. 86.

[38] Hollier, *The College of Sociology*, p. 86.

thing that changes when Stalin is introduced as the signal of this closure is the status of Caillois's inter-war generation of intellectuals: it makes them the immediate heirs of the End of History. Caillois depicts Kojève's relationship with the College as an encounter between a cynical magician and a naïve one, a dialectic appropriate to this post-Historical moment. In the College, philosophy encounters an other who, whilst mirroring it in principle, confronts it with an uncanny inversion of itself; a figure who had crucially misunderstood philosophy's own understanding of its function. Kojève's anticipation of the contented Wise Man was met with a psychotic Conjurer, an allegorical character far better suited to the reality of French Hegelianism, and the exorbitant comedy of errors which shaped it.

Hegel or Hegel: Wahl, Kojève, and Hyppolite on the Unhappy Consciousness

As the following chapters of this book will describe, Marx would be used not only to wound, but also to stabilise this volatile French Hegel. Kojève's reading of Hegel, to be discussed further on, was an attempt to align him with a Marxist version of the progress of History. Georgi Plekhanov's *Fundamental Problems of Marxism* (1908) and Lenin's *Materialism and Empirio-Criticism* (1909), both influential texts which discussed Hegel's significance for reading Marx, were each translated into French in 1928. But there was another critic of Hegel with a great deal of significance in the context of French Hegelianism. The following section of this chapter will focus on a Kierkegaardian theme which was a shared concern amongst several French philosophers who wrote and taught about Hegel in the 1920s and 1930s: that his system is crippled by a devastating fissure, out of which falls—fatally—existence itself. The following section will examine the way in which French writing on the Hegelian figure of the unhappy consciousness circled around the problem posed to the Hegelian system by the ineffable experience of subjectivity. As the remainder of the chapter will then demonstrate, the impasses they encountered formed a matrix to which Lacan would explicitly respond in his reading of Hegel.

In one of the most incisive critiques of Hegel's System, Kierkegaard charges him with an arrogant elision of existence. By 'existence', Kierkegaard means that of the individual living subject, who experiences anxiety, uncertainty, and anguish. Hegel's logic, he argues, would ossify this experience into his logically formulated History which, by resolving subjective experience in its teleological thrust, diminishes it into nothing. For Kierkegaard, Hegel therefore overlooks the immediate yet enduring irresolvability of this existential condition, and the subjects—meaning all subjects—who must bear it. Particularly representative of Kierkegaard's critique of Hegel is his *Concluding Unscientific Postscript* (1846), a satire which from its title onwards confronts Hegel's intended formulation of a rigorously 'scientific' philosophy. This unscientific rejoinder to Hegel's attempt at total systematisation fires back the response that 'no *existential* system is possible'.[39] In leaving out the existence of the individual subject who would need to create it, this greedily parasitic system deprives itself of its host, killing off its necessary foundation and point of origin. Hoist thus with its own petard, 'no logical system may boast of an absolute beginning, since such a beginning, like pure being, is a pure chimera'.[40] Existence may well, Kierkegaard taunts, be 'itself a system for God, but it cannot be a system for any existing spirit', for whilst '[s]ystem and conclusiveness correspond to each other', existence 'is the very opposite', and 'must be annulled in the eternal before the system concludes itself'.[41] Not only self-defeating, then, Hegel's elision of subjective existence is frighteningly repressive, even despotic. This kind of philosophy has 'forgotten that the knower is an existing individual'—for the 'existing individual' it is, in return, 'a chimera'.[42] And so, this 'triumphant victory of pure thought' that Hegel wants to declare is, for its arrogance and its blindness respectively, 'something both to laugh at and to weep over'.[43] It stupidly,

[39] Søren Kierkegaard, *Concluding Unscientific Postscript* (1846), trans. by David F. Swenson (Princeton: Princeton University Press, 1944), p. 102. My italics.

[40] Kierkegaard, *Concluding Unscientific Postscript*, p. 102.

[41] Kierkegaard, *Concluding Unscientific Postscript*, pp. 188, 122. Cited in Merold Westphal, 'Kierkegaard and Hegel', in *The Cambridge Companion to Kierkegaard*, ed. by Alastair Hannay and Gordon D. Marino (Cambridge: Cambridge University Press, 1998), pp. 101–124 (p. 102).

[42] Kierkegaard, *Concluding Unscientific Postscript*, pp. 183, 275.

[43] Kierkegaard, *Concluding Unscientific Postscript*, p. 292.

disastrously, misrecognises as leftover dregs that which was in fact at its own heart, and at the heart of all living beings.

Jean Wahl's writing on Hegel is an extended mediation between Hegel and Kierkegaard. The way in which he performed this mediation was decisive for the following decades of French Hegelianism.[44] If, as Roth and Butler suggest, the publication of Wahl's *Le malheur de la conscience dans la philosophie de Hegel* (1929) was a turning point in French Hegelianism, then it was also a Kierkegaardian turning point. Wahl's writing on Hegel begins in an article from 1926, 'Note sur les démarches de la pensée de Hegel' ('Note on the Stages of Hegel's Thought'), where he identifies behind Hegel's dialectic a logic of paradox and negativity. Wahl argues from the discovery of this underlying nullity that the purpose of philosophy is 'never purely speculative', and that the function of philosophical speculation is to 'brin[g] the highest enjoyment' and allow us 'to fill the void [...] of abstraction which separates reason from the reality of reason as spirit'.[45] The 'beginning of philosophy', he continues,

> as of religion, is less a feeling of wonder than non-satisfaction and torn consciousness. Nothing of that nature, if one has to take as an object of study not the abstract man, but the man determined by his environment, by his circumstances, the man not only reasonable but endowed with a heart, and rise up from him until you reach reason, [it is found to be] closer to the heart than it is to cold understanding.[46]

For Wahl, philosophy must both begin and end in the evanescent anxieties of the individual human person, who suffers from a 'torn conscience', inhabits a 'void', and is prey to their 'environment', 'circumstances', and 'heart'. As if it were the deepest secret of philosophy, Wahl reveals that the subject whose corner was fought so viciously by Kierkegaard lies, in truth, cowering behind any philosophy

[44] And the following century, as Bruce Baugh makes clear in *French Hegel: From Surrealism to Postmodernism* (London: Routledge, 2003), where he finds Wahlian traces lingering as far as Derrida (p. 41).

[45] Jean Wahl, 'Note sur les démarches de la pensée de Hegel', *Revue Philosophique de la France et de l'Étranger* (January–June 1926), 281–289 (p. 288). My translation.

[46] Wahl, 'Note sur les démarches', p. 289.

whatsoever—and the most zealously ambitious the system, the greater the fear and trembling which precipitated it.

When Hegel takes the history of philosophy as his object of study in the *Phenomenology*, then, what he considers are, for Wahl, in truth, 'not philosophies but ways of living'—or at least 'the two are not separated'.[47] Not only does Hegel see philosophies 'as having succeeded one another in history', but also as having a 'rule of succession' that can be generalised from this process, 'so that logic is just as much the germ of the philosophy of history as it is the history of philosophy'.[48] This claim—that the logic that germinates within the historical swell of philosophy is also that which directs its movement—exemplifies the atemporal, paradoxical logic that quivers through Wahl's reading of Hegel. As Wahl is articulating, the historical sequence of different styles of philosophy traced out the contours of a logic which had been there already. This logic could, however, only emerge as such because it was actually struggled through by the historical actors who brought these successive philosophies into being. Destiny and necessity exist, then, but only *after* they are realised. A similar procedure of structural inversion is active in Wahl's collapse of a supposed Hegelian division between the oppositions 'of thought and being' and 'of the essential and the inessential'.[49] The logical core of the Hegelian system is not, Wahl asserts, 'projected on an abstract plane' of logic, but 'thought' and 'the essential' are studied by Hegel 'in the way in which they are felt, lived by humanity'.[50] Hegelian logic, in Wahl's reading, can only come after Hegelian existence. Wahl's prose enjoys this escapade of engulfing the kernel of Hegelian logic within a cocoon of feeling. His writing blends close dialectical thinking with stylistic tenderness and pathos, demonstrating knowingly that the terms of this supposed opposition function remarkably well in co-operation.

Too well, perhaps. If Wahl succeeds in rehabilitating unhappiness into Hegel's system, this comes with its own dialectical antithesis hidden in plain sight, one which will come also to colour Wahl's reading of Hegel

[47] Wahl, 'Note sur les démarches', p. 287.
[48] Wahl, 'Note sur les démarches', p. 287.
[49] Wahl, 'Note sur les démarches', p. 287.
[50] Wahl, 'Note sur les démarches', p. 287.

in *Le malheur de la conscience dans la philosophie de Hegel* (1929). Wahl learned the atemporal rationale that justifies his short-circuit between logic and philosophical history from Victor Delbos, who had lectured on post-Kantian philosophy at the Sorbonne in 1909, and who had given Hegel an unusually fair treatment, anticipating the explosion of popularity Wahl's work was to help precipitate.[51] Delbos interpreted Hegel's dialectic with a similar atemporal logic, reading the moment of synthesis as 'the *reason* for the moments it subordinates and comprises'.[52] If, for Delbos, the concluding synthesis functions as a posterior justification for dialectical conflict—a justification which is, nonetheless, concealed from the present moment in which the conflict is taking place—then, when Wahl transposes the dialectic into affective division, this promise of assured reconciliation becomes sufficient to satisfy the unhappiness of any consciousness.[53] Wahl adopts the perspective whereby the 'principle of antithesis' is regarded as '*necessary* for elevation towards synthesis'—a synthesis which equates, for him, to happiness.[54] '[T]o arrive at this happiness', Wahl reflects allegorically, 'it is necessary to cross misfortune'.[55] The 'misfortune' and unhappiness experienced by any subject is inscribed by Wahl into a logic of *felix culpa*—it is 'necessary' to experience such negativity in order to attain any 'happiness' at all.

Wahl's 1926 article finds the origins of Hegelian logic in unhappy consciousness, and it forms the basis for Wahl's extended reading of the *Phenomenology* in *Le malheur*. In the book, Wahl situates the unhappy consciousness within the development of the sequence of various figures of consciousness Hegel uses to articulate the progress of spirit. In the *Phenomenology*, the precursor of the unhappy consciousness is the sceptic, the subject whose mind is deprived of any certainty, and in which one

[51] See Baugh, *French Hegel*, p. 19.

[52] Victor Delbos, 'Les facteurs kantiens de la philosophie allemande de la fin du XVIIIe siècle et du commencement du XIXe siècle', *Revue de métaphysique et de morale*, 32 (1925), 271–281 (p. 279). Cited in Baugh, *French Hegel*, p. 20. My italics.

[53] Wahl extends this logic of renunciation into a general philosophical principle, that 'reason will emerge from the contradictions of skepticism, from the unreason of unhappy consciousness, as the cogito comes out of Cartesian doubt' ('Note sur les démarches', p. 287); that philosophy will always conform to a comic narrative structure.

[54] Wahl, 'Note sur les démarches', p. 289. My italics.

[55] Wahl, 'Note sur les démarches', p. 289.

thought perpetually changes into another. Manifested in this 'absolute negativity of thought' is, Wahl comments, the 'coming to consciousness' of the dialectical movement of spirit itself.[56] This 'absolute negativity' is sublated in the form of the unhappy consciousness, who manifests negativity which has become conscious of itself as such. Unhappiness is, Wahl writes, the spirit's reflexive understanding of itself 'as transcendental consciousness without content, the perpetual changing from one idea into another, the I opposed to the Not-I, the transition from being to nonbeing and from nonbeing to being'.[57] It is the product of a 'dismemberment of consciousness that derives from its limitations', and is subject to 'a continuous and incessant irony' where it 'ceaselessly ends up with the opposite of what it sought'.[58]

Wahl characterises the unhappy consciousness as pure negativity made subject—as a subject of pure, distilled lack. This allows him to make it the moment of spirit upon which the entire *Phenomenology* pivots. If the book amounts to a 'narration' of the process by which consciousness attempts to 'fill in the separations that it feels within itself', then the negativity that is actualised, made subject, in the unhappy consciousness amounts to the 'driving force' behind this entire movement.[59] As a result, this unhappiness haunts the book as its defining principle:

> The stage of the unhappy consciousness does not occur just once in the life of spirit; it is found at different moments in the *Phenomenology*. Transcended, it nevertheless returns to consciousness at each new bend in the road until consciousness at last feels itself to be united with the object it sought—which is at the same time the subject itself as reality.[60]

---

[56] Wahl, 'Commentaire d'un passage de la "*Phénoménologie de l'Esprit*"', *Revue de Métaphysique et de Morale* 34 (1927), 441–71. Republished as Chapter 3 in Jean Wahl, *Le malheur de la conscience dans la philosophie de Hegel* (Paris: Rieder, 1929), pp. 158–93. Translated by Bruce Baugh as 'Commentary on a Passage from Hegel's *Phenomenology of Spirit*', in *Transcendence and the Concrete: Selected Writings*, ed. by Alan D. Schrift and Ian Alexander Moore (New York: Fordham University Press, 2017), pp. 54–89 (p. 60). Subsequent citations of the article will refer to this English translation.

[57] Wahl, 'Commentaire d'un passage', p. 85.

[58] Wahl, 'Commentaire d'un passage', p. 85.

[59] Wahl, 'Commentaire d'un passage', p. 60.

[60] Wahl, 'Commentaire d'un passage', p. 85.

Yet each of these 'bend[s] in the road'—each crossroads at which we encounter the abject dissolution of unhappy consciousness—only leads gradually towards a 'turning point of cosmic history' in which 'consciousness will find itself in the spiritual daylight of the present':

> However, first of all, it must go through this twilight [*crépuscule*] of morning that is the unhappy consciousness, where the immutable sun sees itself only through the changing colours that are opposed to it. Daylight will reign and there will be peace only when the elements are conceived of not as elements but as notions; not as being opposed but as being both opposed and united.[61]

As romantic as this may sound, it essentially represents a lyrical rendition of the Hegelian logic against which Kierkegaard struggled to save the shadowy recesses of existence from being dazzled away.

Wahl's extensive prioritisation of the unhappy consciousness seems, then, to have been, openly and without exaggeration, directed towards the sole purpose of guaranteeing absolute Happiness, in the bright dawn at the end of Hegel's system. A similar point is made of Wahl, with subtle tact, in a review of *Le malheur* by Koyré, from 1930.[62] What Koyré's review also does is to locate behind Wahl's book a series of conflicting caricatures of Hegel. After a long and appreciative exposition of *Le malheur*, Koyré points out how, due to Wahl's focus on the writings of Hegel's youth, for Wahl,

> even in the most "abstract" works, behind the philosopher we find the theologian, behind the rationalist "the romantic", and behind the satisfied—if not happy—consciousness of the Berlin philosopher, we find "the unhappy consciousness of the romantic, the mystic, the Christian".[63]

---

[61] Wahl, 'Commentaire d'un passage', p. 86.

[62] Alexandre Koyré, 'Review of *Le malheur de la conscience dans la philosophie de Hegel* by Jean Wahl', *Revue Philosophique de la France et de l'Étranger* (July–December 1930), 136–143. Russell Ford takes Wahl's 1933 article 'Hegel et Kierkegaard' as in part a response to Koyré's review of *Le Malheur* (See Ford, 'Introduction to "Hegel and Kierkegaard"', in *Transcendence and the Concrete*, pp. 90–92).

[63] Koyré, 'Review of *Le malheur*', p. 137.

Koyré makes it clear later in the review that he is aware of what is at stake in allowing this young Hegel precedence over the 'satisfied', mature Hegel—and in allowing this at the moment of rebirth in French Hegel studies that Koyré had advocated in his 1930 'Rapport sur l'état des études hégéliennes en France'. 'Such, then', Koyré continues, 'is the new image of Hegel which, in the first of the studies composing his book [...], introduces us to Jean Wahl'.[64] Koyré's interesting choice of phrasing, which makes an 'image of Hegel' act as Wahl's agent, is an apt aside on the drama in which these young philosophers participated, each cutting their teeth on various stages of the life cycle of Hegel's development. Wahl's chosen part is, Koyré recognises, 'this "romantic", this "mystic", this painful soul that he loves in Hegel' and 'it is these opaque and resistant symbols'—of romanticism, mysticism, Christianity, and unhappiness—'which seem to him to form the most precious treasure of Hegelian philosophy'.[65]

Wahl's inclination towards the young Hegel is not in itself a problem for Koyré. What is a problem for him is his suspicion that the young Hegel's insoluble lyricism manifests for Wahl 'the *most* precious' of all of Hegel's abundant treasures. Not only this, but the filaments of Koyré's critique point to there being no little degree of bad faith in Wahl's championing of the early Hegel as the lens through which his entire system should be understood, only to make a furtively teleological argument. If, despite its existential inconsolability, and despite its unyielding intermittence throughout the *Phenomenology*, the unhappy consciousness is, when all is said and done, the dialectical precursor to the 'spiritual daylight' of the *Begriff*, then Wahl's reading of Hegel's life should, Koyré replies, be informed by the same logic. The completed system should then be seen, as Koyré puts it, to be 'the goal that guided the Hegelian meditation' in its entirety.[66] To 'disown' or 'disregard' the 'most profound and powerful impulse of [Hegel's] thought' as it emerges in the *Science of Logic* (1812) or *Naturphilosophie* ('whose role', Koyré remarks, seems 'to be somewhat diminished by Mr. Wahl') would be not only to 'commit an

---

[64] Koyré, 'Review of *Le malheur*', p. 141.

[65] Koyré, 'Review of *Le malheur*', p. 141.

[66] Koyré, 'Review of *Le malheur*', p. 141.

injustice to the philosopher', but also to undermine the principle of resolution on which Wahl's own project sits.[67]

For the older Hegel, the suffering and divisions characteristic of his youthful unhappy consciousness had, as Wahl well knew, been absorbed into the conciliatory movement of the system. 'Does [Hegel] not know', asks Koyré rhetorically,

> that the battle is only a sham battle? And that his God, eternally moving and making himself, is at the same time eternally complete? [...] For God—and also for Hegel—tragedy has already been overcome.[68]

Wahl's reading begins to look like a version of Hegel cherry-picked to suit his taste: even if it is true that 'the fancies, "the hopes, and the despairs" of the young Hegel did not find a place in his system [...] was it not Hegel himself who separated them out?'—on what grounds, then, asks Koyré, to side with one over the other?[69] The mature Hegel of the *Logic* and the *Naturphilosophie* may well not be 'lovable', but, asks Koyré, 'does a romantic Hegel give us anything more than Hölderlin or Novalis? I do not think so'.[70] What makes Hegel either individual or worthy of our attention is, for Koyré, precisely that he moved *beyond* the youthful romanticism which he alleges to be prioritised by Wahl at the expense of Hegel's mature work. Wahl's Hegel may be

> more human; but must we at all costs humanize a Hegel? It is in his inhuman coldness that lies his greatness. Not in the fact that, what he later called "notion", he had first called "love". But on the contrary, in the fact that what he began to call "love", he ended up calling "notion".[71]

Koyré sides, definitively, with the Hegel behind this dialectical progression from "love" to "notion", a Hegel whom he also paints as having estimably 'inhuman coldness'. In fact, the sentimental alternative is

[67] Koyré, 'Review of *Le malheur*', p. 141.
[68] Koyré, 'Review of *Le malheur*', p. 142.
[69] Koyré, 'Review of *Le malheur*', p. 141.
[70] Koyré, 'Review of *Le malheur*', p. 141.
[71] Koyré, 'Review of *Le malheur*', pp. 142–3.

demoted by Koyré into a phoney mannequin; a phantom Hegel with arrested development that haunts the early works—a Kierkegaard in the machine of the dialectic. Schelling, whom Koyré invokes to assist him:

> had discerned it well: in Boehme, he said, the intoxication is real; it is artificial in Hegel. That which in Hegel is true, that which is HEGEL, is the *Logic*, is the eternal cyclic movement of thought, the *Selbstbewegung des Begriffs* [self-movement of the concept].[72]

In a moment of typographical élan, Koyré uses a shift to small capitals to represent the distinction between the young Hegel and the mature HEGEL, a distinction that his review suspects to be at play in Wahl's treatment of the philosopher. And beyond it too: Koyré's creatively typeset letters stage a mise-en-scène of the drama in which the review itself takes part. It performs a burlesque of Wahl's restaging of an internal drama within Hegel; a Punch and Judy where HEGEL bonks Hegel on the head with a stick until he is ejected from a History that can now reach closure. The fight to the death between Hegel and HEGEL is an appropriate textual paroxysm to cap the spectroscopic procedure that was filtering out these Hegelets as his popularity in France began to peak. It condenses too the dialectical criss-crossings that were taking place in the process: siding with the unhappy consciousness, Wahl ends up emphasising the necessity of guaranteed eventual happiness; lauding the fully formed product of Hegel's middle-age, Koyré has to value this 'inhuman coldness' on the romantic fancies it succeeded in fermenting. At the heart of these readings of Hegel is the drama between the young, romantic Hegel of Jena, who anticipated Kierkegaard, and the fully formed *Begriff* of cold-hearted HEGEL.

An 'anthropological turn' made by Koyré, away from both the sporadic French tradition of epistemological work on Hegel, and Wahl's theological version, is often taken to have been continued in Kojève's reading of the *Phenomenology*.[73] His iteration of the Seminar that had originally been taught by Koyré did share with its predecessor both an attempt to

[72] Koyré, 'Review of *Le malheur*', p. 142.

[73] See Baugh, *French Hegel*, p. 27.

perform secular, anthropological revisions of ideas that had previously been treated theologically, and a focus on the phenomenology of time. But it is Wahl whom Kojève follows in making the entire *Phenomenology* turn decisively on what was originally one episode of Hegel's book. The unhappy consciousness that reappeared at each critical moment of the dialectic in *Le malheur* is replaced by Kojève with the dialectic of master and slave from the fourth chapter of the *Phenomenology*, as the mechanism which drives History towards its End.

Kojève makes the struggle of master and slave into a mythical encounter at the origin of History, which he then uses as a structural framework behind the logic of History's subsequent progression. Each of these two primordial subjects seeks recognition from the other of his own superiority; each 'must, therefore, "provoke" the other, force him to start a fight to the death for pure prestige'.[74] Each subject is obliged in this fight 'to kill the other in order not to be killed himself', but when one of them gives up the struggle in order to preserve his life, he will be taken as a slave by the victor, who then becomes his master.[75] The process of the slave's gradual emancipation through his world-transforming work is made by Kojève into a motor propelling History towards its end-state of mutual recognition. The struggle between masters and slaves, occurring continuously through human history and throughout the world, propels Kojève's account of 'historical evolution', which is finally to arrive at 'the universal and homogeneous State' of mutual recognition.[76] This apocalyptic moment is to be precipitated by 'the synthesis of Mastery and Slavery', achieved through the slave's narrative of heroic self-emancipation.[77]

Wahl had acknowledged the struggle between master and slave as a moment in the dialectic prior to the development of unhappy consciousness, in whose self-estrangement, he says, 'it is as if the master and the

---

[74] Kojève, 'In Place of an Introduction' (1939), in *Introduction to the Reading of Hegel: Lectures on the "Phenomenology of Spirit"*, trans. by James H. Nichols, Jr. (London: Cornell University Press, 1969), pp. 3–30 (p. 13).

[75] Kojève, 'In Place of an Introduction', p. 13.

[76] Kojève, 'A Note on Eternity, Time, and the Concept: Complete Text of the Sixth through Eight Lectures of the Academic Year 1938–1939', in *Introduction to the Reading of Hegel*, pp. 100–149 (p. 139).

[77] Kojève, 'In Place of an Introduction', p. 45.

slave had been united in a single mind'.[78] When Kojève comes to address the unhappy consciousness, however, it is not as the key to the entire *Phenomenology*, but as just one moment of tension within it to be surpassed. Kojève takes the unhappy consciousness to be formed on the basis of two divisions which are characteristic of religious belief, both of which derive from the internalisation of the dialectic of master and slave within a single consciousness. The first division is produced by the unhappy consciousness' awareness of its own mortality. Just as the slave surrenders his freedom to save his own life, so the unhappy consciousness 'becomes Slave of God' in order to believe in their immortal soul.[79] The second division comes from the unhappy consciousness' failure to realise their freedom in the mortal world. This leads them to seek their freedom 'beyond the World, in the *Jenseits* [beyond]' of 'religious transcendence'.[80]

The unhappy consciousness attains, along with their false freedom, an equally false knowledge. Kojève envisages absolute knowledge to be possible only in the homogenous State at the End of History. In contrast, the total knowledge of the unhappy consciousness—who is synonymous, for Kojève, with the 'Religious Man'—is proven to itself by a 'universal and homogeneous' God, and independently of any historical conditions or progression.[81] In a process akin to a Kierkegaardian leap of faith, the Religious Man, says Kojève, 'can attain his absolute knowledge at any moment whatsoever of the historical evolution of the World and Man', provided only 'that God reveal himself to (or in and by) a man'.[82] But the unhappy consciousness is forced by their belief to distinguish between their enslaved mortal self and their supposedly free, immortal self. This 'wager on the beyond' backfires disastrously: the transcendent self is *less* free than the enslaved empirical one, because this one is enslaved by 'the

[78] Wahl, 'Commentaire d'un passage de la "*Phénoménologie de l'Esprit*", p. 64.

[79] Kojève, 'Résumé du cours 1934–1935 (Extrait de l'Annuaire de 1935–1936 de l'Ecole Pratique des Hautes Études, section des Sciences religieuses)', in *Introduction à la lecture de Hegel: Leçons sur la "Phénoménologie de l'Esprit professées de 1933 à 1939 à l'École des Hautes Études*, ed. by Raymond Queneau (Paris: Gallimard, 1947), pp. 74–76 (p. 74). My translation.

[80] Kojève, 'Résumé du cours 1934–1935', p. 74. My translation.

[81] Kojève, 'Philosophy and Wisdom: Complete Text of the First Two Lectures of the Academic Year 1938–1939', in *Introduction to the Reading of Hegel*, pp. 75–99 (p. 90).

[82] Kojève, 'Philosophy and Wisdom', pp. 90–91.

absolute Master', God Himself.[83] The advancement of consciousness beyond this state of religious self-enslavement is therefore crucial for facilitating the progression towards freedom narrated by the *Phenomenology*. True liberation is dependent on the unhappy consciousness 'abandon[ing] the idea of the *beyond*'; recognising his 'true and unique reality' in his 'freely performed action in the here-below for the here-below'; and accepting that he is 'nothing outside of his active existence in the World, where he is born, lives and dies'.[84] In doing so, says Kojève, 'he becomes the *Man of Reason* (*Vernunft*), who, according to Hegel, 'has no religion'.[85]

For Wahl, the unhappy consciousness is the manifestation in consciousness of fundamental logical antithesis. Wahl's reading also carries with it an underlying teleology: the negativity incarnated by the unhappy consciousness is a necessary condition for enabling a final synthesis, but it also indicates the possibility of this resolution, because of the way that it yearns towards it. Because it amounts to the subjective experience of a pull towards ultimate synthesis, unhappy consciousness must therefore, for Wahl, 'retur[n] to consciousness at each new bend in the road' throughout the progression the *Phenomenology* describes. Kojève reads the unhappy consciousness very differently, as a single moment of subjective error and wilful slavery which appears within the emancipatory progress of consciousness. That Kojève's unhappy consciousness must be overcome in the path towards freedom, instead of remaining, as Wahl's does, until the very last moment, illustrates the extent of Kojève's departure from Wahl's priorities. Fundamentalising the struggle between masters and slaves, Kojève's materialism roots negativity in an economy of human desire, and in the social conflict it inevitably produces. He therefore scorns unhappy consciousness as a failure to work towards its own emancipatory cancellation. For Wahl, the emotional expression of negativity in unhappy consciousness is more fundamental than the violent struggle prioritised by Kojève, and it appears prior to it. This means that,

[83] Kojève, 'Philosophy and Wisdom', pp. 90–91. My italics.

[84] Kojève, 'Philosophy and Wisdom', p. 75–76.

[85] Kojève, 'Philosophy and Wisdom', p. 76.

for Wahl, there is no way out of unhappy consciousness remotely as straightforward as becoming an atheist.[86]

The fact that Kojève's unhappy consciousness not only should, but can be overcome by atheism, indicates that although Kojève and Wahl both use the same Hegelian term, they each mean very different things by it. Certain properties of the Wahlian unhappy consciousness that do not exist in the Kojèvian rendition find expression, however, elsewhere in Kojève's reading of the *Phenomenology*. The permanence of Wahl's unhappy consciousness as a state of negativity propelling the dialectic is the basic characteristic of Kojève's slave, to whom the unhappy consciousness is reduced in his reading. But Kojève's Philosopher, who anticipates his own transformation into the Wise Man, also carries over several features of Wahl's unhappy consciousness. They resemble one another, firstly, in their negativity, both being defined atemporally by the synthesis which they await, and both signalling, by their very presence, the failure of this synthesis to arrive. Kojève's Philosopher also serves the function of a kind of prophet, who enables the spread of self-consciousness to others by guiding humanity through each stage of the dialectic:

> at each dialectical turning point there must be a Philosopher who is ready to become conscious of the newly constituted reality. Indeed, it is the Philosopher, and only he, who wants to know at all costs where he is, to become aware of what he is, and who does not go on any further before he has become aware of it.[87]

Kojève's Philosopher reappears 'at each dialectical turning point' just as Wahl's unhappy consciousness returned 'at each new bend in the road', as a principle of consciousness whose continual resolution acts as a historical motor. Both represent the leftovers of History that are indispensable

[86] At the heart of this discrepancy is the Nietzschean question, of what exactly it would mean to smash our idols, and whether it is even in our power to do so. Kojève says that this is necessary for emancipation, and is confident that we can. Wahl presents a vital scepticism in this respect (which is far more anticipatory of Lacan's inversion of Dostoevsky that without God *nothing* is possible), which answers that such iconoclasm is itself a fetishised myth. See Lacan, Lesson of 16 February 1955, 'XI. Censorship is not Resistance', in *Seminar II (1954–1955)*, ed. by Jacques-Alain Miller, trans. by Sylvana Tomaselli (London: Norton, 1991), pp. 123–133 (p. 128).

[87] Kojève, 'Philosophy and Wisdom', p. 85.

to its movement, as if Kojève has made the Philosopher the very subject whose broken existence, in Kierkegaard's critique, falls out of Hegel's system, which thereby obliterates its own origin.

Wahl's reading of Hegel takes the Kierkegaardian critique seriously, if only to reabsorb the damage of its impact, and Kojève brushes it aside in his focus on a politically-driven epic of History. Neither, however, are particularly interested in individual, flesh-and-blood people and the development of their personal histories, or in their particular, personal consciousnesses. Even Wahl keeps at arm's length the human feeling whose significance he so ardently affirms, preferring to isolate it in the allegorical figure of the unhappy consciousness, or within the mind of the young Hegel. One philosopher who departs in this key respect from the themes of this emerging episode of French Hegelianism is Jean Hyppolite, particularly in his early articles on Hegel. The most important contribution that Hyppolite—perhaps anyone—made to French Hegelianism was his French translation of the *Phenomenology*, published in two instalments in 1939 and 1941. He had been working on it from 1936, without a publisher, or any guarantee of its publication, and having learned German only by reading Hegel in isolation.[88] Like many of his generation, his 'first real shock' of Hegel came from Wahl, reading *Le Malheur* was 'a sort of revelation', and Koyré's work provided just 'as basic' a foundation for his Hegelianism.[89] He had, on the other hand, 'scrupulously avoided' Kojève's lectures, for fear of 'being influenced'.[90]

Hyppolite's own writing on Hegel achieves a measured, reflective style of interpretation, which often retreads ground covered by Wahl or Koyré in order to add subtle twists or inflections to their more decisive readings of Hegel. His earlier writings combine his inclination towards the study of individual consciousness with aspects of the occult that echo the concerns of Bataille or Caillois. As John Heckman describes, Hyppolite 'occupied a position which was', almost paradoxically, 'distinct from that

[88] Heckman, 'Introduction' to *Genesis and Structure of Hegel's Phenomenology of Spirit*, p. xxvi.

[89] Quoted in Heckman, 'Introduction', p. xx.

[90] Heckman, Interview with Mme Hyppolite, cited in 'Introduction' to *Genesis and Structure of Hegel's Phenomenology of Spirit*, p. xxvi.

of any of the major groupings and at the same time typical'.[91] After publishing his translation, Hyppolite would write several more book-length commentaries on the *Phenomenology* and other areas of Hegel's work.[92] But, as Heckman notes, his 'immediate influence was as much due to his role as a teacher' as to these publications.[93]

In a series of early articles, Hyppolite makes a reorientation of the question of unhappy consciousness by rearticulating it within a quasi-biological framework. In Hyppolite's earliest articles on Hegel from the mid-1930s, there is an emphasis on religion and subjective division that closely follows Wahl's. In Hyppolite's first article on Hegel, 'Les Travaux de Jeunesse de Hegel d'après des ouvrages récents' ('Hegel's Early Work According to Recent Publications', 1935), he agrees with Wahl that Hegel 'sticks to what the subject feels', and that his dialectic 'is only the expression of the oppositions and conciliations which appear in every life of the mind'.[94] But he adds to this an emphasis on the *institution* of religion, finding the contrast between 'subjective' or 'private religion', on the one hand, and 'objective religion' or 'the religion of a people', on the other, to be at stake in the problem of unhappy consciousness.[95] He takes this to manifest the conflict between an individual's relationship, on the one hand, 'with God as pure objectivity' and, on the other, with 'God as subjectivity'.[96] The unhappy consciousness appears in history, says Hyppolite, as a result of this division, 'when the individual isolates himself from the absolute', and 'remains purely passive in his faith'.[97] Hegel wants, says Hyppolite, to resolve this division by 'integrat[ing] private

[91] Heckman, 'Introduction', p. xxvi. Hyppolite served, as his obituary in *Le Monde* put it, as 'the consciousness of our time'. Heckman, p. xxvi, citing *Le Monde*, October 31 (1968).

[92] See Jean Hyppolite, *Genesis and Structure of Hegel's "Phenomenology of Spirit"* (1946); *Introduction to Hegel's Philosophy of History* (1948), trans. by Bond Harris and Jacqueline Bouchard Spurlock (Gainesville: University Press of Florida, 1996); and *Logic and Existence: An Essay on Hegel's Logic* (1953), trans. by Leonard Lawler and Amit Sen (New York: State of New York Press, 1997).

[93] Heckman, 'Introduction', p. xxvii.

[94] Jean Hyppolite, 'Les Travaux de Jeunesse de Hegel d'après des ouvrages récents', *Revue de Métaphysique et de Morale* 3 (July 1935), 399–426 (pp. 399, 404). My translation. Hyppolite is referring to Wahl by 'des ouvrages récents'.

[95] Hyppolite, 'Les Travaux', p. 407.

[96] Hyppolite, 'Les Travaux', p. 424.

[97] Hyppolite, 'Les Travaux', p. 422.

religion into the religion of a people', a synthesis aligned with the 'integration of the citizen into the city' which Hegel took to characterise life in ancient cities, and which amounted, for him, to true freedom.[98] Following Wahl again in the importance he placed on Hegel's religious thought, Hyppolite agrees that the person of Christ manifests a synthesis of the 'historical element' with 'the absolute', and of 'infinity [with] individuality', because Christ is a God who 'teaches and acts', and who 'speaks of his own individuality'.[99] This, says Hyppolite, makes Christ 'the source of the dialectic of Hegel'.[100] But whilst Wahl's Hegel was romantic in the sense of lyrical and impassioned, Hyppolite casts Hegel in the tradition of an arcane, hermetic romanticism, of chthonic energies and psychological speculation. Hyppolite's Hegel wanted 'to grasp not only the living whole of the forces of the soul, but also the depth of the subject'; he 'analyses sleep and dreams, somnambulism, madness, and presentiments', and his work 'complements transcendental psychology by a study of the language and diseases of the soul'.[101]

Hyppolite's following article, 'Vie et Prise de Conscience de la Vie dans la Philosophie Hégélienne D'Iéna' ('Life and the Consciousness of Life in Hegel's Jena Philosophy', 1938), continues this arcane line of enquiry. It discusses Hegel's exploration of how "[t]o think life"; of how life, in an organic, material sense, leads to consciousness of life.[102] Hyppolite states in the article that '[i]n its immediate form self-consciousness is Desire', and that the object of consciousness is 'nothing else than the object of its desire', sounding, far from the spirituality of Wahl, more like Kojève in his description of consciousness as a bloody pursuit of desire.[103] But

[98] Hyppolite, 'Les Travaux', pp. 418, 421.

[99] Hyppolite, 'Les Travaux', pp. 416, 418.

[100] Hyppolite, 'Les Travaux', p. 416.

[101] Hyppolite, 'Les Travaux', p. 425. Hyppolite describes Hegel's system as 'only the deepening of an anthropological metaphysics'. This description is a significant gesture at synthesising several currents of interpretation of Hegel, asserting his philosophy's 'anthropological' character in line with Koyré and Kojève, without abandoning its transformed 'metaphysics', and whilst prioritising the Wahlian theology of unhappy consciousness.

[102] Hyppolite, 'Vie et prise de conscience de la vie dans la philosophie Hégélienne d'Iéna', *Revue de Métaphysique et de Morale* 1 (January 1938), 45–61 (p. 47). My translation. The passage of Hegel Hyppolite refers to here is in G.W.F. Hegel, *Early Theological Writings*, trans. by T.M. Knox (Chicago: University of Chicago Press, 1948), p. 254.

[103] Hyppolite, 'Vie et prise', p. 45.

Hyppolite modulates this with his own added emphasis on the literal 'flesh and blood' of nature in its organic materiality. The experience of 'being other' is, he describes, only an anticipatory moment in 'opposition to the point when it will be resolved in enjoyment [*jouissance*]'; when '[t]he living creature grabs the thing and assimilates it to his own substance', making it 'his flesh and blood'.[104] He goes as far as to find the origins of Hegel's dialectical thought in this relationship between living consciousness and its inorganic environment.[105] In Hegel's early writings, he summarises, the 'relation of the universe and of an organism, of the universal and of the individual' is represented in a 'biological form', and this dialectic of the individual subject and the eternal, infinite universe is depicted by Hegel in 'the relation between the environment and the living'.[106] Life, Hyppolite concludes, 'is itself this dialectic'—and it is also 'life that compels the spirit or mind to think dialectically'.[107] It is highly striking that this account of the origins of the dialectic contains no intersubjective component whatsoever. Hyppolite's Hegel developed the dialectic from the experience of the solitary individual as an organic, material being which is motivated by biological drives.

This relation between the individual organism and the infinite universe allows Hyppolite to recast the unhappy consciousness in a new light. In similar terms to Wahl, Hyppolite describes the unhappy consciousness as an expression of 'a mystical image', of 'an absolute that is divided and torn', which had been 'translated in Hegel by the invention of dialectical thought'.[108] But Hyppolite's focus on the transition from the biological to the conceptual situates organic, bodily experience at the heart of unhappy consciousness. Hyppolite argues, strikingly, that 'the inner contradiction' at 'the very heart of desire', which perpetually orients it towards future satisfaction, 'is felt as pain': physical pain, he says, 'is the

[104] Hyppolite, 'Vie et prise', p. 45.
[105] Hyppolite, 'Vie et prise', p. 45.
[106] Hyppolite, 'Vie et prise', p. 53. In the Jena writings, specifically, Hyppolite says that the 'concept of Life' can be discovered in the way Hegel conceives of infinity, as the dialectic 'between the One and the Many' ('Vie et prise', p. 48).
[107] Hyppolite, 'Vie et prise', p. 48.
[108] Hyppolite, 'Vie et prise', p. 50.

lived contradiction, the biological experience of the dialectic'.[109] Hyppolite goes even further than Wahl in embedding unhappy consciousness at the centre of subjectivity. Not only a consciousness of pure negativity haunted by its alienation from the absolute, and necessary for the fulfilment of this absolute—for Hyppolite, unhappy consciousness is inevitable because of the very embodied nature of human consciousness.[110]

Some time later, in 1946, Hyppolite published an article that reconsiders the relationship between Hegel and Kierkegaard that had been examined thirteen years earlier by Wahl. Hyppolite's 'L'existence dans la phénoménologie de Hegel' ('Existence in Hegel's Phenomenology') begins by retreading in strikingly similar terms the very problematic Wahl had begun with in 1927—but from the other side of the rise of the Existentialist movement and the publication of Sartre's *Being and Nothingness* (1945). Kierkegaard, Hyppolite recapitulates, criticises Hegel for giving 'no place to existence' in his system, and for staging 'a disappearance of the very notion of existence'.[111] Not dwelling on these points, Hyppolite concedes with striking objectivity that 'there is little doubt that in general Kierkegaard is right against Hegel'.[112] Acknowledging, as Wahl had, that in Hegel's early works as well as in the *Phenomenology*, we find 'a philosopher much closer to Kierkegaard than might seem credible', and asking 'whether there is not in this work a conception of existence which is kin to certain contemporary existentialist notions', he then recapitulates the fundamental logic behind the development of self-consciousness in the *Phenomenology*, to generate an account of subjectivity approximating that of the Existentialist philosophy contemporary to the article.[113]

---

[109] Hyppolite, 'Vie et prise', p. 53.

[110] Christ, then, represents the source of the dialectic, not only in the synthesis of individual and absolute that his being represents, but as God incarnated in the *body* of a man.

[111] Hyppolite, 'L'existence dans la phénoménologie de Hegel', *Études germaniques*, 1 (1946), 131–141. Translated as 'The Concept of Existence in the Hegelian Phenomenology', in *Studies on Marx and Hegel*, trans. by John O'Neill (New York: Harper, 1969), pp. 22–34 (p. 22). Subsequent citations of the article will refer to this English translation.

[112] Hyppolite, 'L'existence', p. 22.

[113] Hyppolite, 'L'existence', p. 23.

Hyppolite draws Existentialism back into Hegel through the conflict it restages between 'being-for-itself' and 'being-for-another'. Because 'being-for-itself' has to recognise itself in the other in order to attain human consciousness, it necessarily becomes 'being-for-another', and amounts to 'a vanishing moment' of 'absolute negativity' comparable to 'contemporary existentialist formulations'.[114] This logic manifests not in the struggle that propels Kojève's historical epic, nor in the incessant division of Wahl's unhappy consciousness, but in a Sartrean negativity which reaches freedom only in the face of death.[115] Hegel does not, however, 'stop with this liberty toward death', but provides a pre-emptive critique of the Existential problematic. For Hegel, man transforms his own negativity into substance, in 'struggl[ing] with himself to assume or take upon himself every determination' that overshadows his particular existence: by negating these determinations 'as death negates every living particular', he also 'conserves them and endows them with a new meaning'.[116] This is how human existence generates its own history, where 'the partial moments are continually negated and at the same time always resumed in order to be surpassed'.[117] The 'true life of the spirit', as Hyppolite reads Hegel here, is not in the one who, like the slave, 'recoils from death', nor in the Sartrean existentialist who 'becomes conscious of it so as to confront it authentically', but in 'him who internalizes death'; who makes it, as Hyppolite quotes Hegel, 'the magic power that converts the negative into being'.[118] This 'power' is, says Hyppolite, 'identical with what Hegel calls the Subject'; the subject which both 'contains human history in its development', and is 'not limited to the historicity of a particular being'.[119] This subject overcomes its being-for-itself, says Hyppolite, by generating a history, which then 'interrelate[s]' with other individual existences, and

[114] Hyppolite, 'L'existence', p. 28.

[115] Hyppolite, 'L'existence', pp. 28–9.

[116] Hyppolite, 'L'existence', pp. 30–31.

[117] Hyppolite, 'L'existence', p. 31.

[118] Hyppolite, 'L'existence', p. 31. See Hegel, *The Phenomenology of Mind*, trans. by J.B. Baillie (London: George Allen and Unwin, 1964), p. 93.

[119] Hyppolite, 'L'existence', p. 31.

which, 'as a concrete universality', is 'what judges them and transcends them'.[120]

From a certain perspective, it seems ineffectual for Hyppolite to have retrodden the ground that, as this chapter has been describing, was so well-muddied by this point, by rediscovering in Hegel the Kierkegaardian moment that had frustrated Wahl, Koyré, and Kojève. The 1946 article on 'Existence' appears similarly banal as a defence of Hegel's continued relevance in the context of the rising popularity of Existentialism; a tone that is rung in the article's closing reassurance that '[n]umerous other aspects of th[e] marvellous work' of the *Phenomenology* 'are even more likely to arouse the interest of contemporary philosophers'.[121] The article's true achievement is more subtle. Where it succeeds is in producing a reinscription of the negativity of the Existentialist subject within the debate, by then well-rehearsed, over what becomes of the languishing, miserable existence of unhappy consciousness when it is confronted with the obliterating, forced resolution of Hegel's system. If Hegel would continue to 'arouse the interest' of this new generation, it was because he articulated a problem that was crucial to engage with if any satisfactory account of subjectivity were to be possible, and one which they would encounter, not as a result of Hegelian despotism, but whether they liked it or not. It is Hyppolite's strategy of responding to Hegel—not so much his explicit contribution to the questions raised by unhappy consciousness, but his manner of handling them—that is carried over in Lacan's own reading of Hegel. As the following section will describe, Lacan takes up an argument made by Hyppolite in framing attempts to *escape* Hegel as the truest possible expressions of his philosophy. As Lacan puts it in *Seminar X: Anxiety* (1962–63)—nearly forty years after Wahl first wrote on the unhappy consciousness—Kierkegaard therefore becomes, for Lacan, 'the one who imparts the truth of the Hegelian formula'.[122]

The problem of existence, embodied in the fate of the unhappy consciousness as it was stated and restated by the philosophers rehabilitating

[120] Hyppolite, 'L'existence', p. 31.

[121] Hyppolite, 'L'existence', p. 31.

[122] Lacan, Lesson of 21 November 1962, 'II: Anxiety, Sign of Desire', in *Seminar X*, pp. 16–28 (p. 25).

Hegel in France, honed in on a limit of the Hegelian dialectic that had first been perceived by Kierkegaard. In response to this, the philosophers discussed in this section repeated an attempted suturing of this limit. Each did so, however, by relying on something that only served to exacerbate the limit further. Wahl, raising unhappy consciousness to pre-eminence, stakes everything on the subject's faith in an atemporal synthesis; Koyré rejects this only by arguing that the synthesising leap was already made by Hegel in his own life; Hyppolite gives uncanny prominence to the proto-dialectical, material core of consciousness; and Kojève caps all of these, by explicitly foreshadowing the Hegelian death of philosophy. The *Phenomenology* narrates the progress of knowledge as something always moving, self-sufficiently, through, beyond, and because of its own contradiction. By Wahl, Koyré, Hyppolite, and Kojève, tangents are drawn from individual moments in the movement of consciousness that Hegel describes, in an attempt to prove that his philosophy works. The points that these tangents lead to, however, end up eclipsing the movement of knowledge in the *Phenomenology*, because they make the functioning of Hegel's system dependent on something outside of it. Their attempts to rescue Hegel—and to restore his position in French intellectual life—actually unveiled Hegel's reliance on something that his philosophy does not contain. This had already been demonstrated by Hegel's most famous critics, Kierkegaard and Marx. What the French Hegelians approached, in response, was the idea that these limits could already be found within Hegel, by those who wanted to find them.

This chapter has so far been describing the reception of Hegel in France, with an emphasis on its points of reversal, irony, and confusion. Underlying this reception history was a general conflict between a view of Hegel, on the one hand, as a philosopher who was ridiculous and excessive, and who could be ignored, or even relegated to a position of madness, and a view of Hegel, on the other, as a mysterious, dazzlingly powerful force, whose Messianic potential made his philosophy's illumination a vitally pressing task. What was not appreciated by readers of Hegel contemporary to Lacan was how the conflictual, libidinally cathected position they had given to him was interacting with the way they read and understood his philosophy. The readers of Hegel discussed so far in this chapter were not themselves able to articulate the conflicts that it has been documenting with an awareness of this interaction. The following section of the chapter will describe the development of Lacan's own thinking about Hegel from the 1930s to the 1960s. It presents this as a movement towards the convergence between love and knowledge that is formulated in Lacan's theory of transference. Lacan's precise and delicate thinking about Hegel was, the section will demonstrate, the realisation of something first mimed out in the drama of the French reception of Hegel, and then glimpsed, falteringly, by the French Hegelians. This, it will argue, is why it is insufficient to think of Lacan as a mere 'repetition' of Hegel.

How to Escape Hegel

We know from the École Pratique's registers that Lacan started attending Kojève's seminar sometime in 1934.[123] And there are, most definitely, Kojèvianisms in Lacan's work from this point in the mid-1930s onwards, with the dialectic of master and slave that Kojève placed at the core of Hegel remaining a basis for key elements of his Seminar even in the 1960s. The dominant theme in Lacan's earliest work, of the aggressive psychic parasitism that exists between the subject and their 'semblable', is based on this dialectic. Lacan's development of this theme culminates in his theories of the ego's origins in the mirror stage, and of the 'imaginary register', the zone of subjectivity in which he positions these paranoid relationships to hold sway.[124] But the relationship between Lacan and Kojève was clearly less simple than an encounter between a wise teacher and a patient student. It is not only that, as it begins to appear from the archival research of Elisabeth Roudinesco, Juan Pablo Lucchelli, and Todd McGowan, this relationship was more like one between two equals

[123] See Roth, 'Appendix', in *Knowing and History*; and Juan Pablo Lucchelli, 'The Early Lacan: Five Unpublished Letters from Jacques Lacan to Alexandré Kojève', pp. 332–33, for closer scrutiny of these records.

[124] It extends back, however, to the chthonic sibling pairs that recur in Lacan's early case studies of feminine psychotic crime. See Lacan, 'Motifs du crime paranoïaque: le crime des sœurs Papin', *Le Minotaure*, 3/4, 100–103, and Lacan, *De la psychose paranoïaque dans ses rapports avec la personnalité, suivi de Premiers écrits sur la paranoïa*, (1932) (Paris: de Seuil, 1975) pp. 149–215.

in a productive exchange of ideas.[125] More substantially, Lacan's work can be seen to return, in pervasive and significant ways, to the themes of French Hegelianism as a *whole*, and not just to the reading of the *Phenomenology* that was given by Kojève.

A central component of Lacan's response to Hegel in the 1930s and 1940s—the years coinciding with and directly following Kojève's Seminar—is his association between the formal progression of the *Phenomenology* through its different moments of consciousness, and the structure of psychosis.[126] The clearest manifestation of this argument is in the 'Presentation on Psychical Causality' Lacan delivered in 1946, as a critique of Henri Ey and the organicist aetiology on which his work was based. Here, Lacan draws a 'general principle of madness' from Hegel, as a rebuttal of Ey's organicism that refers directly to the way Hegel writes about madness in the *Phenomenology*.[127] Hegel's madman, as Lacan reads him, imposes 'the law of his heart onto what seems to him to be the havoc [*désordre*] of the world'.[128] The Hegelian madman fails to recognise either that 'this havoc' is 'the very manifestation of his actual being', or that 'what he experiences as the law of his heart is but the inverted and virtual image of that same being'.[129] This double misrecognition leaves only one way out for the madman: to lash out violently against the chaos he perceives, inevitably bringing down upon himself the social repercussions of his own violence. Lacan associates this misrecognition with a disruption

[125] Elisabeth Roudinesco, *Jacques Lacan* (1993), trans. by Barbara Bray (New York: Columbia University Press, 1997), pp. 104–5; Juan Pablo Lucchelli and Todd McGowan, 'The Early Lacan: Five Unpublished Letters from Jacques Lacan to Alexandre Kojève', *American Imago* 73, no. 3 (Fall 2016), 325–341.

[126] There are two texts among Lacan's earlier writings that are particularly important to this emerging response to Hegel: firstly, the 1946 'Presentation on Psychical Causality' (in *Écrits*) (London: Norton, 2006), pp. 123–160; and secondly, 'Aggressiveness in Psychoanalysis', a 1948 paper elaborating on Lacan's earlier exploration of the aggression characteristic of the mirror stage (in *Écrits*, pp. 82–101). The presence of Hegel in both of these pieces is clear, and is far more confidently displayed by him there than it had been a decade earlier.

[127] Lacan, 'Presentation on Psychical Causality', p. 140. Interestingly, Lacan first cites Véra's notoriously imperfect translation *La Philosophie de l'esprit* (Paris: Germer Baillière, 1867) in this chapter of the *Écrits*, as if this were the standard French edition, before also referencing Hyppolite's 'excellent French translation' *La Phénomenologie de l'esprit* (Paris: Aubier, 1939).

[128] Lacan, 'Presentation on Psychical Causality', p. 140.

[129] Lacan, 'Presentation on Psychical Causality', p. 140.

of 'dialectical development'. The mistake of the Hegelian madman represents a 'general formulation' of madness, he describes,

> in the sense that it can be seen to apply in particular to any one of the phases in which the dialectical development of human beings more or less occurs in each person's destiny; and in the sense that it always appears in this development as a moment of stasis, for being succumbs to stasis in an ideal identification that characterizes this moment in a particular person's destiny.[130]

Madness, as Lacan defines it here, results when 'dialectical development' congeals into a 'moment of stasis'. It amounts, Lacan says, to a short-circuiting of dialectical progress. Lacan's madman is fixated on a frozen moment in the dialectical history of his consciousness that eclipses his own being.

Lacan finds in Hegel's *Phenomenology* a playbook for the operations of imagoes—a term he uses in this early work to refer to images that have imprinted themselves on the unconscious—and the sphere of whose operations Lacan names the imaginary. The theory of the mirror stage positions the ego as the cynosure of the imaginary, and as the imago to govern all other imagoes. As is epitomised in the way that Lacan understands the ego, the imago is an eternal compromise between dialectical propulsion, on the one hand, and the undialectical fixation at the heart of madness, on the other. In his 1948 presentation on 'Aggressiveness in Psychoanalysis', Lacan, drawing on Pierre Janet, describes paranoid delusions of persecution as a 'stagnation[s]' that fixate on a single moment of ordinary social behaviour, and which dissect the dialectical fluidity of this interaction into an uncanny, petrified cross-section, 'similar in strangeness to the faces of actors when a film is suddenly stopped in mid-frame'.[131] He also makes a manoeuvre here, one that would become characteristic of his later work, of seeing in this formal stasis not a breakdown of the operation of knowledge, but the truth of its entire function. Lacan identifies this paranoiac formal stagnation as 'the most general

[130] Lacan, 'Presentation on Psychical Causality', p. 141.

[131] Lacan, 'Aggressiveness in Psychoanalysis', in *Écrits*, p. 90.

structure of human knowledge'.[132] He argues that it is this fixation that makes not only the ego, but all objects that exist for the subject, possess for this subject 'the attributes of permanence, identity, and substance', and appear to them as 'entities or "things"'.[133] The imaginary fixation that creates the ego is, Lacan argues, the same process that precipitates the experience of ontological reality—a reality that he therefore presents as equally illusive. Though they characterise paranoid psychosis, the fixations that these dialectical stagnations produce also enable the very recognition of ontological forms out of the flux of sensory experience.

The function of the imago as Lacan describes it is fundamentally contradictory. It is a point of stasis in mental functioning, in a way which interrupts the movement of inevitably-unfolding thought described in Hegel's dialectic. The imago produces, on the one hand, resistance to dialectical progression, acting as a freeze-frame in its movement. On the other hand, imaginary functions are a crucial part of the extended dialectical weaning process: the 1949 paper on the 'Mirror Stage'—the final iteration of a theory that Lacan had been developing since 1936—argues that the ego is a 'primordial form' of a subjectivity that will eventually be 'restore[d]' by language 'in the universal'.[134] Lacan argues, therefore, that being captured in the field of the ego is an essential moment in this process. This theory is not simply reapplying the notion of a synthesising Hegelian *Begriff* to resolve the dialectical tensions of imaginary life. If it were, then it would seem from this that the hazardous effects of imaginary identification might be fully avoided if the subject were to proceed through them to their eventual integration in the universal of language. But Lacan introduces a hugely significant departure in this respect. In the passage below, Lacan describes the consequences of egoic conflict in an extended musical metaphor. He observes that

> the earliest dissonance between the ego and being would seem to be the fundamental note that resounds in a whole harmonic scale across the

[132] Lacan, 'Aggressiveness in Psychoanalysis', p. 90.

[133] Lacan, 'Aggressiveness in Psychoanalysis', p. 90.

[134] Lacan, 'The Mirror Stage as Formative of the *I* Function as Revealed in Psychoanalytic Experience', in *Écrits*, pp. 75–81 (p. 76).

> phases of psychical history, the function of which is to resolve it by developing it.[135]

The function of 'psychical history' is, he says, to 'resolve', in a harmonic sense, a fundamental dissonance between the ego and being, by 'developing it' into a formal cadence. As is made clear in the 1949 paper, the initial dissonance of the ego may well lead to the final harmonic resolution of the *Begriff*. As the passage describes, the function of 'psychical history' is to enable this Hegelian resolution. Lacan qualifies this, however, by adding that:

> Any resolution of this dissonance through an illusory coincidence of reality with the ideal would resonate all the way to the depths of the imaginary knot of narcissistic, suicidal aggression.[136]

This resolution, achieved through 'an illusory coincidence of reality with the ideal', would be no less disastrous than a dialectical stagnation. It would 'resonate', continuing the musical metaphor, to the dark core of 'narcissistic, suicidal aggression', to produce the psychosis that Lacan read in Hegel's 'general formula' of madness.

This is illustrated in Lacan's example, which is only partly satirical, of Napoleon's identification with Napoleon. Napoleon, says Lacan, successfully resolved his egoic dissonance precisely because he did *not* fall into the trap of being 'someone who thought he was Napoleon'.[137] On the contrary, as Napoleon knows, 'man's ego is never reducible to his lived identity'.[138] The rapport between the two—ego and 'lived identity'—can only be an appearance, or in Napoleon's case, a well-crafted deception. For the subject to conflate the two, by maintaining the unity of their ego with this 'lived identity', would result in 'the very delusion of the

[135] Lacan, 'Presentation on Psychical Causality', pp. 152–3.

[136] Lacan, 'Presentation on Psychical Causality', pp. 152–3.

[137] Lacan, 'Presentation on Psychical Causality', p. 140. Knowing, on the other hand, that 'Bonaparte produced Napoleon', and that 'Napoleon sustained his existence at every moment', he restored his subjectivity by making posterity 'think that he had thought he was Napoleon'.

[138] Lacan, 'Aggressiveness in Psychoanalysis', p. 93.

misanthropic beautiful soul' that Lacan saw in the Hegelian madman who casts 'out onto the world the disorder that constitutes his being'.[139]

If there is a critique of Hegel immanent to this early stage of Lacan's work, it is only an implicit one. This period of Lacan's teaching, prior to the Rome Discourse and the beginning of his Seminar in 1953, is characterised by his distinctly positive transference towards Hegel. As the following section will emphasise, however, Lacan's Hegelianism does not exist in a static or constant form. In the 1930s, and in Lacan's 1936 article on 'Family Complexes' in particular, although he uses Hegelian principles to think with, there is a sense that these concepts remain exotic and glamorous to him: he maintains something of a distance to them, offering brief, explicit, slightly clumsy references to what 'Hegel proposed' as vague justifications for an assorted recapitulation of miscellaneous Hegelian ideas.[140] He makes not even remotely clear how his theories might be challenging these, or putting them under pressure. At this point, he is not yet able to envisage the position of his own work towards Hegel as being more than an imprecise calibration to his thought, as if he lacks, understandably, in these early years, self-belief and confidence in his ability fully to master this thought. In the period from the late 1930s to the late 1940s, which is dominated by his discussion of the functions of the imaginary, Lacan's work moves—particularly in the passages of 'Aggressiveness in Psychoanalysis', 'Presentation on Psychical Causality' and the 'Mirror Stage' paper discussed above—towards a more confident paraphrase of Hegel, via an application of Hegel's theories into the zone of psychology.[141] In making this paraphrase, Lacan is extrapolating Hegel's philosophy into a zone where its limits would become almost awkwardly clear, with a touch of satirism that he would later embrace fully and explicitly. He begins there to perform something more like a commentary on Hegel. This progresses, by the watershed of 1953, towards a substantial psychoanalytic unfurling of his thought.

[139] Lacan, 'Aggressiveness in Psychoanalysis', p. 93.

[140] Lacan, 'La Famille', in *Encyclopedie Française*, vol. 8, *La Vie mentale*, ed. by Henri Wallon (Paris: Société de gestion de l'Encyclopédie Française, 1938).

[141] He was following, in this respect, the work of Henri Wallon, which will be discussed in detail in Chap. 4.

Before 1953, Hegel represents for Lacan the key to unlocking a precise theory of madness, by formulating the pathologies of the imaginary. After this, when—wielding his Excalibur of the symbolic—Lacan has inaugurated the return to Freud, the association of Hegel with the imaginary is rephrased, and reframed as Lacan's critique of Hegel's *overemphasis* of the paranoid violence of this register. Lacan's fundamental objection to Hegel is repeated almost every time he mentions him in the Seminar. Hegel, he argues, overemphasises the operations that Lacan consigns to the imaginary, because he positions the fight to the death between the master and slave for pure prestige as the logical basis of the entire *Phenomenology*.[142] Lacan instead reads this dialectic as the apex of the imaginary register. By 1953, Lacan treats Hegel, read in this way, as having offered an account of subjectivity, and of society, which is insufficient. It is insufficient, however, in a way that needs to be understood very precisely. In *Seminar I: Freud's Papers on Technique* (1953–54), Lacan takes the *Phenomenology* to represent a schematisation of the structure of desire 'before language', when desire, restricted to the plane of imaginary, specular relation, is 'projected' and 'alienated in the other'.[143] The formula 'man's desire is the desire of the other'—which could epitomise this phase of Lacan's work—is derived from this mode of relation. Lacan supposes Hegel to teach us that the showdown between master and slave can have 'no other outcome [...] than the destruction of the other'.[144] In response to Hegel, Lacan emphasises that analytic experience emphatically does not occur on this level: that it is 'not a total' experience, because it is 'defined' instead on

[142] See Lacan, Lesson of 9 June 1954, 'XVIII. The Symbolic Order', in *Seminar I: Freud's Papers on Technique (1953–1954)*, ed. by Jacques-Alain Miller, trans. by John Forrester (London: Norton, 1991), pp. 220–236 (pp. 222–226), (where the 'limit-case' claim is made); Lesson of 30 November 1955, 'III. The Other and Psychosis', in *Seminar III: The Psychoses (1955–1956)*, ed. by Jacques-Alain Miller, trans. by Russell Grigg (London: Norton, 1997), pp. 29–43 (pp. 40–43); Lesson of 7 June, 'XXIV. Identification via "*Ein Einziger Zug*"', in *Seminar VIII: Transference* (1960–61), ed. Jacques-Alain Miller, trans. by Bruce Fink (Cambridge: Polity, 2015), pp. 344–359 (pp. 352–53); Lesson of 27 February 1963, 'XI. Punctuations on Desire', in *Seminar X: Anxiety* (1962–63), ed. by Jacques-Alain Miller, trans. by A.R. Price (Cambridge: Polity, 2014), pp. 147–156 (p. 153); Lesson of 10 May 1967, and Lesson of 31 May 1967, in *Seminar XIV: The Logic of Phantasy*, unpublished; and Lesson of 11 June, 'XXIII. Genèse logique de plus-de-jouir', in *Le Séminaire de Jacques Lacan, Livre XVI: D'un Autre à l'autre (1968–1969)*, ed. by Jacques-Alain Miller (Paris: Éditions de Seuil, 2006), pp. 355–374 (pp. 367–373).

[143] Lacan, Lesson of 5 May 1954, 'XIII. The See-saw of Desire', in *Seminar I*, pp. 163–175 (p. 170).

[144] Lacan, *Seminar I*, p. 170.

the symbolic plane.[145] Psychoanalysis, Lacan argues, is based on a break from the imaginary totality underlying the *Phenomenology*.

This theme is developed in the following two seminars. In *Seminar II: The Ego in Freud's Theory and in the Technique of Psychoanalysis* (1954–55), Lacan uses this claim to justify a rejection of the Hegelian notion of absolute knowledge. The plenitude of presence, total coherence, and self-justification referred to by absolute knowledge is, he says, characteristic of the imaginary register, and it is therefore alien to psychoanalysis.[146] Hegel, Lacan puts it enigmatically but succinctly, 'is at the limit of an anthropology. Freud got out of it. His discovery is that man isn't entirely in man'.[147] As opposed to the triumphant path of progressively emerging self-consciousness traced out in the *Phenomenology*, Freud, Lacan says here, thinks of the brain as a machine, and understands it through the lens of thermodynamics, and with the operation of the symbol. Following this, in *Seminar III: The Psychoses* (1956–57), Lacan maps out the break between the Other (as unknown, and as a function of the symbolic) and the other (as the 'I' of consciousness, and the source of all knowledge). He explicitly posits this schema as a heuristic to identify what is missing from Hegel. Hegel's understanding of knowledge remains, he says, on the level of the imaginary other, because it did not parse out the break Lacan identifies here, and did not, therefore, formulate the field of the Other.[148]

Lacan does not merely use the symbolic to enact a rejection or undermining of Hegel in these early seminars, however. What he effects is much more subtle. Lacan makes the symbolic a membrane of Hegel's *Phenomenology* that, through the swerve this register facilitates away from the violence of the imaginary, can be understood to defeat the trajectory it borders, which Hegel maps out in his book. Hegel's philosophy therefore becomes a limit, in the mathematical sense, whose excesses enable

---

[145] Lacan, Lesson 9 June 1954, 'XVIII. The Symbolic Order', in *Seminar I*, pp. 220–233 (p. 222–3).

[146] See Lacan, 'The Function and Field of Speech and Language in Psychoanalysis', in *Écrits*, pp. 197–168 (p. 241): 'But Freud's discovery was to demonstrate that this verifying process authentically reaches the subject only by decentring him from self-consciousness, to which he was confined by Hegel's reconstruction of the phenomenology of mind'.

[147] Lacan, Lesson of 12 January 1955, 'VI. Freud, Hegel and the Machine', in *Seminar II: The Ego in Freud's Theory and in the Technique of Psychoanalysis (1954–1955)*, ed. by Jacques-Alain Miller, trans. by Sylvana Tomaselli (London: Norton, 1991), pp. 64–76 (p. 72).

[148] See Lacan, Lesson of 30 November 1955, 'III. The Other and Psychosis', in *Seminar III*.

Lacan to perform his calculus of subjectivity. The symbolic does not simply develop with a 'relation of succession' out of the impasses of the imaginary. Lacan is clear that, because the Hegelian myth of the encounter between master and slave is structured as a game, and because it treats death as a wager—and not as something 'experienced as such', or even as an imaginable fear—this myth is '*already bounded* by the register of the symbolic'.[149] Though occurring on the level of the imaginary, in other words, this dialectic of master and slave, on which the *Phenomenology* is based, already tends asymptotically towards the symbolic.

It was Kojève who had first made Hegel's philosophy orbit around this mythical encounter of the master and slave. Because Lacan's treatment of Hegel tends to condense his philosophy to this dialectic, it is easy to reduce it—as many of Lacan's readers do—to a sign that his Hegelianism is restricted to Kojève's own reading of Hegel. The present chapter is arguing otherwise. As it has sought to emphasise, the person who first introduced to French Hegel studies the theme—and the anxiety—that there was something in Hegel that, taken to its limit, defeated, or at least transformed Hegel, was Jean Wahl. He and Kojève had each relied, respectively, on either the unhappy consciousness or the dialectic of master and slave, as an episode in the *Phenomenology* that is elevated to such overwhelming significance that its form characterises all human experience, and that is perpetually reiterated as a motor for the progress of history. What Wahl finds in the unhappy consciousness, in publications going back as early as 1926, is a way to square Hegel with Kierkegaard and emerge with spiritual reconciliation. What Kojève finds in the dialectic of master and slave, in the Seminar beginning in 1933, allows him to read the *Phenomenology* as a revolutionary Marxist romance. Lacan responds by declaiming the extrapolation of any tangent from the coordinate of this mythical encounter—whether to absolute knowledge, reconciliation, or freedom—as only ever amounting to wilful submission to an illusion. As a result of this, he is able to take seriously something that was implicit in both Wahl's and Kojève's readings of Hegel, and a theme in common to the general milieu of French Hegelianism described in this chapter. What Koyré articulates so elegantly in the typographical

[149] Lesson of 9 June 1954, 'XVIII. The Symbolic Order', in *Seminar I*, pp. 220–236 (p. 223).

distinction between Hegel and HEGEL is borne out in this early phase of Lacan's work: that there are fissures already in Hegel—before Kierkegaard or Marx exploit them—which can only be discovered by serious, assiduous study of his philosophy and its consequences, but that, when discovered, threaten to distort and undermine the entire edifice constructed upon them.

In a College of Sociology publication from 1939, Wahl describes 'dialectic' as a word that 'young philosophers are too fond of'.[150] Lacan uses it over two-hundred times in the *Écrits*; warranting, it would seem, the charge of Jean-Pierre Cléro, that he shared 'with a great number of men of this generation'—Wahl's 'young philosophers' amongst them—the 'prejudice and the belief' that, when dealing with all and any human phenomena, Hegel's philosophy 'provides the language in which it is appropriate to express oneself'.[151] By the start of his Seminar, however, Lacan is treating Hegel with a compelling ambivalence, which combines a disavowal of responsibility for Hegelian concepts, and an approach to his resident Hegelian, Hyppolite, bordering on patronisation, with a relentless wielding of Hegel as a weapon against his various interlocutors. In an exemplary passage of 'The Subversion of the Subject and the Dialectic of Desire in the Freudian Unconscious' (1960), Lacan acknowledges his own use of Hegel to criticise a contemporary 'degradation of psychoanalysis'.[152] But he also defends himself here against the accusation that he has been 'lured' by the Hegelian promise of 'a purely dialectical exhaustion of being'.[153] Lacan presented this paper at a conference at Royaumont, near Paris, on the theme of '*La Dialectique*'—in which he was invited to participate by none other than Jean Wahl. The extenuation just quoted is, as he elaborates in a footnote in the *Écrits*, Lacan's way of batting off a comment that was made by Wahl in excerpts of his diary that had been published just before in *La Nouvelle Revue française*, which euphemistically finger, in Lacan's words, certain '"psychoanalysts" who

[150] Wahl et al., 'Inquiry: On Spiritual Directors' (1939), in Hollier, *The College of Sociology*, p. 67.

[151] Jean-Pierre Cléro, 'Hyppolite et Lacan', *L'École de la Cause freudienne*, 70, no. 3 (2008), 122–128 (p. 123).

[152] Lacan, 'The Subversion of the Subject and the Dialectic of Desire in the Freudian Unconscious', in *Écrits*, pp. 671–702 (p. 681).

[153] Lacan, 'The Subversion of the Subject', p. 681.

[are] too "Hegelian" for his liking'—as if, Lacan sneers, 'anyone in this group but me could even be associated with Hegel'.[154] From roughly the point of this smear onwards, there is a shift of emphasis in Lacan's reading of Hegel. Before, he is mainly concerned with illustrating how Freud clarifies a swerve away from the pathologies of the imaginary that are illustrated by Hegel. When Lacan discusses Hegel after 1960, however, he is particularly concerned with the theme of knowledge. As he announces at the opening of 'Subversion of the Subject', which was delivered in the September of 1960, at this point he is using Hegel both to situate the subject 'on the basis of a relationship to knowledge', but also, simultaneously, to demonstrate 'the ambiguity of such a relationship'.[155] Through the 1960s, Lacan will develop how absolute knowledge, the apex of Hegel's *Phenomenology*, may, whilst being a mirage, amount nevertheless to a mirage with a function that is operative in all knowledge.

Instead of rejecting absolute knowledge as the acme of Hegelian hubris, from this point onward Lacan is able to begin intuiting that this epistemological limit is a function that characterises all knowledge, and which can be used to understand its operation. In doing so, he picks up a suggestion made by Hyppolite during the sixth lesson of *Seminar II*. If it is understood in a certain way, Hyppolite outlines here, absolute knowledge does not necessarily represent an error, or a hubris, on Hegel's part. Is it really to be understood, as it is traditionally—asks Hyppolite on 12 January 1955—that there is 'a moment, in the wake of experience, which appears as absolute knowledge', that would be an endpoint arrived at after a succession of stages, and that could be reached by Napoleon, or by whoever else has checked each of them off their itinerary?[156] Or is it, instead—and far more subtly—that absolute knowledge lies 'in the whole presentation of experience'—that it is not the end of a temporal process, but a limit immanent to the structure of human consciousness?[157] Are we, in other words, 'always and every moment in absolute knowledge'?[158]

[154] Lacan, 'The Subversion of the Subject', pp. 701–2, n. 3.

[155] Lacan, 'The Subversion of the Subject', p. 793.

[156] Hyppolite's intervention, in Lacan, Lesson of 12 January, 'VI. Freud, Hegel and the Machine', in *Seminar II*, p. 71.

[157] Hyppolite, in *Seminar II*, p. 71.

[158] Hyppolite, in *Seminar II*, p. 71.

Hyppolite refers here to Heidegger's interpretation of Hegel, to suggest that absolute knowledge is 'immanent at every stage of the *Phenomenology*', but that it is 'missed' by consciousness, which makes of it just 'another natural phenomenon'.[159] Absolute knowledge, in this Heideggerian reading, would 'never be a moment in history', and yet 'it would always be', because it would be 'experience *as such*, and not a moment *in* experience'.[160] Absolute knowledge would amount, then, to 'seeing the field' that consciousness cannot see, because experience is situated in and conditioned by its arras. When we understand this, Hyppolite adds—in a comment that resonates through the entire history of French Hegelianism—we understand why 'one doesn't go beyond Hegel'.[161]

Six years later, in *Seminar IX: Identification* (1961–62), Lacan returns to this rendition of absolute knowledge given by Hyppolite in 1955. He inverts it, in this later seminar, to highlight the function, and the fiction, of what he names the 'subject supposed to know'. Hyppolite had identified, in 1955, a 'synchronic' quality in absolute knowledge, and had suggested that it does not pop up at the end of history, but rather cuts through history at every given moment of individual consciousness. In the opening lesson of *Seminar IX*, Lacan attributes an adapted version of this structure to what he calls the 'subject supposed to know'. This subject is, he says, like Hyppolite's version of absolute knowledge, 'always there, from the beginning of phenomenological questioning, at a certain point, at a certain knot of the structure'.[162] For Lacan, however, absolute knowledge is not the limit to knowledge that exists at any and every given moment. Knowledge, for Lacan, is instead always bordered by the supposition that there is a *subject* who contains it. Absolute knowledge is always deferred, for Lacan, to the mere supposition of its being possessed by this other subject, and the possibility of actually attaining this knowledge is thereby torpedoed: this knowledge is only ever *supposed*, in the sense of 'assumed' or 'believed', to be within this other subject.

159 Hyppolite, in *Seminar II*, p. 71.

160 Hyppolite, in *Seminar II*, p. 71. My italics.

161 Hyppolite, in *Seminar II*, p. 71.

162 Lacan, Lesson of 15 November 1961, in *Seminar IX: Identification* (1961–1962), unpublished. See Gallagher's unofficial translation, p. 10.

Understanding this, says Lacan, allows us to 'extricate ourselves from the diachronic unfolding which is supposed to lead us to absolute knowledge'.[163] The subject supposed to know that Lacan refers to can be understood as the other side of absolute knowledge—the mannequin behind the mask of this knowledge, which was made visible after Freud disenchanted the victorious march of self-consciousness that Hegel describes in his *Phenomenology*. What is left behind, as the residue of absolute knowledge, is the edifice of a subject supposed to know, which can now be identified, thanks to psychoanalysis, as a mirage. The hollow, then, that Lacan takes Freud to have carved out of Hegel means that supposed absolute knowledge can truly be attributed to nobody at all, because it has no subject. It is only through an identification—the theme of *Seminar IX*—on an imaginary level, that the subject who is supposed to have absolute knowledge is conjured up. Lacan then portrays the Other, in this lesson of *Seminar IX*, as a landfill for all of the symbolic copulas fastening the subject to this imaginary subject supposed to know. The Other is, he says, a 'refuse dump of the representative representations of the supposition of knowledge'.[164] This, as Lacan points out, is another way of describing the unconscious, 'in so far as the subject has lost himself in this supposition of knowledge'.[165] The subject drags along these husks of knowledge 'without his being aware of it', as 'unrecognisable debris' that 'comes back to him from what his reality undergoes' in this field—as the slips, symptoms, and dreams in which the unconscious appears.[166]

Though clearly a critique of the notion of absolute knowledge, this is much more than the dismissal that characterised Lacan's approach to it in the 1950s. The ego was always a necessary fiction in Lacan's theory, because it amounts to a psychic organ enabling bodily coherence and co-ordination—even if it is also a dangerous fiction, as made clear by paranoiac aggression. In the same way, the subject supposed to know is, in *Seminar IX*, an error that is fundamental for a subject of language, because

[163] Lacan, Lesson of 15 November 1961, in *Seminar IX*. See Gallagher, p. 10.

[164] Lacan, Lesson of 15 November 1961, in *Seminar IX*. See Gallagher, p. 10.

[165] Lacan, Lesson of 15 November 1961, in *Seminar IX*. See Gallagher, p. 10.

[166] Lacan, Lesson of 15 November 1961, in *Seminar IX*. See Gallagher, p. 10.

it functions as a screen, or a dupery, required for the subject's functioning in the field of the symbolic. The point is made even more emphatically in *Seminar XII: Crucial Problems for Psychoanalysis* (1964–65). Here, Lacan stresses the function played by the subject supposed to know in the structure of Newton's theories.[167] A 'completed' knowledge, of which Newtonian knowledge represents the exemplary case, has a distinct effect, he says here, on the status of the subject. As was first pointed out by Leibniz, Newton's concept of gravitational attraction, which is supposed to act over a distance between masses with a force proportional to their magnitude, has a suspiciously occult quality—one which Leibniz went so far as to describe as a 'miracle'.[168] Lacan uses this Leibnizian critique to highlight a hole at the centre of Newtonian knowledge. It shows, he says, that Newton secreted away 'a subject who maintains the action of the law'.[169] The operation of gravity, even to Newton, who famously *hypotheses non facit* when it came to this, is only, says Lacan, able to be supported by a 'pure and supreme subject', an 'acme of the ideal subject that the Newtonian God represents'.[170] Not only does the spectre of the subject supposed to know have a role to play in modern science, then, but this 'nothing' of knowledge—the ghost that haunts the vacuum of knowledge—is in fact revealed in a pure form by modern science. The aim should not be, because it cannot be, to purge this imaginary residue from subjectivity, because the subject is only grounded—not in 'a harmonious group of signifiers'—but 'in so far as somewhere there is a lack [...] of a signifier', into which is projected the subject supposed to know.[171] The 'nerve' of the subject's existence lies, says Lacan, in this 'ambiguity' of its relationship to knowledge, and in the lack that always persists in this knowledge. Psychoanalysis, it can then be understood, is designed to exploit this situation, by introducing the psychoanalyst *as* a deliberately

[167] Lacan, Lesson 18, of 12 May 1965, in *Seminar XII: Crucial Problems for Psychoanalysis* (1964–1965), unpublished. For an unofficial translation, see Gallagher, <http://www.lacaninireland.com/web/wp-content/uploads/2010/06/12-Crucial-problems-for-psychoanalysis.pdf>, p. 239.

[168] Koyré, *Newtonian Studies* (London: Chapman & Hall, 1965), p. 139.

[169] Lacan, Lesson 17, of 5 May 1965, in *Seminar XII*. See Gallagher, pp. 240.

[170] Lacan, Lesson 17, of 5 May 1965, in *Seminar XII*. See Gallagher, pp. 240.

[171] Lacan, Lesson 17, of 5 May 1965, in *Seminar XII*. See Gallagher, pp. 240.

fabricated subject who is supposed to know, in order to gain leverage over the structure in which the analysand is situated.[172]

In characteristically entangled style, Lacan's theoretical apparatus of the subject supposed to know interleaves several perspectives on Hegel that were posed before him by the French Hegelians. Aspects of Lacan's subject supposed to know repeat almost exactly, first of all, Kojève's account of the traversal of unhappy consciousness. For Kojève, the unhappy consciousness was able to 'attain his absolute knowledge at any moment whatsoever'—but only by enslaving himself to God, the 'absolute Master'.[173] This meant that his true liberation would be attainable only through abandoning religion. Like Kojève, Lacan relegates this 'synchronic' kind of absolute knowledge, the kind that would be available at any moment, to redundancy, by unmasking the subject supposed to know as its necessary support. The subject supposed to know can be understood, in light of this comparison, as Lacan's general formula for the same epistemological function that Kojève refers to here as 'God'. Both Kojève and Lacan are identifying, in these different terms, the fictional substrate that supports a subject's knowledge.

The relationship, which Kojève dismantled here, of the unhappy consciousness to an absolute knowledge that would be attainable 'at any moment', was exactly what was described by Hyppolite in *Seminar II* (1954–55). Kojève rejected this version of absolute knowledge as a delusion of the unhappy consciousness. It was, however, only possible for Kojève to reject the absolute knowledge of the unhappy consciousness because Kojève preserved—or because he sought to preserve—the *other* form of absolute knowledge that Hyppolite had rejected. This other form of absolute knowledge is the kind that would be attained at the end of the bloody progress of History. Kojève always understood this to be its true form. Lacan's subject supposed to know is situated in the hollow created by the overlap of these two readings of absolute knowledge. As a theoretical apparatus, the subject supposed to know escapes the idea of a diachronic march towards absolute knowledge. This version of the progress

[172] Lacan, Lesson 17, of 5 May 1965, in *Seminar XII*. See Gallagher, pp. 233–4.

[173] Kojève, 'Philosophy and Wisdom: Complete Text of the First Two Lectures of the Academic Year 1938–1939', in *Introduction to the Reading of Hegel*, pp. 90–91.

of knowledge had already been put firmly out of play by Lacan's reading of Freud as categorically denying the possibility of self-consciousness by articulating a subject of the unconscious. Yet the subject supposed to know also clearly avoids the slavery that Kojève identified in the kind of immediate absolute knowledge available to the unhappy consciousness. Instead of understanding disbelief in the absolute master to facilitate this master's obliteration, as Kojève had, Lacan illustrates how this absolute master's power may not only remain, but even be intensified, if He is not believed in, because belief only takes place on the level of consciousness. The power of the subject supposed to know, in other words, cannot be annulled by a conscious choice not to believe in it. It is not something that is overcome once and for all, by an act as straightforward as becoming an atheist, in the way that unhappy consciousness was for Kojève. Like Wahl, Lacan is making the unhappy consciousness, and the knowledge that it supposes, a motif that has to be repeatedly resolved in the life of the subject, rather than one that is surpassed historically once and for all. Unlike Wahl, and here developing Kojève's reading, Lacan makes the unhappy consciousness the waste object of an absolute master—a master who is, however, already dead, and who is therefore undefeatable in any permanent sense.

At the same time, Lacan definitively rejects the tragi-comic aspect of Kojève's reading of Hegel and, more broadly, the theme of resolution that had been articulated in various forms by the French Hegelians. The reformulations of the dialectic of desire that Lacan gives in *Seminar X: Anxiety* (1962–63) make particularly clear that, for him, there is something that haunts Hegel's philosophy, but which goes unregistered by him. Lacan's reading of Hegel is one on the level of loss and tragedy. There is never, *Seminar X* teaches, a sufficient recognition of the subject by the Other. Instead, the status of desire imposes a fundamental limitation onto mankind, and creates an unfillable hole at the core of every subject. Self-consciousness—the process of *Selbstbewußtstein* narrated in the *Phenomenology*—is treated by Lacan as merely the myth of overcoming this condition. In *Seminar X*, Lacan identifies anxiety as the fallout of this asymmetry, and Kierkegaard as, therefore, 'the one who imparts the truth of the Hegelian formula'.[174] The meaning of the truth of anxiety that Kierkegaard introduced is described by Lacan in *Seminar X* as a choice between two mutually exclusive positions, according to the formula in the title of Kierkegaard's famous book:

> there is *either* the function of the concept as Hegel would have it, that is, the symbolic hold over the real, *or* the hold that we have, the one anxiety gives us, the sole final perception and as such the perception of all reality—and [...] between the two, one has to choose[.][175]

In this passage, Lacan rearticulates the crux that each of the French Hegelians discussed in the previous section of this chapter had attempted to solve. Definitively, however, he is presenting it here as a problem without a solution.

That Hegel is in no way escaped by these formulations is made clear by the bifurcation, articulated by Koyré, between Hegel and HEGEL. As Koyré was so astutely pointing out when he expressed this division, the choice between the—mutually exclusive—options of anxious existential subject, or stony effigy of the concept, is one that occurs on the level of Hegel's philosophy itself. What the French Hegelians discovered is that a serious reading of Hegel would have to be based on gaps within Hegel that explicitly implicated his readers. Their work demonstrates how Hegel pushes his most assiduous, devoted, and serious readers towards a form of paranoia that brings their own practice of reading into anguished question, and that forces them to recognise it as being, not transparent access to his thought, but something internal to it; a moment already inscribed within it.

---

174 Lacan, Lesson of 21 November 1962, 'II. Anxiety, Sign of Desire', in *Seminar X*, pp. 16–28 (p. 25).

175 Lacan Lesson of 3 July 1963, 'XXIV. From the *a* to the Names-of-the-Father', in *Seminar X*, pp. 324–338 (p. 333). In the following year's seminar, Lacan articulates this in the logic of the 'vel', which imposes on the subject the choice between 'meaning' or 'being'. As a result, the subject can emerge at the level of meaning 'only from its *aphanisis* in the Other locus, which is that of the unconscious'. See Lesson of the 27 May 1964, 'XVI. The Subject and the Other: Alienation', in *Seminar XI: The Four Fundamental Concepts of Psychoanalysis* (1964–1965), ed. by Jacques-Alain Miller, trans. by Alan Sheridan (London: Norton, 1998), pp. 203–215 (p. 221).

Lacan's response to this was to treat Hegel as a cipher, that could be reduced to a set of logical gestures, and then approached from an angle that would allow him to exploit each of their faultlines at once. When Lacan claims that Kierkegaard realises, ultimately, the 'truth of the Hegelian formula', he is describing the kind of reading that he himself aspires to: the realisation of a truth that would overturn a formula through pure, limitless assent. Hyppolite was laying the ground for this strategy by claiming that his reading of absolute knowledge demonstrates that we do not 'go beyond' Hegel. Hegel's pattern of thought, this is to say, is one into whose operation we fall even when we seek to escape it: rejecting absolute knowledge as an end-state, we simply discover its operation—as something never fully grasped, which is perpetually on the horizon of consciousness—in every moment of living experience. This chapter has been attempting to demonstrate how Lacan realises the truth of this Hegelian nexus more completely than his contemporaries. He understands that Hegel's consistency depends on the betrayal of his system; on a recognition of the ultimate obstacles to its completion, and on its humiliation as a machine of *Selbsbewußtstein*, which marks its product as a mere counterfeit—a *Selbsbewusßt*-stain.

This is why Lacan—and not readers of Hegel contemporary to him—is regarded by Žižek as his 'repetition'.[176] If, however, in trying to escape Hegel, we inevitably repeat him, this need not press us into the position of awful submission that Foucault articulates when he famously portrays Hegel as an infinite oral drive swallowing up his antecedents.[177] Beneath this lies the phantasmatic, but common portrait of Hegel as the architect of an eternal subterfuge or trap; as an ancient puzzle to be solved by a worthy adventurer. The reason this is not necessary is because the opposite is also true: if the attempt is made to repeat Hegel faithfully, something

[176] Žižek, *Less Than Nothing: Hegel and the Shadow of Dialectical Materialism* (London: Verso, 2013), p. 5.

[177] See Michel Foucault, 'Discourse on Language', in *The Archaeology of Knowledge and the Discourse on Language*, trans. by A.M. Sheridan Smith (New York: Pantheon, 1972), pp. 215–237 (p. 235): 'But truly to escape Hegel involves an exact appreciation of the price we have to pay to detach ourselves from him. It assumes that we are aware of the extent to which Hegel, insidiously perhaps, is close to us; it implies a knowledge, in that which permits us to think against Hegel, of that which remains Hegelian. We have to determine the extent to which our anti-Hegelianism is possibly one of his tricks directed against us, at the end of which he stands, motionless, waiting for us'.

about his philosophy remains imperceptible, which only appears when, with Lacan's reading of Freud, this missing piece is rigorously formulated.

The detail of the history of French Hegelianism, and the detail of Lacan's texts, make it seem inadequate to describe Lacan as having performed an unintentional 'repetition' of Hegel. His work was a response to the application of far more critical, and far more subtle pressure onto Hegel than is captured by this formula. For Lacan, something was traced out by Hegel about the function of knowledge—which is that it does *not* function, and certainly not in the elegant way that Hegel set out to demonstrate. The strategy Lacan develops to read Hegel forms a vital component of the reading of Marx that he carries out in the late 1960s and early 1970s. Based on how Lacan reads him, Hegel cannot be pitted against Marx in any straightforward way, because this reading aims at something about the nature of knowledge that is just as fundamental for Marx's dialectic. As subsequent chapters of this book will show, Lacan was therefore able to make an intervention in the question of the relationship between Hegel and Marx that was different to those made by the French Marxists contemporary to him who were so obsessed by it. Rescued from the reductive position that he had been given historically, of Marx's nemesis, Lacan's redeemed version of Hegel is also crucial to Žižek's philosophical project. It attains this status for Žižek, though, only through neglect for the historical narrative that made this reading of Hegel possible. As the present chapter has shown, Lacan's response to Hegel cannot be fully understood without attention to this historical passage. Its elision leads Žižek to produce an unintentionally pre-Lacanian reading of Hegel, when he attempts to make a Lacanian one.

How to Repeat Hegel

At the centre of Žižek's seminal book *Less Than Nothing* (2013) is an extended analysis of the supposed limits of Hegelian thought. He includes there a list of concepts that can be thought either by Marx or by psychoanalysis, but that are usually considered to be beyond Hegel. The potentially super-Hegelian concepts he lists are: 'repetition; the unconscious; overdetermination; *objet a*; matheme/letter (science and mathematics);

lalangue; antagonism (parallax); class struggle; [and] sexual difference': each of these resists, on some level, the movement towards synthesis-without-exclusion that is supposed—wrongly, for Žižek—to be the form of Hegelian thought.[178] One by one, however, each of these obstacles is shown by Žižek to be metabolisable, without too much effort, by the more sophisticated reading of Hegelian logic that Žižek is committed, across his writings, to elaborating. If there is one unifying argument that galvanises Žižek's entire theoretical career, it is the claim that Hegel is capable of thinking the dialectical materialist break epitomised by the concept of the symptom in a more truly 'symptomatic' way than Marx. The manoeuvre by which Žižek makes this possible is, as laid out much earlier, in *The Sublime Object of Ideology* (1989), a revision that shrewdly rescues Hegel from what Žižek dismisses as the 'good old Marxist reproach' according to which Hegel 'resolves antagonisms only in "thought", through conceptual mediation, while in reality they remain unresolved'.[179] Instead, says Žižek, 'for Hegel, the point, precisely, is to not "resolve" antagonisms "in reality", but just to enact a parallax shift by means of which antagonisms are recognized "as such" and thereby perceived in their "positive" role'.[180]

Recuperated in Žižek's reading of Hegel are the old anxieties about the significance of Hegel for Marx that surfaced after the publication of the *1844 Manuscripts* in 1932.[181] Here, though, secure from the paranoia and strictures of the Stalinist-era PCF that contextualised these debates in the mid-twentieth century, they are dealt with through Žižek's characteristically brusque rhetorical style: the measure of Hegel's distance behind Marx is refound by Žižek to be his greatest strength, rather than his greatest failure. To suggest that there is something that Hegel 'can't think' always has to be followed by a "yes but", if we read the Hegelian totality,

[178] Žižek, *Less Than Nothing: Hegel and the Shadow of Dialectical Materialism*, p. 455.

[179] Žižek, (1989) *The Sublime Object of Ideology* (London: Verso, 2009), p. xvii. For an example of this criticism of Hegel contemporary to Lacan, see Trần Đức Thảo, 'Le "noyau rationnel" dans la dialectique hégélienne', *La Pensée* (January–February 1965), 4–5. Trần's work is discussed in more detail below in Chapter 4, pp. 181–182, n. 77.

[180] Žižek, *Less Than Nothing*, p. 403.

[181] The *1844 Manuscripts* were translated into French by Henri Lefebvre and Norbert Guterman in 1933.

as Žižek does, to designate 'the Whole plus all of its "symptoms"'.[182] This Hegel—unlike the 'ridiculous textbook figure of an absolute idealist who [...] claims to integrate the entire wealth of the universe into the totality of rational self-mediation'—is able to think the notion that, 'according to Lacan, condenses all the paradoxes of the Freudian field, the notion of the non-All'.[183] In terms of what Hegel "cannot do", it is, for Žižek, never a question of simple impossibility or inability', but there is 'in all these cases, a tiny, imperceptible line of separation which compels us to supplement the assertion of impossibility with a qualifying "yes, but..."'.[184] This extends to Hegel's value as a political thinker: rather than being dismissed as the philosopher of a naïve bourgeois liberalism, his central contemporary value lays, for Žižek, in his relevance for a world where Communism is not inevitably on the horizon, but where its twentieth-century attempts to resolve social antagonism ultimately failed. Hegel is uniquely able, when read in this way, to depict, through the very *limits* of his system, the points where cracks emerge in the edifice of liberal democracy—which Žižek identifies as having been revealed more fully by a world post-End of History.[185]

Lacan plays a significant role in this argument. Žižek claims that neither Lacan, Marx, nor anyone else has thought anything that cannot be located as a moment in the Hegelian system—not, however, because Hegel's work is a totalising sphere that encircles everything, but because his thought, anticipating the dimension of the symptom, inscribes these post-Hegelian concepts within its own structure; in its gaps, its points of crisis, and its failures. The concepts listed above that at first appear to exceed Hegel are in fact, Žižek shows, mere opportunities to demonstrate, and to emphasise the significance of, a reading of Hegel in which these concepts always had their place. These supposedly post-Hegelian concepts merely reveal the true nature of Hegel, as freed from the naïve idea of a totalising 'All'. Hegel never did make, Žižek argues, such claims to wholeness or completion, except on the basis of this redeemed idea of

[182] Žižek, *Less Than Nothing*, p. 455.
[183] Žižek, *Less Than Nothing*, p. 455.
[184] Žižek, *Less Than Nothing*, p. 455.
[185] Žižek, *Less Than Nothing*, p. 436.

the 'non-All'. Even the most sophisticated of attacks on Hegel's philosophy serve, for Žižek, if made on this basis, merely to reveal this about it. For this reason, not only does Lacan represent a 'repetition' of Hegel, but Lacan amounts to the only way to 'save Hegel', because he provides the theoretical tools to make this reading.[186]

The present chapter began by describing the reception of Hegel in France as a chain of mistransmission, paranoia, and caricature. It then demonstrated how an approach to reading Hegel was developed in France precisely out of this inability to access his philosophy as a stable, complete object. Lacan's own use of Hegel, the chapter has shown, performed an extensive formulation of Hegel in response to the character of his work that was acknowledged in this context. Žižek also reads Lacan as capturing—in the idea of the 'non-All'—this dimension of Hegel as none had before him. But he positions Lacan as therefore being a 'repetition' of Hegel. Whilst attempting to offer a new way to think about Lacan, as an extension of, an articulation of, or a formula for, complexities and paradoxes that exist in Hegel's philosophy, this reading of Lacan itself unintentionally repeats the questions that concerned the figures on whose work this chapter has been focused. Describing Hegel as 'not-All' uses Lacanian terminology to refer to what Koyré had begun to articulate as a conflict between different versions of Hegel: for Koyré, commenting on the state of French Hegelianism in general, Hegel's system was also already based around its own incompleteness and lack of identity. Without attention to this history of French readings of Hegel, the more subtle repetition being made by Žižek, and the way his work itself is conditioned by this history, remains invisible.

Since the 1920s, French philosophers had discerned that there was something in Hegel's philosophy that sabotaged and undermined itself when taken to a certain limit; a consequence of contradiction that did not lead towards absolute knowledge, but which turned that knowledge into something that was different to anything Hegel had articulated. Žižek's reading of Hegel can be situated in this lineage of questions about Hegel. This chapter argues, however, that Žižek responds to the concerns of the French Hegelians conservatively, by attempting to draw their

[186] Žižek, *Less Than Nothing*, p. 5; and Žižek, *The Sublime Object of Ideology*, p. xxxi.

consequences back into a reading that would 'save' Hegel. Žižek can therefore only read Lacan as the messenger of something that had already been laid out before Lacan. For Lacan, it is not a case of having to use intellectual ingenuity, or the ruses of reason, to resolve Hegel's problems. What Lacan instead argues is that there are historical reasons why something came to appear unstable in Hegel in the way the French Hegelians discerned.

The later chapters of this book will describe this point, and its consequences for reading Marx, in greater detail. This chapter, in conclusion, is not arguing that either Žižek or Lacan are right or wrong in their responses to Hegel. It is arguing that Lacan's position is different to Žižek's, and that it is a position that he took in response to, and as a development of, work by his contemporary readers of Hegel. The following three chapters of this book will build on the history of French Hegelianism narrated in this chapter, to discuss in much further detail the relationship between Marxist and Hegelian thought in France contemporary to Lacan. The conflict between materialism and idealism in which Marxist thinkers understood themselves to be conscripts forms the backdrop to the discussions, in the following two chapters, of materialist psychology, and of structuralist theories of history. Hegel will appear in these chapters with much less vibrancy and detail than he appears in Lacan's reading of him, and almost exclusively as an idealist bogey of the committed Marxist scientists and philosophers whose work these chapters will describe.

The present chapter's close attention to Lacan's reading of Hegel, and to his position in the context of French Hegelianism, is important in this context. It explains why, whilst Lacan, as these later chapters will emphasise, offers a very precise critique of idealism, he clearly does not reject Hegel. This chapter has shown how Lacan's theory of transference uses Hegel to articulate a new way of thinking about the undialectical core of knowledge; something which he thinks Marx did not account for. On this basis, the subsequent chapters will describe, Lacan makes a compelling critique of materialism itself as a philosophical position. The following chapter will illustrate this through an analysis of Lacan's critical responses to attempts, made by his contemporaries, to produce a materialist psychology. In his estimation, what was intended by them to be a break from idealism unintentionally reverted into a degraded, idealistic spiritualism. Psychoanalysis alone, for Lacan, is able to make this failure visible.

3

'Reflex to a Reflex': The Unconscious Between Idealist and Materialist Psychology

After the October Revolution, a project was begun in Russia to transform all areas of human life, culture, and thought, in order to enable the emergence of a new kind of human being—the "new man" of Communism.[1] As part of this project, the mystifying remnants of morality, spirituality, and metaphysics—and with them, any notion of the soul—were to be purged from all fields of science. Those who sought a materialist theory of psychology in this context, however, ran up against a set of serious, recurring problems, because psychology is a science more haunted than any other by these metaphysical revenants. From its etymology onwards, in being prefixed by the Greek *psyche*, it is structured around the locus of the soul. Historically, the science had emerged from an attempt to study a plane of human life that preserved and translated religious and metaphysical ideas into a form that was palatable in an increasingly secular, scientific Europe.[2] Psychology's very function, from a critical, Marxist

[1] See Raymond A. Bauer, *The New Man in Soviet Psychology* (London: Oxford University Press, 1952).

[2] For this historical context, see David Joravsky, *Russian Psychology: A Critical History* (Oxford: Basil Blackwell, 1989); and John McLeish, *Soviet Psychology: History, Theory, Content* (London: Methuen, 1975).

M. Maher, *Symptom Invented*, The Palgrave Lacan Series,
https://doi.org/10.1007/978-3-032-12267-4_3

perspective of its history, could very easily be viewed a means merely to smuggle spirit into science.

For this very reason, the science of psychology came to occupy a privileged position in the context, described in the Introduction of this thesis, of the less monochrome view of idealism that Marxist philosophers outside of the Soviet bloc—such as Hyppolite, Maublanc, and Lukács—began to take from the late 1920s onwards. Because the object of psychology is completely transformed depending on whether or not the psyche can be envisaged materially, psychology became a terrain on which the question of the equilibrium between idealism and materialism could be played out, and potentially transcended.

The position of Freud in these debates was distinctly inconsistent. He appeared in them as a figure in perpetual flux. In Lev Vygotsky's writings, for instance, he is just as much a remnant of mystified, bourgeois consciousness as he is a vital, razor-sharp force for renewal, poised on the edge of radical dialectical materialism.[3] For Georges Politzer and Henri Wallon, in France, Freud's theories in general represented an instrument that could rescue the pursuit of a materialist psychology, because they bridged a gap—and occupied a captivatingly paradoxical position—between a naïvely mechanical materialism, and a mystified idealism. This chapter will describe how the unconscious appeared as a useful, important, but also dangerous, concept for several psychologists who were invested in Marxism in the early twentieth century. As it will point out, their efforts to enlist Freud in the pursuit of a Marxist psychology were characterised by a tension between a vague, ill-defined, but emerging awareness of the possibilities that might be facilitated by what Freud had attempted to achieve, matched with shock and revulsion towards some of these attempts. In general, these figures give a sense of not knowing what to do with Freud, or where he was to be located factionally. For Lev Vygotsky and Alexander Luria, as they put it in their preface to the Russian translation of *Beyond the Pleasure Principle*, Freud was part of the 'difficult and prolonged' labour through which 'bourgeois science is

[3] In addition to the work of Vygotsky, Politzer, and Wallon described in detail below, see Henri Lefebvre and Norbert Guterman, *La Conscience mystifiée* (Paris: Gallimard, 1936).

giving birth to materialism'.[4] But where was this 'difficult and prolonged' labour leading to? And what kind of science would it produce?

This chapter points to a set of questions and contradictions that were encountered by the psychologists and philosophers who sought a materialist theory of psychology, and describes how they independently encountered similar points of crisis within the conceptual basis of psychology as a science. It argues that, as a result, psychology came to act as a screen for the most significant pressure-points of the relationship between idealism and materialism. It follows this by identifying these impasses as central foundations for Lacan's own theories. The chapter narrates a movement between two theoretical objects: the reflex which dominated Russian psychology from the 1860s onwards, and the Lacanian signifier, as he poses it from the early 1950s. Rather than arguing, with some, that Lacan amounts to the heroic heir of this materialist tradition, the chapter will suggest that, when read in the context of attempts to formulate a materialist psychology, Lacan's theories press towards a new way of answering the question of what, fundamentally, materialism *is*.[5] As it will demonstrate, the instabilities at the conceptual basis of the reflex theory are rewritten in Lacan's theory of the instance of the signifier in the unconscious, as instabilities which, for him, lay at the conceptual basis of materialism itself.

Lev Vygotsky and Psychology's *Capital*

When the Russian psychologist Ivan Mikhailovich Sechenov published his book *Reflexes of the Brain* in 1866, it had provoked moral indignation. It was described by state censors as reducing 'even the best of men to the level of a machine devoid of consciousness and free will, and acting automatically', and was publicly denounced as being morally corruptive as a result.[6] In the book, Sechenov argues that all conscious and unconscious

[4] Lev Vygotsky and Alexander Luria, 'Introduction to the Russian translation of Freud's *Beyond the Pleasure Principle*', in *The Vygotsky Reader*, ed. by René van der Veer and Jaan Valsiner (Oxford: Blackwell, 1994), pp. 10–18 (p. 17).

[5] See, for example, Alenka Zupančič, *What is Sex?* (London: MIT Press, 2017), p. 16.

[6] McLeish, '3. The Origin of Objective Psychology', in *Soviet Psychology*, unpaginated e-book.

acts are reflexes—impulsive nervous responses to stimuli—which do not require conscious thought or awareness. The 'higher mental processes' of humans, he argued, could be understood on this basis as mere products of the inhibition of these various reflexive motor-responses. Sechenov was an important figure in introducing materialism to psychology in nineteenth-century Russia.[7] At the time when he published *Reflexes of the Brain*, psychology was still only being studied in Russian philosophy and theology departments, and it was dominated by idealistic, spiritualistic theories. It would only attain independence in universities as a science in its own right after the October Revolution in 1917. This did not, however, produce a conclusive break from the conservatism evident in the reception of Sechenov's work; the Revolution would instead spur decades of retrospective consolidation of all kinds of historically existing strands of psychological thought. There was, nonetheless, a distinct, if not uniform, shift at this revolutionary moment, to what Nikolai Krementsov describes as a 'new lexicon and a new polemical style' that centred around a set of particular figures and ideas.[8] These materialist psychologists would cleave, in particular, to seeds of a psychology left in the writings of Marx and Engels, which argue that the development of all human mental functions was dependent on the history of labour practices, and which lay out the significance of 'revolutionary', 'practical-critical' mental activity.[9]

---

[7] B.G. Anan'yev ed., *Psychological Science in the USSR, Vol. 1* (1959), trans. by US Joint Publications Research Service (1961), p. 2. Sechenov was a student of Helmholtz and Brücke, who extended their shared theoretical principle, that forces operating within organisms were exclusively physical and chemical in nature, to a theory explaining the mechanism of physical activity. See McLeish, '3. The Origin of Objective Psychology', in *Soviet Psychology*.

[8] Nikolai Krementsov, *Stalinist Science* (Princeton: Princeton University Press, 1997), p. 23.

[9] For the former, see Friedrich Engels, 'The Part Played by Labour in the Transition from Ape to Man', *Die Neue Zeit* 14, 545–556. 'The reaction on labour and speech of the development of the brain and its attendant senses, of the increasing clarity of consciousness, power of abstraction and of conclusion, gave both labour and speech an ever-renewed impulse to further development. This development did not reach its conclusion when man finally became distinct from the ape, but on the whole made further powerful progress, its degree and direction varying among different peoples and at different times, and here and there even being interrupted by local or temporary regression'. Cited in Peter E. Langford, *Vygotsky's Developmental and Educational Psychology* (New York: Psychology Press, 2005), p. 1.

For the latter, see Marx and Engels, 'Theses on Feuerbach', in *The German Ideology*, trans. by C.J. Arthur (New York: International Publishers, 1973), pp. 121–3 (p. 121): 'The chief defect of all hitherto existing materialism (that of Feuerbach included) is that the thing, reality, sensuousness, is conceived only in the form of the object or of contemplation, but not as sensuous human activity,

Psychoanalysis, and theories of the unconscious more generally, would have a complicated fate in this context. Older accounts of the history of Soviet psychoanalysis tend to emphasise the staunch rejection of Freud under Stalin, but, more recently, others have identified this Stalinist rejection of psychoanalysis as a later development, that followed its much more ambivalent treatment amidst the general chaos of immediate post-revolutionary thought.[10] The story of psychoanalysis in the Soviet Union is usually given a somewhat flawed protagonist in the psychologist Alexander Luria, whose youthful precocity was central in setting up the first psychoanalytic institute in Russia, but who later renounced Freud under the grip of the restraint that Stalinism placed on all of the sciences.[11] Freud enjoyed a period of evident popularity amongst Russian psychologists in the early 1920s.[12] Luria describes his writings as an alternative to the 'lifeless, impersonal [...] boring, oppressive, vacuous' forms of psychology dominant in the universities, making them, as Hannah Proctor suggests, 'equal', for him, 'to the vitality of the revolutionary moment'.[13] Luria saw psychoanalysis as a break from the metaphysics and idealism of the old psychology, towards 'the perspective of an

practice, subjectively. Hence, in contradistinction to materialism, the *active* side was developed abstractly by idealism—which, of course, does not know real, sensuous activity as such. Feuerbach wants sensuous objects, really distinct from the thought objects, but he does not conceive human activity itself as *objective* activity. Hence, in *Das Wesen des Christentums,* he regards the theoretical attitude as the only genuinely human attitude, while practice is conceived and fixed only in its dirty-judaical manifestation. Hence he does not grasp the significance of "revolutionary", of "practical-critical", activity'.

[10] For examples of these older accounts, see Anan'yev ed., *Psychological Science in the USSR*; and Alex Kozulin, *Psychology in Utopia: Toward a Social History of Soviet Psychology* (Massachusetts: MIT Press, 1984). As examples of the latter, more recent histories, see Martin A. Miller, *Freud and the Bolsheviks: Psychoanalysis in Imperial Russia and the Soviet Union* (New York: Yale University Press, 1998); and Hannah Proctor, '"A Country Beyond the Pleasure Principle": Alexander Luria, Death Drive and Dialectic in Soviet Russia, 1917–1930', *Psychoanalysis and History*, 18, no. 2 (2016), 155–182.

[11] See Proctor, '"A Country Beyond the Pleasure Principle"'. Kozulin also appreciates the ambiguity of any supposed act of criticism under the restrictions of the Stalinist USSR, which could well manifest a 'concealed method of propagation' of its object, where no less covert means for this existed. See Kozulin, *Psychology in Utopia*, p. 89.

[12] Kozulin, *Psychology in Utopia*, p. 83.

[13] Luria cited in Karl Levitin, 'A Criminal Investigation', *Journal of Russian and Eastern European Psychology*, 36, no. 5 (1998), 46–75 (p. 62). Proctor, '"A Country Beyond the Pleasure Principle"', p. 161.

organic process which unfolds in the human organism taken as a whole', and which he hoped would facilitate—when applied alongside reflexology—'a solid basis for the monistic theory of materialist psychology'.[14] Another figure of note here is the philosopher Bernard Bykhovsky, who agreed with Luria, writing in 1923, that psychoanalysis, 'despite its subjectivist appearance', is 'infused with monism, materialism, and dialectics, that is, with the methodological principles of dialectical materialism'.[15] Bolsheviks in the highest levels of power were, says Alexander Etkind, 'enchanted by the possibilities thrown open' by psychoanalysis 'for the scientific transformation of life'.[16] This, Etkind notes, was borne out by the fact that most of the leadership of the Russian Psychoanalytic Society in the 1920s consisted of Bolsheviks. Martin A. Miller goes as far as to argue plausibly that 'no government was ever responsible for supporting psychoanalysis to such an extent, before or after' these early days of the Soviet Union.[17] Even if, however, the demise of psychoanalysis in Russia can be generally blamed on Stalin's expulsion of the left opposition in 1928, the post-revolutionary 1920s did not simply amount to a Freudian utopia.[18] Freud came under public criticism by Lenin himself in 1920 for his 'exaggeration of sexual matters' and 'bourgeois views on women'.[19] There were then several contingent forces that contributed to the decline of psychoanalysis in the Soviet

[14] Alexander Luria, 'Psikhoanaliz Kak Sistema Monisticheskoy Psikhologii', in *Psikhologija Marxizm*, ed. by Konstantin Kornilov (Moscow and Leningrad, 1925), p. 79; translated in English in *Soviet Psychology*, 16 (1977/78), pp. 6–45. Cited in Kozulin, *Psychology in Utopia*, p. 87.

[15] Bernard Bykhovsky, 'O Metodologicheskih Osnovaniyah Psikhoanaliticheskogo Ucheniya Freuda', *Pod Znamenem Marxizma*, 11/12 (1923), p. 169. See also Lawrence Kubie, 'Pavlov, Freud and Soviet Psychiatry', *Behavioural Science*, 4 (1959), pp. 29–34; and Kozulin, *Psychology in Utopia*, p. 91.

[16] Alexander Etkind, *Eros of the Impossible* (London; Routledge, 1997), p. 242.

[17] Miller, *Freud and the Bolsheviks*, p. 68.

[18] Proctor, '"A Country Beyond the Pleasure Principle"', p. 162. Freud was famously critical of the Soviet project in his thirty-fifth Introductory Lecture. See Freud, 'Lecture XXXV: The Question of a *Weltanschauung*' (1933), in *The Standard Edition of the Complete Psychological Works of Sigmund Freud, Vol. XXII*, trans. by James Strachey (London: Hogarth Press, 1964), pp. 158–184.

[19] See Kozulin, *Psychology in Utopia*, p. 91. Lenin made these comments during his talks with Klara Zetkin, an activist of the Women's Chapter of the Komintern. Zetkin's memoirs were later published in *Pravda*, where she included the following remark: 'Those who like to connect Freudism with Marxism and to use the "achievements" of Freud, should think seriously about the words [of Lenin]'. See *Pravda*, 14 June 1925.

Union in the late 1920s: the departure of some promising members of the Psychoanalytic Society as their research interests changed, and the closure of a children's home run by Vera Schmidt attached to the Psychoanalytical Institute, for example.[20] But Kozulin notes, more generally, that psychoanalysis shared the common fate of all independent psychological movements in being silenced after the 1920s.[21]

As is borne out by the work of Soviet psychologists at this time, Marxism appeared to many scientists as a general science that could connect potentially all and any loose ends and discrepancies existing in specific fields, and transform them in all kinds of beneficial ways.[22] The readings of Marx made by Soviet psychologists in these years was, however, not always of a high quality, and nor was their knowledge of Marx particularly sophisticated. Most can justifiably be accused, as Aleksei Leont'ev does, of having done 'no more than [to] illustrate the laws of dialectics with psychological material'.[23] In this context, the psychologist Lev Vygotsky is significant for his ambition, clarity, and precision. Vygotsky did not, like many of his contemporaries, just paste abstracted versions of Marx's ideas onto psychology; he approached the forging of a Marxist psychology by engaging in a serious reading of Marx.

One of the main concerns of Vygotsky's work was to rehabilitate the phenomena of language and consciousness into a theory of reflexology. Reflexology had, in the form it had been given by Ivan Pavlov, become

---

[20] Kozulin, *Psychology in Utopia*, p. 94.

[21] Peter E. Langford, *Vygotsky's Developmental and Educational Psychology* (Hove: Psychology Press, 2005), p. 104.

[22] See R.W. Rieber and Jeffrey Wollock, 'Prologue: Vygotsky's "Crisis" and its Meaning Today', in *The Collected Works of L.S. Vygotsky, Vol. 3: Problems of the Theory and History of Psychology*, trans. by René van der Veer (New York: Springer, 1997), pp. vii–xii (pp. viii–ix). The debate, described above, between materialist and idealist psychologists continued in the Soviet Union in the post-Revolutionary 1920s. Their movements were headed by Konstantin Kornilov and Georgii Chelpanov, respectively. See A.N. Leont'ev, 'On Vygotsky's Creative Development', in *The Collected Works of L.S. Vygotsky, Vol. 3*, pp. 9–32 (p. 11). Kornilov represented the movement that was attempting to develop a Marxist psychology. He sought to assimilate contemporary psychology within a Marxist conceptual framework, rejecting a view of human nature which ignored class, and to cleave it to Marx and Engels's views on human mental processes. See McLeish, 'Chapter 4: The Revolution and its Effects: 1917–1929', in *Soviet Psychology*.

[23] Leont'ev, 'On Vygotsky's Creative Development', p. 11.

the basis for Soviet psychology by the early 1920s.[24] Pavlov's theory of conditional reflexes was famously demonstrated by his experiments with dogs, which he trained to salivate, not only at the sight of food, but in response to various other stimuli. Pavlov's version of the theory aimed to understand all animal behaviour, including even the most complex and varied behaviour of humans, as automatic, nervous responses to stimuli. The methodological and ideological benefits of the theory are clear, in removing the need for an introspective approach to psychological research, and in expunging from psychology an idealist zone of a soul or psyche supplementary to this material network of stimulus and nervous response. It would be reductive, however, despite the materialist standpoint that Pavlov took even in relation to the phenomena of speech and thought, to view him as a mechanical materialist of the likes of Ludwig Büchner, Carl Vogt, or Jacob Moleschott.[25] Although he argued, initially, that the fundamental laws of the reflexological signalling system must govern even the higher human functions, because they stemmed from the same nervous tissue, he would later, in 1932, put forward a 'second signalling system', which reserved at least the possibility that there may, at this higher level, be special laws in operation.[26]

Vygotsky writes with precision and clarity in the 1920s about the limitations of the reflex theory—limitations that Pavlov would try to solve only later, in the early 1930s, by introducing the second signalling system. Because of the apparent success of reflexology as a materialist theory,

---

[24] It is easy to see how the theory of reflexes took its impetus from the Marxist-Leninist theory of "reflection", which puts forward that mental processes are functions of the brain in a material sense, because its matter is able to "reflect" reality (See Anan'ev, *Psychological Science in the USSR*, p. 2). There are also identifiable proximities and correlations between Pavlov's theories and Engels's (McLeish, '2. The Origins of Russian Psychology', in *Soviet Psychology*). Lenin recognised this in a 1921 edict, which ascribed to Pavlov exceptional privileges 'in consideration of these extraordinary scientific services which have enormous significance for the workers of the whole world' (Lenin, edict on Pavlov (January, 1921), printed in E.A. Asratyan, 'Switching in Conditioned Reflex Activity as a Basic Form of its Changeability', *Voprosy Psikhologii* 1 (1955), 49–57. Cited in McLeish, '(iii) Pavlov and Lenin: The Theoretical Basis of Soviet Psychology', '3. The Origin of Objective Psychology', in *Soviet Psychology*).

[25] See McLeish, 'Pavlov's Fifth Phase (1919–1935): Application to Man', '4. The Revolution and its Effects: 1917–1929', in *Soviet Psychology.*

[26] 'No doubt we will reduce thinking by experiments to molecular and chemical motions taking place in the brain, but is the essence of thinking completely explained by this?' Engels, *The Dialectics of Nature* (London: Lawrence and Wishart, 1955), p. 72.

Vygotsky argues, Pavlov had taken it to limits that put it under a degree of strain. He had posed, for example, a 'reflex of freedom' and a 'reflex of purpose' in the late 1910s, in an attempt to explain various behavioural phenomena that were outside the remit of his original physiological postulations.[27] In Vygotsky's 1925 article 'Consciousness as a Problem for the Psychology of Behaviour', he criticises this use of the reflex as an all-purpose explanatory device, and is at pains to emphasise how significant it is that the reflex remains, fundamentally, an abstract concept. In reality, Vygotsky observes, 'we are [not] a leather bag filled with reflexes and the brain is not a hotel for complex groups, combinations and systems built according to the most diverse types'.[28] Lumping together—as Vygotsky illustrates parodically—sensations, gestures, mimicry, instincts, slips of the tongue, emotions, the 'higher processes of thought discovered by the Würzburg school', and the interpretation of dreams, as mere species of reflex, neither 'shed[s] light and clarity on the phenomena under study', nor 'help[s] to differentiate and delimit the objects, forms and phenomena', but 'forces us to view everything in a dim twilight where everything is blended together and no clear boundaries between the objects exist'.[29] The inept conceptual extension of the reflex beyond certain limits, Vygotsky illustrates, had produced an obfuscating, mystifying effect, compromising its ability to act as the clarifying scientific theory that a materialist psychology needed it to be.

[27] The esoteric theories of Vladimir Bekhterev, who had extended the theory of the reflex to a general theory of cosmic energy in his book *Psychology, Reflexology, and Marxism* (1925), would come under particular scrutiny by Vygotsky. Thanks to Bekhterev, Vygotsky mockingly observes, 'it turned out that everything in the world is a reflex. Anna Karenina and kleptomania, the class struggle and a landscape, language and dream are all reflexes'. L.S. Vygotsky, 'The Historical Meaning of the Crisis in Psychology', in *The Collected Works of L.S. Vygotsky, Vol. 3*, pp. 233–344 (p. 245). Citing Vladimir Bekhterev, *Kollektivnaja refleksologija* (Petersburg, 1921); and Bekhterev, *Obshchie osnory rejleksologii cheloveka* (Moscow–Petersburg, 1923).

[28] Vygotsky, 'Consciousness as a Problem for the Psychology of Behaviour' (1925), in *The Collected Works of L.S. Vygotsky, Vol. 3*, pp. 63–80 (p. 66). 'Indeed, the reflex, as it is conceived of in Russia, very much resembles the story of Kannitfershtan whose name a poor foreigner heard each time he asked a question in Holland: who is being buried, whose house is this, who drove by, etc. In his naivete he thought that everything in this country was accomplished by Kannitfershtan whereas this word only meant that the Dutchmen he met did not understand his questions.'

[29] Vygotsky, 'Consciousness as a Problem', p. 66. A better picture, for Vygotsky, is one viewing behaviour as 'the system of *victorious* actions' from the complex and chaotic net of stimuli and reflexes present in the organism.

Vygotsky's response to Pavlov amounts to an insistence that the internal limits of the reflex theory had to be confronted head-on in order to preserve the theory's usefulness. A central example of the kind of limitation Vygotsky emphasises is the 'crisis of methods' that occurs when reflexology turns from 'the foundation, from the elementary and the simple, to the superstructure, to the complex and subtle'.[30] In light of this, Vygotsky takes very seriously the problem that the mind, as the ultimate superstructural, complex, subtle object, poses to the theory. He points out how, whilst reflexology is designed to do away with an idealist understanding of the mind, still 'not even the most extreme physiologists', like Pavlov or Vladimir Bekhterev, are prepared to outright deny that the mind exists.[31] To accommodate for mental phenomena, reflexes should, Vygotsky argues, be understood as bound together in complicated, referential, reflecting systems, in which '*[t]he response part of each reflex (movement, secretion) becomes itself a stimulus for a new reflex for the same system or another system*'.[32] In light of this, Vygotsky gives consciousness a new definition in terms of reflexes: it is 'the experience *of* experience in precisely the same way as experience is simply the experience *of* objects'.[33] Consciousness, as Vygotsky defines it here, 'is merely a reflex to reflexes'.[34] It is the illusion of a separate order, created by an interference effect of reflexes upon each other.

As part of his revision of reflexology, and continuing the emphasis he places on the position of consciousness, Vygotsky would later go on to elaborate the complex dialectical relationship he takes to exist between thought and language. His book *Thinking and Speech* (1934) sets out a psychological theory of language, which challenges Pavlov's first signal system by presenting language as an external mediator for reflexes. Vygotsky argues that language and concepts are mediators of the direct stimuli that could be explained by the mechanism of Pavlov's earlier theories, and he argues that these mediators require their own special place

[30] Vygotsky, 'The Methods of Reflexological and Psychological Investigation' (1926), in *The Collected Works of L.S. Vygotsky, Vol. 3*, pp. 35–50 (p. 45).

[31] Vygotsky, 'The Methods', p. 44. For Vygotsky's critique of Bekhterev, see n. 27 above.

[32] Vygotsky, 'The Methods', p. 40.

[33] Vygotsky, 'The Methods', p. 40. My italics.

[34] Vygotsky, 'The Methods', p. 46.

in a reflexological theory. Speech is not continuous with thought, he argues, like 'a simple mirror image of the structures of thought' which can be 'placed on thought like clothes on a rack', nor does it 'merely serve as the expression of developed thought'.[35] Thought and speech have a relationship of delicate interdependence, but they are not two sides of the same thing: thought is, rather, he says, 'restructured as it is transformed into speech', and it is 'not expressed but completed in the word'. Thought, he says, begins as a 'fused, unpartitioned whole' which is gradually given form by language, and speech is at first a function disconnected from it. Thinking and speech initially develop in isolation from each other, until '[a]t a certain point, the two lines cross: thinking becomes verbal and speech intellectual'.[36] Vygotsky's understanding of the psychology of language explicitly incorporates a historical materialist account of the labour form: he describes language as a 'psychological tool' that 'alters the entire flow and structure of mental functions', by 'determining the structure of a new instrumental act just as a technical tool alters the process of a natural adaptation by determining the form of labour'.[37] Language is split, for Vygotsky, between being both an object of thought and a vessel for it. Instead, however, of siding with one of these perspectives over the other, the way Vygotsky envisages the process of language acquisition is as a developing synthesis of these two functions. Thought, for Vygotsky, 'does not express itself in a word but *takes place* in a word'.[38] Meaning then emerges as a third term, out of the dialectical relationship between the two different entities of thought and word.[39]

[35] L.S. Vygotsky, *Thinking and Speech* (1934), in *The Collected Works of L.S. Vygotsky, Vol. 1: Problems of General Psychology*, ed. by R.W. Rieber and A.S. Carton, trans. by N. Minick (London: Plenum Press, 1987), pp. 39–288 (p. 251).

[36] Vygotsky, *Thinking and Speech*, pp. 251, 110, 112.

[37] Vygotsky, 'The Instrumental Method in Psychology' (1930), in *The Concept of Activity in Soviet Psychology*, ed. by J.V. Wertsch (New York: Armonk, 1981), pp. 134–143 (p. 137).

[38] Vygotsky, *Thinking and Speech*, p. 307. Cited in Vladimir P. Zinchenko, 'Thought and Word: The Approaches of L.S. Vygotsky and G.G. Shpet', in *The Cambridge Companion to Vygotsky*, ed. by H. Daniels, M. Cole and J.V. Wertsch (Cambridge: Cambridge University Press, 2007), pp. 212–245 (p. 224).

[39] Vygotsky, 'The Historical Meaning of the Crisis in Psychology: A Methodological Investigation', p. 133.

A particularly significant component of Vygotsky's critique of reflexology is his identification of its unintentional proximity to a spiritualistic idealism. Vygotsky alleges that, though scientific psychology had attempted to escape subjective, introspective psychology by excluding the question of the psychological nature of consciousness, it indirectly preserves the very dualism and spiritualism that was so problematic about subjective psychology in the first place.[40] The problem, he says, goes as deep as reflexology's basic assumptions, firstly, 'that it is possible to fully explain all of man's behaviour without resorting to subjective phenomena', and secondly, that it could 'build a psychology without a mind'.[41] This, Vygotsky alleges, amounts to 'the dualism of subjective psychology turned inside out': it has produced, he says, 'the counterpart of subjective psychology's attempt to study the pure, abstract mind', because in both cases 'mind and behaviour are not one but two'.[42] In making, with Pavlov, mind consist of 'nonspatial and noncausal phenomena', or taking it, with Bekhterev, to possess 'no objective existence *whatsoever* as they can only be studied on oneself', the mind, in either case, becomes 'something which must be studied separately, and independently of which we must study the reflexes'.[43] This effacement of the mind from science is materialistic only insofar as it 'isolat[es] the mind and its study from the general system of human behaviour'.[44] Vygotsky can thereby claim quite tidily that psychologies that perform this isolation amount to 'idealism of the highest order', and to 'a dualism that might more correctly be called an idealism turned upside down'.[45] Vygotsky notes Bekhterev's panpsychism, and his refusal to 'repudiate the hypothesis about a soul', as symptomatic of reflexology's constraint by this 'physiological materialism'. Not a single psychologist, he adds elsewhere, 'not even an extreme spiritualist and idealist, disclaimed the physiological materialism of reflexology', but '[o]n the contrary, all forms of idealism always invariably presupposed it'.[46]

[40] Vygotsky, 'Consciousness as a Problem for the Psychology of Behaviour' (1925), p. 65.
[41] Vygotsky, 'Consciousness as a Problem for the Psychology of Behaviour' (1925), p. 65.
[42] Vygotsky, 'Consciousness as a Problem', p. 65.
[43] Vygotsky, 'The Methods of Reflexological and Psychological Investigation' (1926), p. 46.
[44] Vygotsky, 'The Methods', p. 46.
[45] Vygotsky, 'The Methods', p. 46.
[46] Vygotsky, 'Consciousness as a Problem', p. 65.

Reflexology, embarrassingly, and treacherously, had been secretly in league with a backward, spiritualistic idealism. It had unwittingly slipped, Vygotsky alleges, into a new idealism, precisely in its efforts to escape the old idealism.

Building on the critique of reflexology described above, from at least the early 1930s Vygotsky depicts the science of psychology as being in the midst of a crisis, embodied by a proliferation in the science of competing, contradictory theories, and the absence of either a unifying, general psychology, or of the principles with which the latter could be created. Each new discovery of empirical data, he describes in *Thinking and Speech* (1934), rather than contributing to a coherent development of the science, cannot even be comprehended by its various branches in a common way, and instead necessitates the formation of a new psychological theory in order to make sense of it. This, says Vygotsky, has left psychology in a mess of contradictory positions; with an ever-expanding mass of knowledge, but lacking the direction or coherence that he deems to be the necessary basis for a mature science. Dualism, he says in 1934, is the 'stamp' of this crisis, because it 'reflects the fact that when psychology takes a step forward in the accumulation of empirical data it consistently takes two steps back in its theoretical interpretation of this material', leaving its vital new discoveries 'bemired in prescientific concepts which shroud them in *ad hoc*, semi-metaphysical systems and theories'.[47] Psychology, as Vygotsky frames it in the 1930s, exists in a futilely self-defeating state, embedding theoretical bunkum deeper and deeper into itself with each stride it takes forward empirically.

The Freudian unconscious is, for Vygotsky, a symptom of this situation. It exists, as he portrays it, on the faultline between, on the one hand, the 'refusal to study the mind' epitomised by reflexology, and on the other, 'the "study" of the mind through the mental' epitomised by

[47] Vygotsky, *Thinking and Speech*, Ibid., p. 54. Vygotsky explicitly positions Freud in the context of this conflict between progressive, monistic materialism and regressive idealism—but he does so, notably, because of Freud's association with Piaget, who used the pleasure principle as a model for what he identified as a primary autistic phase in child development. The 'metaphysic', as Vygotsky puts it, of the pleasure principle, leads to Piaget erroneously casting realistic thinking, governed by the reality principle, '*as pure thought*' divorced from 'needs, interests, and wishes' that govern the pleasure principle (*Thinking and Speech*, p. 77).

descriptive psychology.[48] The Freudian path of 'knowledge of mind *through* the unconscious' represents, as Vygotsky presents it, a third option to these two, because it puts forward a different way to approach the mind.[49] Nevertheless, the 'attempt to create a psychology by means of the unconscious' remains, for Vygotsky, ambiguous: it is allied both with idealist psychology, 'insofar as it fulfils the ordinance to explain mental phenomena *by mental phenomena*'—*and* with materialism, 'inasmuch as [Freud] introduces the idea of the strictest determinism of all mental manifestations and reduces their basis to an organic, biological drive, namely the reproductive instinct'.[50] Freud offers a way out of the fundamental conflict that is dividing psychology, between introspective idealism and organicist materialism, only because his option, as far as Vygotsky is able to understand psychoanalysis here, contains elements of both.

The impoverished state of psychology as Vygotsky saw it in the 1920s and 1930s is the subject of an unpublished manuscript of his, which he titled 'The Meaning of the Historical Crisis in Psychology'. This long essay performs a thorough critique of what Vygotsky saw as the failures of the science.[51] In it, Vygotsky develops his analysis of Freud's position in psychology. As a result of Freud's contradictory function, Vygotsky argues, the merging-together of Freud's and Marx's theories—at least in the deficient way that it had been attempted by this point—had produced only impotent chimeras, or 'monstrous combinations'.[52] These eclectic attempts, in which 'the tail of one system is taken and placed against the head of another and the space between them is filled with the trunk of a third', are not incorrect per se.[53] But 'the question they wish to answer is stated incorrectly', because they 'reply to a question raised by Marxist philosophy with an answer prompted by Freudian

[48] Vygotsky, 'Mind, Consciousness, the Unconscious', in *The Collected Works of L.S. Vygotsky, Vol. 3*, pp. 109–122 (p. 112).

[49] Vygotsky, 'Mind, Consciousness, the Unconscious', p. 112.

[50] Vygotsky, 'Mind, Consciousness, the Unconscious', p. 112.

[51] Because the manuscript went unpublished during his lifetime, it is not possible to pinpoint exactly at what point this critique was motivated.

[52] Vygotsky, 'The Meaning of the Historical Crisis in Psychology', in *The Collected Works of L.S. Vygotsky, Vol. 3: Problems of the Theory and History of Psychology*, trans. by René van der Veer (New York: Springer, 1997), pp. 233–244 (p. 259).

[53] Vygotsky, 'The Meaning of the Historical Crisis', p. 259.

metapsychology'.[54] The method taken thus far, Vygotsky summarises satirically, is one that 'by analogy with geometry might be called the method of the logical superposition of concepts': Marxism is defined as being monistic, materialistic, and dialectical, then the same attributes are identified in Freud, and finally 'the superimposed concepts coincide and the systems are declared to have fused', with any contradictions being simply smoothed out.[55]

The impotence of such attempts is identified by Vygotsky in his question of why, if Freud had accidentally created a Marxist doctrine of the mind, would psychoanalysis need to be merged with Marxism in the first place?[56] Attempts at finding identity between Marx and Freud overlook, Vygotsky is at pains to point out, the contradictory genesis of their ideas, and the different philosophical foundations of their theories: Freud is firmly situated by Vygotsky as an inheritor of Schopenhauerian idealism; Freud's 'doctrine of the primary role of blind drives, of the unconscious as being reflected in consciousness in a distorted fashion', he says, 'goes back directly to Schopenhauer's idealistic metaphysics of the will and the idea'.[57] Even in its 'more "concrete" works', psychoanalysis, Vygotsky alleges, 'displays not dynamic, but highly static, conservative, anti-dialectic and anti-historical tendencies', and 'reduces the higher mental processes—both personal and collective ones—to primitive, primordial, essentially prehistorical, pre-human roots, leaving no room for history'.[58] Psychoanalysis effectively commits the same offence of which Vygotsky had accused vulgar reflexology, in reducing everything—'the creativity of a Dostoyevsky and the totem and taboo of primordial tribes; the Christian

[54] Vygotsky, 'The Meaning of the Historical Crisis', p. 259.

[55] Vygotsky, 'The Meaning of the Historical Crisis', p. 260. Freud, for example, is de-sexualised by these botched Freudo-Marxisms. Vygotsky specifically mocks this enlisting of Freud as an unwitting historical materialist in papers by Luria and Fridman. See Luria, 'Psikhoanaliz, kak sistema monistieheskoj psikhologii' (1925), in *Psikhologija* i *rnarksizm*, ed. by K.N. Kornilov (Leningrad: Gosudarstvennoe Izdatel'stvo), pp. 47–80; and B.D. Fridman, 'Osnovnye psikhologicheskie vozrenija Frejda i teorija istoricheskogo materializma' (1925), In *Pstkhologija i marksizm*, ed. by K. N. Kornilov, pp. 113–159.

[56] Vygotsky, 'The Meaning of the Historical Crisis', p. 261.

[57] Vygotsky, 'The Meaning of the Historical Crisis', p. 263.

[58] Vygotsky, 'The Meaning of the Historical Crisis', p. 263.

church, communism, the primitive horde'—to 'the same source'.[59] Freud's contradiction of the methodology of Marxism is borne out in the works of psychoanalysis that deal with culture, sociology, and history. 'To reduce personality[,] money[,] cleanliness, stubbornness and a thousand other, heterogeneous things to anal erotics', says Vygotsky, is 'not yet monism'.[60] But, '[w]ith an uncritical approach, everybody sees what he wants to see and not what is: the Marxist finds monism, materialism, and dialectics in psychoanalysis' which is, for Vygotsky, definitively 'not there'.[61]

There remain, however, two sides to Vygotsky's reading of Freud. In 1925, Vygotsky and Luria wrote an introduction to the 1925 Russian translation of *Beyond the Pleasure Principle*, which prefaces the text with much hope for the materialist potential of its theories. Vygotsky recalls in the 'Crisis' how, despite the death drive being a 'fictitious', 'speculative' construct, with a 'giddy paradoxical nature' which 'contradict[s] [...] generally accepted ideas', and despite Freud's conclusions which 'coincide with the philosophy of the Nirvana', the death drive nevertheless represents a step towards the capacity of biology to register death in a positive sense, rather than just as non-being.[62] The death drive, he says, 'satisfies the need of modern biology to master the idea of death, just like mathematics in its time needed the concept of the negative number'.[63] In Vygotsky and Luria's 1925 introduction to the text, they depict the death drive as a profoundly materialistic theory, and one that reverses the traditional scenario in which psychology had tended to borrow its concepts from the biological sciences. In *Beyond the Pleasure Principle*, as they read it, Freud begins to theorise a biology in the form of a psychological theory, and, in the process, to invent a means to reintegrate organic life with the surrounding world.[64] Vygotsky and Luria stop short of a total

[59] Vygotsky, 'The Meaning of the Historical Crisis', p. 263.

[60] Vygotsky, 'The Meaning of the Historical Crisis', p. 265. Vygotsky is specifically responding to Luria, 'Psikhoanaliz, kak sistema monistieheskoj psikhologii'.

[61] Vygotsky, 'The Meaning of the Historical Crisis', p. 265.

[62] Vygotsky, 'The Meaning of the Historical Crisis', p. 265.

[63] Vygotsky, 'The Meaning of the Historical Crisis', p. 265.

[64] Vygotsky and Luria, 'Introduction to the Russian translation of Freud's *Beyond the Pleasure Principle*' (1925), in *The Vygotsky Reader*, ed. by René van der Veer and Jaan Valsiner (Oxford: Blackwell, 1994), pp. 10–18. See also the passage below, for example:

endorsement of Freud's theories, conceding that 'it is not necessary to share all his hypotheses'.[65] But they treat his work as part of an extended transition between bourgeois science and materialism, a 'difficult and prolonged' process, whose heralds in Freud's work should, they say, be acknowledged and developed accordingly.[66]

The criticisms of Freudo-Marxism in the 'Crisis' manuscript are made in service of Vygotsky's broader project, of outlining what is, in effect, his manifesto for a new, general psychology that could replace all the disparate strands he identifies and satirically attacks in the text. The applications of Marxism to psychology that had been attempted so far were inadequate, he argues, because they failed to transform psychology fundamentally, on the level of method. No philosophical system, he says, 'can take possession of psychology directly, without the help of methodology, i.e., without the creation of a general science'.[67] The only 'rightful application' of Marxism to psychology would amount to the creation of a 'general psychology', in which the concepts of psychology would be 'formulated in direct dependence upon general dialectics, for it [would

> Once and for all it completely breaks with any teleological concepts in the spheres of psychology and biology. Every instinct is causally dependent on its previous condition which it strives to reinstate. Every instinct has a conservative character and it is impelled backwards and not forwards. And this is how a bridge (a hypothetical one) is thrown across from the science of the origins and development of organic life to that dealing with inorganic matter. For the first time in this hypothesis, the organic whole is so decisively integrated into the general context of the world (pp. 14–15).

The death drive does not, then, represent a 'throwback to pessimist philosophy' (p. 14). Aswell as traversing the barrier between biology and psychology, and eschewing the 'mystical specificity' of psychology (p. 17), it presents the human psyche as a dialectic of biological conservatism and sociological progress:

> So, according to Freud, the history of the human psyche embodies two tendencies, the conservative–biological and the progressive–sociological. It is from these factors that the whole *dialectic of the organism* is composed and they are responsible for the distinctive 'spiral' development of a human being. This book represents a step forwards and not backwards along the path to the construction of a whole, monistic system, and after having read this book a dialectician cannot fail to perceive its enormous potential for a monistic understanding of the world (pp. 16–17).

[65] Vygotsky and Luria, 'Introduction', p. 17.

[66] Vygotsky and Luria, 'Introduction', p. 17.

[67] Vygotsky, 'The Meaning of the Historical Crisis in Psychology', in *The Collected Works of L.S. Vygotsky, Vol. 3*, pp. 233–344 (p. 330).

be] the dialectics of psychology'.[68] The diffuse nature of the existing alternative, and its failure to reorient psychology on this fundamental level, leads only to 'scholastic, verbal constructions', to the 'dissolution of dialectics into surveys and tests'; to 'judgement about things according to their external, accidental, secondary features', and to 'the complete loss of any objective criterion and the attempt to deny all historical tendencies of the development of psychology'.[69] This would amount to 'a gross distortion of both Marxism and psychology'. The approach to psychology that Vygotsky is scornfully describing embodies, he alleges, the opposite of Engels's formula 'not to foist the dialectical principles onto nature, but to find them in it'.[70] Vygotsky sees existing psychology as having, in other words, forced dialectical logic onto its object, rather than subtly identifying this logic in its empirical observations.

Vygotsky is resolute, however, that the '*direct* application of the theory of *dialectical materialism* to the problems of natural science', and 'in particular to the group of biological sciences or psychology'—in the way that, he says, these reductive theories attempt—'is *impossible*'.[71] *The problem of psychology's relationship to Marxism cannot be solved, he says, merely by conjuring a 'psychology which is up to Marxism'. What is needed, Vygotsky prescribes, is an* 'intermediate *special theory* of historical materialism which explains the *concrete* meaning, for the given group of phenomena, of the abstract laws of dialectical materialism'.[72] *This 'special theory', he describes, would be a mediator between the specific object of psychology, on the one hand, and the general premises of dialectical materialism on the other: it would amount to a* 'theory of biological materialism and psychological materialism', and would explain 'the concrete application of the abstract theses of dialectical materialism to the given field of phenomena'.[73] This 'dialectics of psychology' or 'general psychology' would, he says, 'reveal the *essence* of the given area of phenomena, the laws of their change, their

68 Vygotsky, 'The Meaning of the Historical Crisis', p. 330.

69 Vygotsky, 'The Meaning of the Historical Crisis', p. 330.

70 Vygotsky and Luria, Vygotsky, 'The Meaning of the Historical Crisis', p. 330. Citing Engels, *Dialektik der Natur* (1925) (Berlin: Dietz Verlag, 1978), p. 348.

71 Vygotsky, 'The Meaning of the Historical Crisis', p. 330.

72 Vygotsky, 'The Meaning of the Historical Crisis', p. 330.

73 Vygotsky, 'The Meaning of the Historical Crisis', p. 330.

qualitative and quantitative characteristics, their causality', and would 'create categories and concepts appropriate to it'.[74] *This, Vygotsky announces, would amount to 'our own Capital'—it would be the equivalent to Capital in the field of psychology.*[75] *This theory would supply the intermediary terms that would be counterparts, in the field of psychology, to value, class, commodity, capital, interest, production forces, base, and superstructure. And just as Capital is a critique of political economy, this would also be a 'critique of psychology'.*[76] *Such a text would escape the method of "logical superposition" that Vygotsky finds to govern contemporary attempts at a Marxist psychology. It would instead develop what can be found in '[n]either Marx, nor Engels, nor Plekhanov': a unified method of how to build a science of psychology.*[77]

Vygotsky's prescription for a 'general psychology' implicitly makes a sophisticated point about the position of *Capital* in Marxist thought generally. Vygotsky implies here that Marx's *Capital* does not represent an endpoint, supplying an armoury of terms and concepts that can be lumped together inelegantly with those of psychology, or of any other science. *Capital* should instead, for Vygotsky, be regarded as a *model*, with respect to economics, for the kind of transformation he deems to be required in the field of psychology. At the conclusion of the 'Crisis' manuscript, Vygotsky is identifying a blank space—one that all number of psychologists had been filling with lame squibs—in which the psychological equivalent of Marx's book could distil and portion-out the specific terminology and concepts of the science. Merely importing terms from Marx's theories into psychology—in what Vygotsky mocks as a geometrical 'superimposition of concepts'—represses what *Capital* truly represents: a transformation, on a fundamental, epistemological level, of the way science is able to operate. Vygotsky presents Marx as having unlocked an entirely different mode of thought to that which was still guiding the sciences at the time of his own work. *Capital*, for Vygotsky, was a

[74] Vygotsky, 'The Meaning of the Historical Crisis', p. 330.
[75] Vygotsky, 'The Meaning of the Historical Crisis', p. 330. Amended to *Capital* from *Das Kapital*.
[76] Vygotsky, 'The Meaning of the Historical Crisis', p. 330.
[77] Vygotsky, 'The Meaning of the Historical Crisis', p. 331.

conceptual event that must be observed assiduously by all sciences, with regards to each of their own phenomena of study.[78]

It is easy to see why Vygotsky fell out of favour with Stalin, because the position he gives to Marx here is antithetical to a treatment of Marx's theories as mere dogma. Vygotsky's Marx is an interlocutor demanding obligatorily critical dialogue. Roman Jakobson would assert years later that Vygotsky's approaches to psychology and to language were far more in the 'high Russian intellectual tradition' prioritising higher functions, than were the 'bottom-up' approaches of the Pavlovian reflexologists—and Jerome Bruner, comparing Vygotsky's Marxism with other co-ordinates, describes him as being 'closer to Althusser, Habermas, and the Frankfurt School than to the Soviet Marxism of his times'.[79] Questions about the functioning of the human psyche forced Vygotsky to press towards a more fundamental enquiry, into how entire fields of science would need to be reformulated in light of Marx. Vygotsky already balked, in the 1920s, at attempts to perform a reductive stitching-together of Marx with psychoanalysis. Despite Vygotsky's considerable ambivalence towards Freud, the positions that the 'Crisis' give to him and to Marx are similar: neither Freud nor Marx, for Vygotsky, provide any definitive answers to the form psychology must take, but both open up a path—an evidently problematic, difficult path—towards its future development, by indexing it onto a set of unavoidable dilemmas.

[78] The question of politics therefore becomes far from straightforward—this reading of Marx justifies leaving concepts like 'exploitation' (along with the others listed by Vygotsky) out of the picture, because these concepts only represent the 'mediation' of Marx on the level of economics. In another field, like psychology, a whole new set of 'abstract and historical categories' would be required to operate with the 'general principles and categories of dialectics, like quantity-quality, the triad, the universal connection, the knot [of contradictions], leap etc.' in the field of psychology ('The Meaning of the Historical Crisis in Psychology', p. 330).

[79] Jermone Bruner, 'Prologue to the English Edition', in *The Collected Works of L.S. Vygotsky, Vol. 1*, pp. 1–16 (pp. 2–3).

Georges Politzer's 'Concrete Psychology': Psychoanalysis Without the Unconscious

Reflexology, as Vygotsky's critique shows, created at least as many problems for materialist science as it had appeared to solve. In France, the question was much more open than it was in the Soviet Union as to what form a materialist psychology would take, because reflexology had not become the panacea there that it had in Russia. Reflexology did not, as a result, hold the same synonymity with psychology in France; it appeared as one component of the armoury at the disposal of psychologists in their struggle towards materialism, but not as the endpoint of that process. Vygotsky's sharp critique of reflexological theory found, partly as a result of this more varied French perspective, echoes and recipients amongst the French psychologists working in this context, and also took some clear influence from them.[80]

One of the clearest indicators of the positions of both psychology and psychoanalysis within French Marxist thought of the late 1920s is the work of the philosopher Georges Politzer. Politzer wrote extensively about psychology, from the mid-1920s up until his execution in occupied Paris in 1942. Starting in two articles, 'Médecine ou philosophie?' and 'Le mythe de l'antipsychanalyse', published in the journal *Philosophies* in 1924, he both applauds Freud for developing a scientific method able to study the individual in their singularity, but also criticises him for the

[80] There were, of course, different co-ordinates framing French psychology in the 1920s and '30 s, which had its own way of registering the conceptual focal points dominating the science in the Soviet Union. For example, the principle of historicism—of the interdependency of the mind and the history of society—that was central in Soviet, Marxist psychology, had its influence in France largely in connection with the question of the social determination of the mind. Durkheim is a central figure here, for his treatment of society as an aggregate of collective representations, along with the anthropologist Lucien Lévy-Bruhl, who proposed that it was not just the content of human thought, but human logic, and the pre-logical aspects of human thought, that develop historically. The most important psychologist in France by the end of the 1920s, however, was Pierre Janet, who hypothesised that child development was driven by the child's internalisation of the behaviour of adults around them. Janet's theories are representative of French psychology in general, including that of Piaget, in being based on the anti-Marxist assumption that a child is initially asocial, and that socialisation is forced upon them from the outside. Janet, again in opposition to Marx, viewed society as fundamentally based on co-operation, rather than on economic relationships. See A.N. Leont'ev, 'On Vygotsky's Creative Development', in *The Collected Works of L.S. Vygotsky, Vol. 3*, pp. 9–32 (p. 20).

strains of abstract, classical psychology that remain in his theories.[81] This began an ambivalent approach to psychoanalysis that would last throughout Politzer's career. Politzer was born in Hungary in 1903, and met Freud and Ferenczi in Vienna when he attended Psychoanalytic Society seminars, before coming to Paris in 1922.[82] After translating Schelling into French in 1926, he published a detailed and compelling critique in 1928 of the contemporary theoretical basis of psychology. *Critique of the Foundations of Psychology* acts as a manifesto for the renewal of psychological science out of its classical mystifications, into a new, materialist form, which he names 'concrete psychology'.

The *Critique* was envisaged by Politzer as the first of a series of three volumes which were to lay out the co-ordinates of this revival of psychology. It takes the form of a detailed reading of Freud's *The Interpretation of Dreams* (1900). At the core of Politzer's denunciation of 'classical psychology' is his accusation that it projects metaphysical abstractions onto a reified 'inner life', which it seeks through methods of introspection.[83] As opposed to physics, which is a 'science of the third person', psychology is, he describes, a chimerical science, which wants to study the facts of the first person *in* the third person.[84] Thus far, however, as Politzer claims in 1928, classical psychology has only been able to 'consider the same thing twice in the third person', by projecting 'the outside into the inside, from which it tries later, but in vain, to make it get out', and by attempting an alchemy through which 'it divides the world to make of it first an illusion and then to try to make of this illusion reality'.[85] Though claiming to enlighten the psyche by bringing it into the realm of scientific study, what psychology has actually been doing, Politzer alleges, is inventing a fictional psychic mechanism on the model of other sciences. As a result, it

---

[81] Republished in Georges Politzer, *Écrits II: Les Fondements de la Psychologie*, ed. by J. Debouzy (Paris: Editions Sociales, 1969).

[82] Elisabeth Roudinesco, *Jacques Lacan & Co.: A History of Psychoanalysis in France, 1925–1985*, trans. by J. Mehlman (Chicago: University of Chicago Press, 1990), p. 60.

[83] Politzer, *Critique of the Foundations of Psychology: The Psychology of Psychoanalysis*, trans. by M. Apprey (Pittsburg: Duquesne University Press, 1994), pp. 8, 12.

[84] Politzer, *Critique*, p. 29.

[85] Politzer, *Critique*, p. 30.

is continually slipping back into the metaphysics that it had attempted to escape.[86]

Against this backdrop of the history of psychology, Politzer presents Freud's theories as a turning-point that had made possible a new, 'concrete psychology'. Psychoanalysis is crucial for Politzer's vision of concrete psychology because it seeks 'the comprehension of psychological facts *in terms of the subject*', from the first-person account of a 'dramatic life', which had previously been blotted out by the metaphysical hydraulics of classical psychology.[87] Hence the privileged place of *The Interpretation of Dreams* in Politzer's project: in Freud's theory of dreams, he stays resolutely faithful to the contextualisation of the symptom within the dreamer's experience, as a cipher that is unlocked only by reconnection with this experience.[88]

But Politzer does not spare Freud his own share of harsh criticism. At the heart of Politzer's complaint with Freud is his dissatisfaction with the notion of the unconscious itself. He sees it as merely the shadow of the dregs that remain in Freudian psychoanalysis of classical psychology. Despite the manifest importance of psychoanalysis in developing the concrete, first-person psychology that Politzer envisages, he notices several signs that 'deep within its heart [psychoanalysis] conceal[s] the old psychology that it was mandated to eliminate' as well as feeding an 'unimportant romanticism and speculations that solve only obsolete problems'.[89] Freud falls back, for Politzer, into classical psychology and naïve psychologism, by shuttling the knowledge contained in dreams away into an unconscious that he assumes to be an inaccessible realm. The hypothesis

[86] Politzer, *Critique*, p. 31.

[87] Politzer, *Critique*, pp. 28, 35. My italics.

[88] Politzer, *Critique*, p. 38.

[89] Politzer, *Critique*, p. 14. Classical psychology's methods of introspection are redundant, for Politzer, to the extent that they can, by definition, never reveal the meaning of something that has been forgotten; to progress beyond this, Politzer claims, the act of forgetting must be made to appear as such by contextualisation in a 'story', the kind constructed in psychoanalysis, in a dialectical approach that replaces the inadequacy of a reliance on introspection (p. 52). A gap is then revealed between the 'conventional collective significations' used to tell this story, and the 'individual significations' that enmesh the subject's symptom or dream, revealing the irreducible, and heretofore obscured, network of personal meaning bestowed upon it (p. 59). Politzer says nothing, however, of the significance of Freud's own introspective self-analysis for his theory of dream interpretation.

of the unconscious is, as Politzer describes, produced not from the 'human' facts of an analysis, but from 'an interpretation of these facts consistent with the point of view of abstraction'.[90] Politzer illustrates neatly how, if the recovery of memories is taken as proof of the existence of the unconscious, this also assumes that 'the memory is real before its conscious realization'.[91] This assumption would be acceptable to a realist, classical model of psychology, but it preserves a metaphysical fiction that is anathema to Politzer's desired turn to the 'concrete'. The term 'unconscious' serves for Politzer as the indication that the objects of psychoanalysis remain 'purely fictitious psychological entities', which turn human experience—the 'drama' of life Politzer privileges—into a mystified cosmological circuitry.[92] He also sees the unconscious as a kind of infallibility clause, a sleight-of-hand that saves Freud from having to substantiate his assumptions. When Freud declares that his interpretative constructions, whatever they may be, are a product of the unconscious, he thereby makes them immune to doubt—and the unconscious itself thus simultaneously becomes an irrefutable component of his theory: 'the unconscious makes the postulate irrefutable, and the postulate makes the unconscious irrefutable'.[93]

Politzer takes the notion of the unconscious in general as condemning psychoanalysis to 'theoretical powerlessness'.[94] At the same time, he also deems the unconscious to be as unimportant to psychoanalysis as it is debilitating: it appears in psychoanalysis, he says, not due to empirical necessity, but to a priori necessity, and 'due to the fact that psychoanalysts use it in the elaboration of the facts of classical psychology'.[95] Politzer sees the unconscious as the residue in psychoanalysis of a redundant classical psychology—but, for this very reason, the unconscious is also, for him, the manifestation of a historical shift *away* from classical psychology. Its appearance in psychoanalysis is therefore a sign of progress, that represents 'a decisive moment of the dissolution of classical psychology, to a

[90] Politzer, *Critique*, p. 109.

[91] Politzer, *Critique*, p. 103.

[92] Politzer, *Critique*, p. 112.

[93] Politzer, *Critique*, p. 121.

[94] Politzer, *Critique*, p. 122.

[95] Politzer, *Critique*, pp. 121–2.

moment when, while still wanting to save abstraction, psychology started to detach itself away from it'.[96] Politzer opts to exploit these conditions, by taking hold of exactly this negativity in order to bring about a true concrete psychology. The 'duality' of psychoanalysis—which is, for him, both progressively dialectical and mystifyingly conservative—was, he says, 'necessary for an enterprise like ours to be born', and its 'abstract speculations present a paradox that imperiously calls for a critique'.[97] Politzer sides with the more dialectical unconscious that can be preserved from Freud, most evidently in the concept of identification, a psychic act which, in that it 'concerns *being* someone else or something else than himself', amounts to 'conforming to a model by adopting so to speak all its dialectics'.[98] Taking the best of the combination of psychoanalysis, behaviourism, and the third component of Gestalt psychology—the latter two of which were to be objects of each of further volumes of Politzer's *Critique*, which he did not start writing before his death—would, he believes, enable the development of true concrete psychology, liberated from the abstractions of the science's classical form.

Politzer's critique teeters in this way between accepting, on the one hand, the long-term strategic importance of psychoanalysis—or its 'dramatic' component at least—for facilitating the science he wants to bring into being, and, on the other hand, castigating Freud for failing to carry out this revolution already. After joining the Communist Party in 1929, Politzer's approach to Freud becomes less equivocal, and more straightforwardly critical, and he makes less reference to the roots that the 'drama' of concrete psychology have in psychoanalysis. These slightly later writings depart significantly from the *Critique*'s appreciation of Freud's successes: in them psychoanalysis no longer appears as a necessarily flawed revolutionary movement, but instead as a bourgeois fad that is only useful in spite of itself.[99]

---

[96] Politzer, *Critique*, p. 131.

[97] Politzer, *Critique*, p. 139.

[98] Politzer, *Critique*, p. 62.

[99] Politzer renews his criticisms of psychoanalysis in 'Le crise de la psychanalyse' ('The Crisis of Psychoanalysis', 1929), an article published in *La Revue de psychologie concrete*; 'Un faux contre-révolutionnaire, le freudo-marxisme' ('A False Counter-Revolutionary, Freudo-Marxism', 1933), published in *Commune*; and, under the pseudonym Th. W. Morris, 'Le fin de la psychanalyse' ('The

Politzer continues this critique in *The Crisis of Contemporary Psychology*, published posthumously in 1947. In the book, Politzer identifies—over two decades after Vygotsky wrote with precision on the same theme—the science of psychology as being in the grip of a crisis; afflicted with regressive, contradictory theories, and torn between materialism and idealist abstraction. He also renews his claim for the significance of 'concrete psychology', by situating it as the way out of this crisis that psychoanalysis was not able to find. Politzer identifies the crisis in 1940s psychology as the result of its theories being torn between the two conflicting foundations of materialism and idealism.[100] The crisis in psychology, Politzer states clearly:

> consists only in the fact that psychology is idealist when it should be materialist, or, if one likes it better, that [psychologists] are idealists who would like to work as materialists: psychology can only become a science by renouncing idealism, while current psychologists are unable to renounce it.[101]

Politzer records how idealism, on the contrary, is not only widespread, but even enjoying a covert renaissance. He identifies the occurrence of a 'general fusion in idealism' and a 'great idealistic liquefaction' of various groups: in the theological-Bergsonian psychology that had appeared in France, the *Geisteswissenschaftliche Psychologie* and idealistic metaphysics of the Leib-Seele-Einheit in Germany, the psychoanalytic theories of Otto Rank, and even non-physiological behaviourism—the latter of

End of Psychoanalysis', 1939), published in *La Pensée*. These articles are republished in Politzer, *Écrits II*. Many of his complaints in these articles amount roughly to repetitions of the classic criticism that psychoanalysis is a therapy and an ideology of the petite bourgeoisie. Freud committed the dual transgressions, says Politzer in 'La fin de la psychanalyse', of eclecticism and dogmatism—which, he says, are not opposed procedures, but necessary companions—and psychoanalysis's sole interest, he claims, lies in its historical existence, and in the 'social facts of which it contains the reflections', and not in either its theories, or its claims to being a scientific movement. Politzer 'Le fin de la psychanalyse', *La Pensée*, 3 (October–December 1939), 13–23 (p. 14). My translation.

[100] Politzer, *La Crise de la Psychologie Contemporaine* (Paris: Éditions Sociales, 1947). Like Vygotsky, Politzer highlights the importance of overcoming 'individual or regional arbitrariness' when posing the science's problems (p. 18). Concrete psychology, he says, is not '*a* psychology', but '*the* psychology' (p. 77). My translation.

[101] Politzer, *La Crise*, p. 90.

which is, he remarks, 'more or less strongly idealistic'.[102] Politzer points out the spectacle of idealist psychology changing its form with the fashions of the science, even going as far as attempting to accommodate itself to materialism to save itself, whilst preserving exactly the theories and frameworks which it had always propagated. Since he published his *Critique*, Politzer comments wryly, this technique of rebranding has made it seem as if 'there has never been anything but concrete psychology in the world'.[103] Materialism, however, as it currently exists in psychology, fares no better, he says, because it merely 'tries to express the "spiritual"', by the 'classic means' of 'the nervous system; viscera; the glands with internal secretion', or 'the organism considered as a whole'.[104] Medical, physiological, or biological materialism is, Politzer claims, 'still only a negative reaction against spiritualism', and is 'cast on the mold of spiritualism'.[105] Psychology is therefore locked in an opposition from which it had been, up until this point, impossible for it to escape, because all psychologists 'have been looking for was the image of the thesis', in the absence of a true antithesis.[106] Both the spiritualists and the existing materialists, he claims, share the same objectives, have one common campaign plan, and rely on the same "formal equipment".

It seems a distant memory, at this point in Politzer's writings, that the panacea to which concrete psychology is supposed to amount initially emerged out of his reading of Freud. Politzer's ambivalence is another indication that it was not clear exactly where Freud stood with respect to materialism, or what could be done with this rogue element of psychoanalysis within a materialist framework. Like Vygotsky, Politzer identifies a tension in Freud, between elements that point towards dialectical

[102] Politzer, *La Crise*, p. 90.

[103] Politzer, *La Crise*, pp. 92–3. The theologians, he says, 'put on white coats and hid Saint Thomas in the recording cylinders', and "calculation and measure" became passwords in place of "spirituality-liberty-immortality", as theologians masqueraded as scientists in order to save the domain of the soul. It is, he says, 'exactly the same tactic' that inclines them towards concrete psychology, which 'they think, is in fashion'. Each would like, he says, 'the name "concrete psychology", because each one would like to appear the saviour of the old treasure, and all want it simply for the old theology of the soul, because it is she who they would all like to save' (p. 96).

[104] Politzer, *La Crise*, p. 103.

[105] Politzer, *La Crise*, p. 103.

[106] Politzer, *La Crise*, p. 103.

materialism, and others that regress into idealism. Neither Vygotsky nor Politzer knew exactly what to do with Freud. Both go through a similar movement, from excitement about and endorsement of psychoanalysis, to a much more dismissive view of Freud, articulated in their later work, when both attempt to evaluate seriously the state of psychology as a science, and to pave a way out of its contradictions. To both, Freud appears on the cusp between idealism and materialism, and his position between the two is an object of profound contention.

There are some important limitations to the way Politzer envisages concrete psychology as a project—especially considering the extent of the redeeming mission that he imparts to it. In 1963, Althusser would find in Politzer's *Critique* an impressive yet flawed false-start of French psychoanalysis, which he identifies as having triggered an encounter between psychoanalysis and philosophy that was then to pass through the existential humanism of both Sartre and Merleau-Ponty.[107] Althusser had planned, in 1955, to republish the *Critique* with a 'theoretical preface'. In a letter to its would-be publisher, Guy Besse, he outlines how, despite both the *Critique*'s brilliance, and Politzer's appreciation of Freud's importance at a time when it was unrecognised in France, the *Critique* remains 'profoundly idealist', making 'an exposition and critique [...] that was *100% idealist*, and very precisely existentialist'.[108] The decadent Freudianism of Sartre and Merleau-Ponty, he adds, followed directly from what they learned from Politzer. Despite Althusser's dissatisfaction with these attempts, he acknowledges that it was nonetheless 'through Politzer that psychoanalysis became an object of philosophical reflection' in France.[109] Politzer's errors, as Althusser sees them, come down to the uncritical redundancy of the concept of the "concrete". Politzer's 'proclamation of the arrival of "*concrete* psychology" was never followed by any works', Althusser charges, because '[a]ll the virtue of the term "concrete" was in fact exhausted in its critical use, without ever finding the slightest amount of knowledge which only exists in the "abstraction" of con-

[107] Louis Althusser, 'The Place of Psychoanalysis in the Human Sciences' (1963), in *Psychoanalysis and the Human Sciences* (New York: Columbia University Press, 2016), pp. 1–45 (p. 12).

[108] Althusser, 'The Place of Psychoanalysis in the Human Sciences', p. 12, n. 4.

[109] Althusser, 'The Place of Psychoanalysis in the Human Sciences', p. 12, n. 4.

cepts'.[110] Althusser alleges that Politzer, in fetishising the empty notion of the "concrete", repeated the errors of Feuerbach, who 'tried desperately to free himself from ideology by invoking the "concrete", i.e., the ideological concept which confuses knowledge and being'.[111] Marx's earlier works—still not having broken fully with the concepts from which he would later fully depart—contain, Althusser notes, the same ambiguous references to the 'concrete', to the 'real', and to 'real, concrete' men. Yet, for Althusser, in both Marx and in Feuerbach these terms remain empty, ideological mannequins; ones that Politzer also still uses to sweep aside the commitment to theoretical rigour and ingenuity that Althusser deems necessary to escape idealism. Concrete psychology does not, for Althusser, escape the proximity to idealism that Politzer was so committed to eliminating from psychology.

The value of Politzer's work on psychological theory lies not so much, then, in its prescription of a redeeming concrete psychology. Despite manifesting a fascinating attempt to synthesise existent conflicts in psychology—conflicts which, as his own *Crisis* made clear, were certainly evident in the science—concrete psychology appears as something of a magic bullet, or as Politzer's messianic prophecy. Althusser also identifies in 1963 how concrete psychology ended up forming the basis for the psychoanalytic existentialism that he finds so disappointing. In 1964, Althusser would challenge Politzer's reproach of psychoanalysis 'for its *abstractions*', and would criticise Politzer's subsequent rejection of 'the unconscious, the Oedipus complex, the castration complex, and so on' for supposedly amounting, as Politzer claimed, to remnants of idealist, metaphysical psychology.[112] Althusser defends here the abstract components of psychoanalytic theory: no science, he argues, 'can do without abstraction, even when', like psychoanalysis, 'it is dealing in its "practice" [...] solely within those singular and unique variations constituted by the "dramas" of individuals'.[113] Some aspects of Freud that Politzer dismisses

[110] Althusser, 'From *Capital* to Marx's Philosophy', in *Reading Capital*, trans. by B. Brewster (London: New Left Books, 1970), p. 39, n. 18.

[111] Althusser, 'From *Capital* to Marx's Philosophy', p. 39, n. 18.

[112] Althusser, 'Freud and Lacan' (1964), in *Writings on Psychoanalysis*, (Columbia University Press, 1999) pp. 7–32 (p. 28).

[113] Althusser, 'Freud and Lacan', p. 28.

were also given at least the benefit of the doubt by Vygotsky and Luria, in their introduction to *Beyond the Pleasure Principle*, for instance. In his later writings, Politzer loses sight of an idea he voiced earlier on: that Freud was so valuable exactly *because* of the contradictions at work in his theories. In light of this earlier observation, what was required was a more subtle, creative way of negotiating what were, as so many had acknowledged, serious conflicts within psychoanalysis.

Henri Wallon's Psychology of Idealism

Although Politzer wrote extensively about psychology, and was heavily engaged in working on its theories, he was not himself a psychologist who conducted empirical research. Partly for this reason, the psychologist Henri Wallon made possible a more virtuosic integration of Freud with a dialectical materialist psychology, which preserves close attention both to organic processes, and to the phenomenology of perception in child development. Presumably, this was not beyond the remit of what Politzer envisaged for concrete psychology. Because of his attention to the theoretical foundations of the science, however, Politzer does not articulate the practical applications of his theories in the way that Wallon is able to when working with results from his own experiments. The idea that an infant's reality is socially mediated is a central aspect of Wallon's developmental schema, which he lays out most extensively in his 1938 study of child development, *La Vie mentale*. This idea also informs Vygotsky's theories of language acquisition. Vygotsky, in one instance of the attachment to western ideas and theories that earned him disrepute in the Soviet Union, appears to have taken this idea from Wallon. He had read Wallon's work in the early 1930s, and both he and Wallon attended the 7th International Congress on Psychotechnics in Moscow in 1931, where they may also have met in person.[114] What is clear in their theories, just as it is in Politzer's, is the way in which a reading of Marx could press

[114] See René van der Veer, 'Henri Wallon's Theory of Early Child Development: The Role of Emotions', *Developmental Review*, 16 (1996), 364–390 (p. 377); and Henri Wallon, 'Sur la septième conférence internationale de psychotechnique' (1932), *Revue de Psychologie Appliquée de l'Est* (September 1931), 3–12.

towards a confrontation with faultlines in the theoretical foundations of psychology. Wallon shared with Vygotsky a propensity towards theories that could encompass empirical observations elegantly, as opposed to research that would isolate a diffuse set of observations before reassembling them into a psychological theory. Wallon was also concerned, like Vygotsky, with the need to develop a more subtle mechanism to account for the higher functions of human life than that which had been offered by Pavlov.

In 1938, Wallon published *La Vie mentale*, an expansive and comprehensive study of child development, in the volume of the *Encyclopédie Française* that he also edited.[115] As Wallon presents it there, psychology is the dialectical science par excellence, because it makes possible a hybrid between 'the sciences of nature' and 'the science of the mind'.[116] Wallon announces as his project here the repositioning of psychology on the threshold between the idealism and organicism that had polarised it in the past.[117] The division, then, between idealism and materialism that both Vygotsky and Politzer considered to be an impediment of psychology, is reframed by Wallon as the very mark of its significance. The science was, in his hands, to form a bridge between the organic and the social, and between the physical and mental dimensions of human life, by taking the individual as the intermediary in either case.[118] The title of the study itself was supposed to represent 'something of a hybrid'; mental life was, it prescribes, to be seen as a living mind, poised between organic processes and a diverse external milieu.[119]

It is well known, and evident, that the foundations for what Lacan would call the 'mirror stage' were laid in Wallon's own studies of mirror recognition in young children, Wallon having written extensively about the developing relationship between young children and their reflections

---

[115] Wallon ed., *Encyclopédie Française, Vol. 8: La Vie mentale*, (Paris: Société de gestion de l'Encyclopédie Française, 1938).

[116] Henri Wallon, *La Vie mentale* (Paris: Editions Sociales, 1982), p. 114.

[117] Wallon, *La Vie mentale*, p. 114.

[118] Wallon, *La Vie mentale*, p. 119.

[119] Wallon, *La Vie mentale*, p. 114.

years before Lacan turned his attention to it in 1936.[120] Several studies exist in English condemning Lacan for stealing from Wallon without citation. This is despite the fact that the first written version of Lacan's mirror stage theory was published *by* Wallon, in Wallon's edition of the *Encyclopédie Française*. None of these studies, however, make clear that Wallon is also one of the most evident points of contact between Lacan and dialectical materialist thought. Wallon's leading role in the 'Cercle de la Russie', a group of scientists working to reformulate their fields in light of Marx, makes clear his commitment to and prominence in this effort.[121] Lacan learned from Wallon not just the mirror stage, but also the notion of a 'symbolic' register acting a threshold in psychic development. These were both products of decades of effort by Wallon in pursuing a materialist theory of psychological development. His work is a crucial context, therefore, for Lacan's position in the history of Marxist thought more generally. Wallon's theories were the clearest source Lacan had access to of a thorough, expansive account of psychic functioning and development that took very seriously the challenges that Marx posed to any attempt to formulate these. Wallon's work is also an important document of another, alternative way to those described earlier in this chapter, to envisage Freud's position in the conflict between idealism and materialism. In a clear precursor to Lacan's rendition of the imago as a congealed moment of the dialectic, Wallon uses Freud as a means to metabolise idealism as a psychological misfiring; a moment to be superseded in the process of psychic development.[122]

---

[120] In Wallon, 'Comment se développe chez l'enfant'. As mentioned in the Introduction to this thesis, some damnatory texts have been written about Lacan's use of Wallon. See Elisabeth Roudinesco, 'The Mirror Stage: An Obliterated Archive', in *The Cambridge Companion to Lacan* (Cambridge: Cambridge University Press, 2010), pp. 25–34 (p. 27); and Michael Billig, 'Lacan's Misuse of Psychology: Evidence, Rhetoric and the Mirror Stage', *Theory, Culture & Society*, 23, no. 4, 1–26.

[121] A collected edition of the Cercle de la Russie's writings was published in 1935, with a follow-up in 1937, both edited and introduced by Wallon under the title *A la lumière du Marxisme* (Editions Sociales Internationales, 1935 and 1937). Other contributors to the first edition included the mathematician Paul Labérenne; the astronomer Henri Mineur; the linguists Marcel Cohen and Aurélien Sauvageot; and the philosophers Jean Langevin, Marcel Prenant, René Maublanc, Charles Parain, Georges Friedmann, and Jean Baby. The second edition included texts by the philosopher Lucie Prenant, Marx's biographer Auguste Cornu, and the journalist Armand Cuvillier.

[122] See Chap. 2 above, pp. 57–62.

Wallon writes about Freud from the 1920s onwards, and draws extensively on psychoanalytic theory in his account of psychological development.[123] Freud appears in Wallon's work as a source of significant insights, but ones that are also in need of rehabilitation by experimental psychology. In a study of *The Interpretation of Dreams* from 1927, Wallon describes the essential themes of psychoanalysis as being 'more romantic than scientific in origin', but he also argues that the first contact of these psychoanalytic concepts 'with objective and scientific psychology must be gathered, verified, and used by' this rigorous psychology.[124] He makes it clear, however, that his reservations with Freud lead him not to the anti-Freudianism that was standard in France at the time, but to a recontextualisation of Freud into a more subtle, epistemologically shrewd, and dialectical narrative of mental development than those that were being offered by his contemporaries.

Wallon borrows the notion put forward by Freud, that 'mental representations' govern the thought of both 'primitive' humans and infants, and situates this as a moment in the process of language acquisition. His short 1930 article 'De l'image au réel, dans la pensée de l'enfant' ('From the image to reality, in the thought of the child') is a comprehensive sketch of the mental development of ontological stability in children's perception, and of how this leads them into a universe of abstract, disembodied symbols. Wallon gives homage to Freud for showing that desire is actively involved in perception, and how it is therefore also involved in the precipitation of a child's experience of ontological reality. If an object may exist for a child 'only through his desire and the satisfactions he finds in it', then even the 'actual, immediate and concrete experience of things, far from giving a true image, begin to be an essentially subjective and

[123] In a 1920 article, 'La conscience et la vie subconsciente' ('Consciousness and Unconscious Life'), Wallon makes it clear that he considers it definitive progress 'to have affirmed, in the face of conscious representations, the existence of psychical states which are not conscious', as this changed the meaning of 'the previously established opposition between consciousness and the unconscious' (Wallon, 'La conscience et la vie subconsciente', p. 393). In a study of *The Interpretation of Dreams* from 1927, he describes the essential themes of psychoanalysis as being 'more romantic than scientific in origin', but he also argues that the first contact of these psychoanalytic concepts 'with objective and scientific psychology must be gathered, verified, and used by it' (Cited in Roudinesco, *Jacques Lacan & Co.*, p. 69).

[124] Roudinesco, *Jacques Lacan & Co.*, p. 69.

momentary reaction'.[125] Consequently, for Wallon, we also find in Freud a sceptical challenge that 'the real, instead of being given by the image', which is always refracted by desire, 'should be sought outside of it'.[126]

Wallon's dialectical materialist account of mental development takes the division between subject and object to be only an acquired, rather than an original one. Wallon describes how, before this division occurs in mental life, reality is in a state of ontological elasticity, a 'global' primordial state of confused intermingling, which 'unites' subject and object before their division. In the phase where this protean mode of reality holds sway, a child is unable to relate to objects as having consistency and permanence beyond any given moment of sensory perception. Their world is one of continual metamorphosis, where objects are indistinguishable, but where representations of them in thought are also irreducible to one another. This state will only be fully rectified by the child's developing ability to name objects, and to manipulate these symbols. Gradually, he postulates, children are able to perform the mental process of 'doubling'—also identified by Lévy-Bruhl in his anthropological studies of 'primitive mentality'—in which an abstract mental image is formed 'by elimination of all the sensible qualities which make the experience concrete, particular, [and] lived'.[127] The 'double' acts as an intermediary between raw sensory perception, on one hand, and the formation of an immaterial, symbolic network of association on the other. It allows a child to conceptualise both the 'passage from one individual or object to another', and also the 'reciprocal action' between objects, which could not have been formed before this initial level of abstraction.

This developing capacity to think abstractly, and to form dematerialised networks of association between objects, presses the child towards the symbolic exchanges of language use, a phenomenon Wallon takes to be 'universal' in humans.[128] The effect of language is to shift a child's mode of engagement with reality, opening up an entirely new dimension of existence. For Wallon, when a child is curious about the names of

[125] Wallon, 'De l'image au réel, dans la pensée de l'enfant', *Revue Philosophie de la France et de l'Étranger* (January–June 1930), 446–458 (p. 448).

[126] Wallon, 'De l'image au réel', p. 448.

[127] Wallon, 'De l'image au réel', p. 453.

[128] Wallon, 'De l'image au réel', p. 456.

objects, it is not merely in the interest of expanding their vocabulary, but in response to 'the need to realise fully the existence of the object' itself.[129] Wallon is clear that knowledge of words does not immediately cast a child into a virtual, symbolic register, and he takes this to be only gradually distilled out of an original state of fusion between word and object. A name begins, for a child, 'by being identical to the thing itself', to the extent that 'the existence of the thing without knowledge of the name will seem inconceivable to him'.[130] At this stage, he says, things 'exist because the child knows their name', a name that appears 'in some cases to be the creator of the object'.[131] Gradually, he outlines, the name will become dissociated from the object, allowing the filtering out of the 'sensible appearance' of a thing from the occult appendage of its 'double'. By its 'progressive dematerialisation', the word 'emigrates towards the more abstract domain of the idea', and acquires the 'mystical efficiency' of the *Logos*.[132] At this point, words, still located by children in physical space, are imagined by them to be more and more diffusely located, up to a point when language exists 'everywhere', so that the 'virtual' dimension it conjures up takes on the quality of 'ubiquity'. Words are then imagined by children, Wallon describes, to be sequestered in the 'hidden parts of visible and tangible space'—'the name is in the little corners', as a child says in one of Jean Piaget's studies cited by Wallon.[133] At this point, Wallon envisages the child to be 'very close to inaugurating the ideal and virtual environment of pure mental evocations, where it, the symbol, takes the place of encounters with the sensible'.[134]

A Freudian view of symbolic mental life is the hinge about which Wallon turns this transition. At the point in a child's early understanding of language when words begin to detach from their earlier state of fusion with objects, he identifies two correlative schemas taking precedence as ways for them to conceive of language. On one hand, they imagine language as a presence existing, with the diffuse ephemerality he has already

[129] Wallon, 'De l'image au réel', p. 456.
[130] Wallon, 'De l'image au réel', p. 456.
[131] Wallon, 'De l'image au réel', p. 456.
[132] Wallon, 'De l'image au réel', p. 456.
[133] Wallon, 'De l'image au réel', p. 456.
[134] Wallon, 'De l'image au réel', p. 456.

noted, in the 'air and space', in which speech is felt to the child to 'vibrat[e] in a sort of impalpable way'. On the other hand, speech also becomes associated with the 'mouth from which it exhales', and the child imagines all language to be concentrated into the tongue or the lips. At this point, he identifies a particular symbolic logic to take operation:

> There is a displacement of that which animates a whole ensemble onto a single organ or a part of an organ, and a condensation onto this organ of an intuition, or a global and complex notion, a notion whose existence totalises its active ingredient. In the same way, after displacement of language into one of its organs, the lips, they will find themselves having condensed into them all that which touches on language, including thought, which has not yet been distinguished [from language as a whole].[135]

In Wallon's sketch of this moment in mental life, he explicitly invokes what he refers to as 'logical processes' discovered by Freud. Once this 'last adhesion' of language to the material of the lips is diminished, he says, 'it will be released from all attachment with the sensible' and 'the distinction comes to be effected between language which is spoken or heard and immaterial thought'.[136] This amounts to the last surge of development towards the conditions of mature language use:

> Then the child finds himself, as does the adult, between two closely conjugated universes, but with radically different forms and developments: that of the senses and that of thought. And it is henceforth in the latter that he will look for all explanation, and in which he will place all reality. Thus, he will have completed the conversion, which extracts the sensory image from the real, to transpose it onto the plane of mental representation and of its symbols.[137]

It is significant to Wallon's overall account of mental development that he makes condensation and displacement—the axes of the Freudian dream-work and symptom—such privileged mechanisms for a child's movement

[135] Wallon, 'De l'image au réel', pp. 457–458.

[136] Wallon, 'De l'image au réel', p. 458.

[137] Wallon, 'De l'image au réel', p. 458.

into the symbolic. This follows Wallon's earlier stated appreciation of Freud, for opening paths, in his accounts of desire and of the pleasure principle, that allow perceptive deformations to be understood as interminglings of subject and object. So, following this, the Freudian dreamwork—the mechanism that fixes hallucinations onto the infrastructure of desire—comes to Wallon as the ideal cantilever for articulating the symbolic logic he takes to preside over sensory perception. Wallon gives much greater accord to these Freudian mechanisms than they could have acquired whilst veiled by the notion, which he finds so reductive, of their 'primitivity'. Wallon demonstrates how, in the right hands, these mechanisms could be mobilised to solve the most pressing epistemological aporias that arise within a dialectical materialist schema of mental development. They allow him to explain coherently, without recourse to spiritualism, the transition between the perception of objective reality, and mental representation

Wallon's account of mental development does not view it, like Piaget's developmental psychology, as a gradual discovery of external objectivity by an originally autistic ego. Instead, Wallon depicts it as a conversion, a modal shift, from the synesthetic confusion of sheer exposure to the 'real', towards the gradual extraction of discrete objects from mental images, and finally to a virtual layer of symbols which allow these objects to be manipulated in social life. In doing so, he enlists not the Freud of solipsistic, epistemological isolation invoked by Piaget, but the Freud who discovered a symbolic logic of condensation and displacement that come to be expressed in the anatomy.

In *Thinking and Speech*—which was structured in part as a polemic against Piaget—Vygotsky pits his own perspective on Freud against the Piagetian uptake of psychoanalysis.[138] Like Wallon, Vygotsky is also concerned with dissolving the division between the social and the biological, which he takes to be a lapse into semi-metaphysical idealism. But Vygotsky, as described above, does so not, like Wallon, by attention to sensory perception and its organisation from the perspective of the developing child, but through his commitment to establishing an experimentally valid, monistic theory of psychology. The context of reflexology, and the politics of Russian experimental psychology, led to Vygotsky's work

[138] See A.N. Leont'ev, 'On Vygotsky's Creative Development', in *The Collected Works of L.S. Vygotsky, Vol. 1*, p. 26.

making some very different emphases to Wallon's. The developmental schema in *La Vie mentale* is clearly more phenomenological, and more Hegelian, in the way that it gives shape to a romance of the choreography of subject and object as these form and change position in early human life. Vygotsky did not share these concerns, and his work built much more clearly on Marx's and Engels's writings on the relationship between labour and psychology.[139]

Vygotsky was carving out a position for the higher functions in the field of reflexology that was central to Russian psychology in the 1920s and 30s, and in the wake of the materialist revolution that reflexology represented. Most of Wallon's observations would have been regarded as too idealistic in post-revolutionary Russia, because it would not have been possible to verify them with the same experimental opacity and precision as Pavlov's, which had set the standard for Russian experimental psychology. For Wallon, idealism is not strictly the enemy, in the sometimes paranoid way it became for Russian psychologists. The task, as Wallon articulates in *La Vie mentale*, is not endlessly to hunt down the idealisms remaining in psychology, but instead to situate psychology at the faultline *between* materialism and idealism, in order to make the science the unique vantage point from which the relationship between these positions could be scientifically assessed, and then strategically mediated. Wallon's developmental narrative demonstrates how idealism need not be the eternal nemesis of materialism, but that it can be absorbed, subsumed, and neutralised by a materialist psychology. His definitive shift is to make idealism into a mode of psychic operation, which can be indexed onto a period of mental development. The spiritualism, mysticism, or occultism that frustrated Vygotsky and Politzer are reframed by Wallon, as episodes in a process of psychological development that can only be understood fully by a framework that can supersede them; they are each components or moments of the rich mental life whose development Wallon narrates. This amounts, in part, to a new, inventive way of applying Freud. Wallon is not as deterred by the Freudian idealism that was so

[139] In, for example, his view of language as a tool for thinking. He took language to impact on thought in the same way technology shapes labour historically. See Vygotsky, 'The Instrumental Method in Psychology' (1930), in *The Concept of Activity in Soviet Psychology*, p. 137.

offensive to Vygotsky and Politzer, because even the dimensions of Freud that are less materialist allow Wallon to neutralise a more extreme, more problematic form of idealism.

This solution contrasts with that put forward by Vygotsky's theories, which consign idealism to the status of a methodological error—one that threatens to raise its head and appear unexpectedly if a psychological method has an unsound and leaky theoretical basis—a position more directly anchored in Marx's *The German Ideology* (1932 [1846]) and 'Theses on Feuerbach' (1888 [1845]). In the 1930s, Wallon was already writing in a climate with a different understanding of the relationship between Marx and the idealism that was taken to be epitomised by Hegel. Vygotsky, on the other hand, wrote in the wake of the world's first Communist revolution, where the stakes were understandably high as to what form psychology would take in the new world it had made possible—hence the rigour and intensity with which he approached formulating a new basis for his science, and the brittle and confrontational tone of his writings. For Marxists in France, Communism remained a fantasy, and the form it might have taken could be explored theoretically by them—until occupation at least—in an environment of relative freedom. For Vygotsky, on the other hand, Communism was a very real and present political project, and it urgently required a psychology to make sense of questions around the "new man" that its society aimed to produce. At the same time, this context pressed Russian psychology to confront both its own disparateness, and what those like Vygotsky viewed as its regressive tendencies—two attributes attested to in his 'Crisis' manuscript—as well as, when the Stalinist era arrived, forcing its psychologists into a struggle for livelihood, reputation, and survival.

Shortly after Wallon outlined the development of a child's mind as a movement from the imaginary to the symbolic in general terms, he made a much longer study of one pivotal moment in this process. The growing awareness a child has of its own body, and its developing means of conceptualising it, offer Wallon an exceptionally befitting junction between all the elements of mental development that concern him the most. It represents a special case in the broader process of psychogenesis, when a convergence takes place between, on one hand, the needs and activities of the body, and on the other, a sense of exteriority. This moment acts, as he presents it, as an essential platform for the further development of consciousness.[140] The evolving response a child has to their mirror image serves for Wallon as a privileged index for this development. It indicates, in a way that is easily available to empirical observation, a child's ability to abstract mental images from their perception of space. It also amounts to a process with clear consequences for a child's entrance into symbolic life and social relationships. Wallon makes an extended discussion of this process in a 1931 article, 'Comment se développe chez l'enfant la notion du corps propre' ('How the notion develops in the child of their own body'), which closely follows the research of Charles Darwin, the physiologist William Preyer, and the psychologist Paul Guillaume, into infants' reactions to their mirror images.

One broad aim of Wallon's paper on the concept of the body is to demonstrate that the notions out of which consciousness is constituted—even some of the most apparently simple and immediately assumed ones—are products of a juddering and intricately complex dialectical progression.[141] Wallon's developmental schema has the effect of levelling out the hierarchy of validity between images, by making an image always already 'a differentiated result, and not an element of psychic life'.[142] This revokes the simple designation of any image as hallucinatory or unreal, because the virtual system of representations that arranges images has necessarily already departed from stark reality in order to deal with virtual spaces—the ones that are epitomised, and fastened to the image of one's own body, by a mirror's reflection.

Lacan first described his own rendition of the mirror stage in an unpublished paper he read at the 1936 conference of the IPA in Marienbad.[143] He then made reference to the theory in his long article *La Famille*, published alongside *La Vie mentale* in the volume of the

---

[140] Wallon, 'Comment se développe chez l'enfant la notion du corps propre' (1931), *Enfance*, 16, nos. 1–2 (1963), 121–150 (p. 149). Originally published in *Journal de Psychologie* (November–December 1931).

[141] This follows the same concern of the article 'De l'image au réel, dans la pensée de l'enfant' (1930).

[142] Wallon, 'Comment se développe chez l'enfant', p. 150.

[143] The earliest remaining record of the theory is a set of notes made by Françoise Dolto at a lecture Lacan gave in June 1936, which have since been published in French. See Françoise Dolto, 'Notes de Françoise Dolto à la S.P.P. le 16 juin 1936', in Gérard Guillerault, *Le miroir et la psyché. Dolto, Lacan et le stade du miroir* (Paris: Gallimard, 2003), pp. 267–272.

Encyclopédie Française that was edited by Wallon. Wallon's *La Vie mentale* takes up roughly a quarter of the 324 pages of the volume. The other contributors included Pierre Janet, Charles Blondel, Georges Dumas, Benjamin Logre, Eugène Minkowski, the psychoanalysts Paul Schiff and Édouard Pichon, and Daniel Lagache—the only other one from Lacan's own generation.[144] Lacan had met Wallon several times between 1928 and 1934 at the Société de Psychiatrie, during which time Lacan read Wallon's book *Origines du caractère chez l'enfant* (1934), which reprinted Wallon's article on mirror recognition.[145] Lacan's entry in the *Encyclopédie*, *La Famille*, serves as an introduction to Freud that attempts to rehabilitate several of his ideas.[146] It is also an accompaniment to Wallon's own narrative of mental development, and places it in the context of the Freudian family romance.[147]

Whilst this publication represented Lacan's explicit entry onto the scene of the conversations surrounding Marxism and psychology in France, he had already been greeted by several members of the Surrealist

---

[144] Lagache would be the object of a 1958 article published in Lacan's *Écrits*. See Lacan, 'Remarks on Daniel Lagache's Presentation: "Psychoanalysis and Personality Structure"' (1960), in Écrits, trans. by B. Fink (London: Norton, 2006), pp. 543–574

[145] Roudinesco, *Jacques Lacan & Co.*, p. 142.

[146] Republished as Lacan, *Les Complexes familiaux dans la formation de l'individu. Essai d'analyse d'une fonction en psychoanalyse* (Paris: Navarin, 1984). For an unofficial translation, see Cormac Gallagher, <http://www.lacaninireland.com/web/translations/ecrits/>

[147] Two priorities of the leading figures behind the project were interdisciplinarity and accessibility. Febvre hoped for the encyclopaedia to be more than just a catalogue of terms, and wanted to create a sophisticated whole that would allow the reader to survey the knowledge presented for its interconnectedness and affinity (Jalley, 'Introduction a la lecture de *La Vie Mentale*', in *La Vie Mentale*, pp. 21–96 (p. 40)). Febvre was something of a hero of historical universality, who had fought throughout his career against an erudite historicism concerned only with individual figures or events, envisaging a 'total' history built 'at the crossroads of all the social sciences' (p. 39). He was naturally interested in Wallon's approach to psychology, which treated the individual as a fundamentally social being produced through their interactions with an environment. Wallon and Febvre both describe psychology as being directed towards a 'psychic paleontology' (p. 41), the study of layers of the mind in which historical environments have been inscribed. Psychology, from this perspective, amounted to a 'history of affective life' and of its 'emotional equipment' (p. 41). The convenor of the *Encyclopédie française* shared with Wallon, firstly, a vision of intimate dialogue between the human sciences (the kind of dialogue that Wallon, in *A la lumière du Marxisme*, finds to have been realised in the Soviet Union), and secondly, a view of the human individual as an organism animated by such a dynamic, unlimited confluence of events and ideas. For them, psychology was a means of building up this perspective of the human as being entirely composed of an interplay between organic substrates and historical events. Wallon had demonstrated that this synthesis could be achieved without any risk of either idealist mystification or materialist reduction.

movement as a revolutionary new voice in dialectical materialism, after the publication of his doctoral thesis, *On Paranoid Psychosis in its Relation with the Personality*, in 1932. The main aim of the book is to argue and explain the relationship described in its title, between paranoid psychosis and the personality, by demonstrating it through a case study of a woman Lacan treated at Saint-Anne, to whom he gives the pseudonym 'Aimée'. Lacan attempts to understand Aimée's psychosis as a reaction to events in her life, and a result of conflicts these events produced in the structure of her personality. He explains her psychosis purely from these psychological sources, rather than from organic ones, posing intelligible, meaningful psychological connections between her psychotic symptoms and her life history. As part of the 'phenomenology of madness' that he begins to develop from the case study, Lacan pays a great deal of attention to the copious writing that accompanied Aimée's psychosis. The poet Paul Éluard, one of the founders of the Surrealist movement, would later publish some of Aimée's poems in a collection of "involuntary" poetry in 1942.[148]

Lacan's thesis was popular amongst several other figures associated with Surrealism. Dalí praised it in the first issue of *La Minotaure* for transcending the 'mechanical miseries' of contemporary psychiatry, and Paul Nizan saw in it a 'definite and conscious influence of dialectical materialism', pitted against psychological and psychiatric idealism.[149] Lacan's thesis was received with particular enthusiasm by René Crevel, who, in the article 'Notes en vue d'une psychodialectique' ('Notes for a Psychodialectic')—published in 1933 in *Le Surréalisme au service de la révolution*—presents it as a bastion of progress towards the rejuvenation of psychoanalysis by dialectical materialism. In the article, Crevel

[148] Paul Éluard, *Poésie involontaire et poésie intentionnelle* (Villeneuve-les-Avignon: Seghers, 1942).

[149] Salvador Dalí, 'Paranoiac-Critical Interpretations of the Obsessive Image of Millet's "Angelus", in *The Tragic Myth of Millet's Angelus*, trans. and ed. by A. R. Morse (The Salvador Dalí Museum, 1986), pp. 215–16. Nizan cited in Roudinesco, *Jacques Lacan*, p. 59. Before this, though, Lacan had published a paper on the '"Inspired" Writings' of schizophrenic patients, which draws an explicit connection between these disordered writings and the automatic writing practised by the surrealists, difficult to read without sensing an ironic testing of the limits between madness and poetic talent. This dialogue would continue in a publication in the surrealist journal *La Minotaure* in 1933. See Lacan, J. Lévy-Valensi and Pierre Migault, 'Écrits "inspirés": schizographie', *Les Annales Médico-Psychologiques*, II (1931), 508–522. Available online at <http://aejcpp.free.fr/lacan/1931-11-12a.htm>

describes the decadent state of philosophy, and the uselessness of Freudian psychoanalysis, which, as he perceives it, exists in a state of geriatric impotence. Psychoanalysis, he says, 'appears ready to turn the most complex complex into a uniform for an abstract mannequin'.[150] He mocks Freud and Einstein's dialogue in 'Why War?' (1931–32), and lambasts Freud's denunciation of Communism in *The Future of an Illusion* (1927) as hypocrisy.[151] But Lacan's thesis is credited by Crevel as demonstrating a ray of hope, and the necessary antidote to a 'mechanical materialism' into which he accuses Freud of lapsing: '[m]aterialist science', he says 'for its psycho-dialectic, has need of monographs which are [as] detailed, precise, complete' as Lacan's.[152] The article is as vehemently animated as all Surrealist writing, and it ends with a rousing call-to-arms for dialectical materialist psychoanalysis. Freud, writes Crevel, may be 'tired enough to want no more than to busy himself with his trinkets. We can excuse that. But which young psychoanalyst will take over to speak up?'.[153]

If it seems clear from his championing of Lacan, who receives essentially as much attention in the article as Freud, whom Crevel has in mind to take up this mantle, it is also true that at this stage Lacan had only just begun to read Freud, and only in the context of psychiatry. Lacan clearly offered much for those of his readers inclined to dialectical materialism to be aroused by. But his interest in their politics or theory was in no sense explicit, particularly in light of how bombastic the political rhetoric of many of these readers was. It was not even really implicit either: Lacan does not address politics at all in the writings that impressed these Surrealists, and makes none of the gestures of devotion to dialectical materialism, or to the writings of Marx and Engels, that so many of his contemporary scientists—not just in psychology, but across a range of fields—routinely did.[154] So what did they see in Lacan which directed

[150] René Crevel, 'Notes en vue d'une psychodialectique', *Le Surréalisme au service de la révolution* 5 (May 1933). Reprinted in *Le Surréalisme au service de la révolution: Collection complete* (Paris, 1976), pp. 48–52 (p. 48). '[A]pparait prête à faire du complexe le plus complexe un uniforme pour mannequin abstrait'.

[151] Crevel, 'Notes en vue', p. 50.

[152] Crevel, 'Notes en vue', p. 50.

[153] Crevel, 'Notes en vue', p. 52. Cited in English in Roudinesco, *Jacques Lacan & Co.*, p. 56.

[154] See the work of the Cercle de Russie published in *A la lumière du Marxisme* (Editions Sociales Internationales, 1935 and 1937).

their hopes towards him, rather than towards the more obvious candidates of Politzer, or Wallon, or the Soviet psychologists? Was it the enthusiasm and sympathy he shared with the Surrealists for the experience of madness, and particularly for the madness of women?[155] Was it his mutual fascination with writing and poetry, and especially with the writings of the mad? Was it more a result of Lacan's deliberate courtship of the Surrealists' circles?[156] Or was there something genuinely exciting on the level of Lacan's *theories* at this stage—something that singled him out even from those of his contemporaries who were often explicitly invested in Marx, and in revolution?

There is an important similarity between the Surrealists, Althusser, and the philosophers of the Ljubljana School in this respect. Around half a century before Žižek published *The Sublime Object of Ideology* (1989), and thirty years before Althusser wrote 'Freud and Lacan' (1964), several politically-committed Surrealists had also wanted to press Lacan into the service of revolution, apparently in spite of the absence of revolutionary Marxism from his work. His status for each—as the 'young analyst' who would be the heir apparent to Freud, or as the herald of a new materialism-without-matter—could be so Messianic seemingly because he did not ask for this position, which allowed they themselves to discover him in the bullrushes. His appeal for them lies, maybe, in him being a revolutionary, to paraphrase Žižek, 'without knowing it'.[157] Lacan clearly does not commit the error made in the bids—botched by Luria, Politzer, Fridman, Reich, and a string of others—openly to press Freud into line with a Marxist project. This attempt had, as the present chapter has documented, always backfired, and backfired in ways that appeared to the

[155] See Lacan, J. Lévy-Valensi and Pierre Migault, 'Écrits "inspirés": schizographie', *Les Annales Médico-Psychologiques*, II (1931), 508–522. Available online at: <http://aejcpp.free.fr/lacan/1931-11-12a.htm>; and Lacan, 'Motifs du crime paranoïaque: le crime des sœurs Papin', *Le Minotaure* 3/4, 100–103. Available online at: <http://aejcpp.free.fr/lacan/1933-12-12.htm>

[156] See '3. Baltimore in the Early Morning', in Macey, *Lacan in Contexts* (London: Verso, 1988), pp. 44–74.

[157] See Žižek, *The Most Sublime Hysteric: Hegel with Lacan* (2011), trans. by T. Scott-Railton (Cambridge: Polity Press, 2014), p. 4, where he claims that Lacan 'was fundamentally Hegelian, but did not know it'.

most attentive observers to undermine the fundamental premises of that very project.[158]

In the 'Notes en vue' article, Crevel positions himself equivocally, as both despondent with psychoanalysis, and eager for its renewal. He echoes Politzer and Vygotsky in this sense. Their position is emblematic of the way Freud appeared to those who stood in the name of a philosophically-minded dialectical materialism. For them, psychoanalysis could only be trusted as far as it was capable of reform, but it was only worthy of reformation to the extent that it could already be seen to have borne fruit. Lacan's reading of Freud would make it much clearer where psychoanalysis stood in this context. The complexity of his reading of Freud made possible a different way to manage the equivocations and difficulties encountered by so many Marxists when they attempted to enlist Freud to their political and scientific projects. As the following section will demonstrate, Lacan reads Freud in a way that *preserves* the conflicts these Marxists had discovered in him. Instead of Freud being regressive, contradictory, or having attempted a materialist break that lapsed unintentionally into idealism, Freud, in Lacan's reading, presses towards an entire reorientation of the relationship between materialism and idealism.

Reflex and Signifier

The present chapter has been documenting crises in the theoretical basis for psychology that were encountered by materialist psychologists in the early twentieth century. These, it has showed, traced out fundamental impasses in the relationship between materialism and idealism. Vygotsky and Politzer, as the chapter has documented above, identified how the science of psychology lacked the conceptual equipment that was crucially

[158] It is not difficult to see Lacan's tableau of the mirror stage in the late 1930s performing the combination of perspectives Politzer had in mind for concrete psychology: it includes a Freudian family drama, a constructive critique of Gestalt psychology, and even elements of a redeemed behaviourism, in its charting of the body's physiological response to mirror-identification. Lacan would pay direct homage to Politzer in his 1946 'Presentation on Psychical Causality', where he admits how far away from 'concrete psychology' he and his audience still remain at that point. *Écrits*, trans. by B. Fink (London: Norton, 2007), pp. 123–160 (p. 131).

needed to approach these questions effectively. Something else was also made clear, though, by their extensive critiques of psychology's theoretical and methodological bases: that the questions punctuating psychology as a science pressed, in addition, beyond the usual limits of a philosophical approach to this relationship. Psychology, as Vygotsky and Politzer portrayed the science, was fumbling in a darkness where existing philosophy seemed to be able to offer it no truly helpful co-ordinates. Psychoanalysis was identified by them as a field that could provide these co-ordinates. Nobody, however, had been able to apply Freud in this way without either producing, like Vygostky's adversaries, an impotent theoretical miscellany, or being dissuaded, like Vygotsky, by the risks of doing so.

Lacan, as the following section will describe, makes his own version, in the 1960s, of the classic critical manoeuvre made by Vygotsky and Politzer, that pulls the mask from a materialist theory to unveil, beneath its outward appearance, a secret idealism. What he adds, however, to the condemnation of idealism that was routine in these critiques, is an assertion that this recognition also holds significant consequences for materialism itself. Lacan positions psychoanalysis as the field capable of acknowledging and articulating a more subtle status for materialism. Lacan approaches the questions that concerned Vygotsky, Politzer, and Wallon, in a way that clearly attempts to reduce them down to more fundamental co-ordinates than had previously been attempted. He rearticulates the limitations of reflexology as questions about the status of scientific knowledge itself.

Pavlov I: The Signifier against the Stimulus

The following section of this chapter identifies three phases to a reading of Pavlov made by Lacan in his writings and Seminar. In these three phases, Lacan works through the position that he envisages for psychoanalysis with respect to reflexology. The first time Lacan mentions reflexology is in the Rome Discourse of 1953, published in the *Écrits* as 'The Function and Field of Speech and Language in Psychoanalysis', part of which is an attack on existing attempts to wed psychoanalysis to Pavlov's theories. In its second section, Lacan stages a critique of an article published in 1944 by the psychoanalyst Jules H. Masserman, 'Language, Behaviour and Dynamic Psychiatry'.[159] Masserman's article is a good example of the kind of theory that could dribble out of an uncritical incorporation of psychoanalysis into reflexology. The article pays lip service to the problem—described in the opening section of this chapter—that language had always posed to Pavlov's first signalling system. Masserman adds that, in order for language to be understood as a stimulus unproblematically, all symbols have to be recognised as having a 'personalised significance' for any given individual.[160] Masserman explains how the effect of language on, and the use of language by a patient can be understood as the result of a process of 'conditioning' that has taken place throughout their life. As a result of this conditioning process, elements of language, viewed as stimuli, will always be refracted through the past emotional experiences that the patient associates with them. An element of language, in other words—like the bell that made Pavlov's dogs drool—produces a physiological response in a person depending on the associations this linguistic element has been given by the events of that individual's life.

Masserman's article is obviously announcing the significance of language for psychoanalysis in a way that is absolute anathema to Lacan's return to Freud. But the specific target of Lacan's scorn is Masserman's description of an experiment by the British psychologist C.V. Hudgins, in which Hudgins successfully made a human subject associate the projection of a bright light into their eyes with the instruction "contract".[161] This, Masserman recounts, produced the effect in the subject's autonomic

---

159 Lacan, 'The Function and Field of Speech and Language in Psychoanalysis' (1953), in *Écrits*, trans. by B. Fink (London: Norton, 2006), pp. 197–268 (pp. 225–228). See Jules H. Masserman, 'Language, Behaviour and Dynamic Psychiatry', *International Journal of Psychoanalysis*, 1944, 1–7. Lacan's critique of Masserman in that paper is continued from the lecture 'The Symbolic, the Imaginary, and the Real', given just before, in the same year. See Lacan, 'The Symbolic, the Imaginary, and the Real', in *On the Names-of-the-Father*, trans. by B. Fink (London: Polity, 2015), pp. 1–52.

160 Masserman, 'Language, Behaviour and Dynamic Psychiatry', p. 3.

161 Misspelt rustically in the English translation of the *Écrits* as "Hudgkins". C.V. Hudgins, 'Conditioning and the Voluntary Control of the Pupillary Light Reflex', *Journal of General Psychology*, 8, no. 3 (1933), 3–51.

nervous system, of their pupils contracting upon them merely hearing this word. In response, Lacan asks, with satirical but serious derision, whether the same effect was produced when the word "contract" was used in different lexical categories than the imperative—when it was used as a noun, or a negative imperative—or when it was progressively shortened down to its first syllable.[162] The reason Lacan makes this point is because these material changes would have given the word an entirely transformed meaning, even if it remained exactly the same word phonetically; the semanteme would be entirely different, even if the phonemes (kənˈtrakt) remained identical. The effects of the experiment clearly require further elaboration: either, says Lacan, the physiological response 'would no longer be produced' by these alternative forms of the word, 'thus revealing that they do not even conditionally depend on the semanteme', or 'they would continue to be produced, raising the question of the semanteme's limits'.[163] If the physiological effect had no longer been produced, then it could never have had anything to do with the word "contract", as a semanteme, in the first place. If the physiological effect *had* still been produced by the alternative forms of the word, then this would have demonstrated that, even as a stimulus, a word has a dimension of meaning operating on a level that cannot be studied within a reflexological framework. Either way, neither Masserman nor Hudgins are able even to conceptualise this distinction.

Lacan uses the porousness of this framework, which he reveals here so briskly, to demonstrate the necessity of a structuralist theory of language. He illustrates that it is not possible to explain Hudgins's experiment without this structuralist theory. This is because there is something of the nature of language that is missing from the account given by Masserman, which Lacan specifies as the dimension of the signifier. Any effects on a subject of an 'element of language', detected experimentally or otherwise, must, Lacan argues, be understood as a result of the status of this element of language as 'distinguished […] in the supposedly constituted set of homologous elements'—in the structuralist grid of signifiers—prior and

[162] The 'control test required by strict scientific method would then be supplied all by itself as the French reader muttered this syllable' (i.e., the expletive '*con*'). Lacan, 'The Function and Field of Speech and Language in the Unconscious', p. 226.

[163] Lacan, 'The Function and Field of Speech and Language in the Unconscious', p. 227.

independently 'to any possible link with any of the subject's particular experiences'.[164]

Lacan develops this critique of reflexology further a few years later, in *Seminar V: Formations of the Unconscious* (1957–58). In the nineteenth lesson of the seminar—titled 'Signifier, Bar and Phallus' by Jacques-Alain Miller—Lacan asserts that there remains great value in Pavlov's experiments, but not in the place where it had previously been recognised. The experiments amount, he describes here, to a demonstration that the field of the Other, which is created by language, is operative for the animal in the experiment. Each of the artificial stimuli—'the little electrical signals, the little buzzers and little bells'—are, he says, 'actually signifiers, really, and nothing but', because they amount to 'fabrications' created by the experimenters, whose world is 'very clearly' formed by the dimension of the signifier.[165] What cannot, however, be discovered by this kind of experiment is, he argues, 'the *law* by which the signifiers involved are organised', because this law does not exist for animals, despite there being for them a dimension of the Other.[166]

The experiment, as Lacan dismantles it, proves something that can be easily observed simply by witnessing the behaviour of domestic dogs: that the dimension he calls the Other is operative for them. The experiment cannot, however, for Lacan, discover anything about the nature of the signifying field, because—even if animals have been drawn into the field of the Other by domestication—its *laws* are not operative for the experiment's animal subject. According to Lacan's critique, Pavlov's experiment proceeds as if Galileo had proven an object's time of descent to be

[164] Lacan, 'The Function and Field of Speech and Language in the Unconscious', p. 227.

[165] Lacan, Lesson of 23 April 1958, 'XIX. Signifier, Bar and Phallus', in *The Seminar of Jacques Lacan, Book V: Formations of the Unconscious*, ed. Jacques-Alain Miller, trans. Russell Grigg (London: Polity, 2017), pp. 315–332 (p. 320). Putting pressure at the same point Vygotsky had, of the gap between Pavlov's first and second signal systems, Lacan adds that the dimension of the signifier is what constitutes this distinction.

[166] Lacan, *Seminar V*, p. 320. My italics. Lacan adds that what is lacking in the discourse of animals is an aspect of 'concatenation' (*Seminar V*, p. 320). As he adds in 1962, in *Seminar X: Anxiety*, this presence of the Other for a dog is clear merely from observing its behaviour towards its master. The presence of the researcher 'as a human figure, handling a certain number of things around the animal' should therefore be counted as part of the experiment'. Lesson of 12 December 1962, 'V. That Which Deceives', in *Seminar X: Anxiety* (1962–63), ed. by Jacques-Alain Miller, trans. by A.R. Price (Cambridge: Polity, 2014), pp. 55–68 (p. 58).

independent of its mass, and then sought to discover the laws of gravity by studying the material composition of the falling objects themselves. This would have elided the field of gravity in the same way that Lacan alleges Pavlov to have elided the laws and function of language. Lacan catches Pavlov in a trap: he positions Pavlov's famous experiment as proof of a field—the Other—whose study Pavlov himself, along with all classical materialists, simultaneously elides.

In these passages from the 1950s, Lacan is feeling out the limits of Pavlov's theory of reflexes, whilst also not doing away with what is useful about reflexology. This has much in common with Vygotsky's critical procedure from the 1920s and 30 s. Lacan makes only one substantial reference to Vygotsky in either his writings or his Seminar, in the second lesson of *Seminar XII: Crucial Problems for Psychoanalysis* (1964–65), from 9 December 1964.[167] It is a fairly—perhaps conspicuously—vague appeal, which lasts just a few paragraphs in print. But Lacan speaks very favourably of him, and implores the seminar's participants to read Vygotsky's work. In the lesson, Lacan uses Vygotsky to criticise Piaget's theory of language development, which had envisaged it as a gradual externalisation of concepts that existed in the child's mind. Vygotsky, as Lacan appeals to him here, appreciated, on the other hand, the way children actually spontaneously use words at a moment that is clearly prior to these words being attached to a concept. The anticipatory use by young children of particles of language—like "perhaps not", or "but still", for example—demonstrates that, in Lacan's words, 'grammatical structure is absolutely correlative to all the first appearances of language'.[168] Words observably are not externalised concepts, then, but phonetic fragments which children start to arrange around grammatical structures. Lacan uses Vygotsky to illustrate how words have another level for a child than as vehicles for concepts, and how in the speech of children signifiers are often, and first, used independently of this level of the concept.

---

[167] He mentions him once more the following year, in a summary of this previous mention, in Lesson 14, of 20 April 1966, in *Seminar XIII: The Object of Psychoanalysis* (1965–1966), unpublished.

[168] Lacan, Lesson 2, of 9 December 1964, in *Seminar XII: Crucial Problems for Psychoanalysis* (1964–65), unpublished. For an unofficial translation, see Gallagher, <http://www.lacaninireland.com/web/wp-content/uploads/2010/06/12-Crucial-problems-for-psychoanalysis.pdf>, p. 21.

Lacan is, unsurprisingly, siding with Vygotsky against Piaget's idealism. On levels that Lacan does not refer to, however, there are other significant, and more fundamental parallels between his and Vygotsky's critical handling of reflexology. Vygotsky, in the theoretical writings of the 1920s and 1930s discussed in the first section of this chapter, monistically flattens out the nature of consciousness, the function of language, and introspective methods of self-observation into phenomena that could be easily metabolisable by an extended theory of reflexes. Reflexes had to be understood, for Vygotsky, not as blind, unilateral spasms of the flesh—nor, equally, as Bekhterev's cosmic hydraulics—but as arrays of elegantly interconnected systems that constantly adapt and co-ordinate themselves into place around each other, and which respond to each other so precisely, in this way, that they could appear to the naïve observer to be beyond the limits of empirical enquiry, of even of a spiritual nature. The reflex, for Vygotsky, was not something that was *in* either the body or the brain; it was an experimental technology that existed to aid precise empirical enquiry, so that previously untraversable planes of human life could become traversable and observable by science. If applied in this way, there was no reason, to him, why reflexology should not be able to formulate an elegant and sophisticated theory of language. Vygotsky conceives of language as an external mediator to physiological reflexes, with which any individual's thinking exists in a developing, dialectical relationship. In Vygotsky's redeemed reflexology, both idealist subjectivity, on the one hand, and materialist automatism, on the other, are replaced by a grid of co-ordinates—external to the subject and pre-existing them—that are mapped onto the body, and that create, through their interrelationships, the mirages of consciousness and thought that had been wrongly identified as extra-material. Viewed in this way, Vygotsky's axiom that 'consciousness is merely a reflex to reflexes'[169] has a more than aesthetic proximity to Lacan's formula 'the signifier represents a subject for another signifier'. There is an innovative and logically similar squaring in both formulas of, on the one hand, the idealist ephemera of consciousness, identity, and subjectivity, with, on the other, a materialist reduction to a set of automatic causes and responses. Vygotsky's amended reflexology approached the same limit to the relationship between subject and

[169] Vygotsky, 'The Methods of Reflexological and Psychological Investigation' (1926), p. 46.

structure that Lacan articulates in the 1960s with the aid of structuralist theories and vocabulary.

Pavlov II: Another Way Out of Idealism

In *Seminar XI: The Four Fundamental Concepts of Psychoanalysis* (1964)—the watershed in Lacan's teaching that followed his departure from the IPA—he makes another reading of Pavlov. Here, Lacan identifies Pavlov's experiment as offering a different way out of idealism than that which Pavlov himself, and all other reflexologists, had understood it to. From the 1950s—and even up to the previous year's seminar—Lacan had presented Pavlov's experiment as an unintentional demonstration that the field of the Other is operative for its animal subject.[170] In the seventeenth lesson of *Seminar XI*, from 3 June 1964, Lacan expands on what the experiment, understood in this way, tells us about subjectivity. After making a dog salivate at the sight of a piece of meat, Lacan summarises, reprising the reading of Pavlov from *Seminar V*, the experiment demonstrates that 'the Other is there' by 'interrupt[ing] the process [of salivation] at the point of secretion'.[171] This shows, he repeats, that the dog's salivation can be produced by 'something that functions as a signifier'; by a fabrication, created by the experimenter, that acts as a signifier.[172] At this point in *Seminar XI*, Lacan is able to formulate how the true value of the experiment lays in what it tells us about the perception, not of the animal, but of the experimenter:

> The main interest of these experiments is to show us that differential range of the animal at the level of a perception that cannot in any sense be a representation, for there is no other subject here than the subject of the experimenter. And this goes much further still. In fact, we interrogate the animal about our own perception. This way of limiting the scope of the Pavlovian experiments restores to them, at the same time, it can be seen, their very great importance.[173]

---

[170] See Lacan, *Seminar X*, p. 58.

[171] Lacan, Lesson of 3 June 1964, 'XVII. The Subject and the Other: Aphanisis', *Seminar XI*, pp. 216–229 (p. 228).

[172] Lacan, *Seminar XI*, p. 228.

[173] Lacan, *Seminar XI*, p. 228.

The signifiers in play in the experiment are those of the human experimenter, says Lacan, because it is this experimenter who 'order[s] them in perception'.[174] The value of the experiment is, he says, that it shows how, in the animal, the signifiers 'express among themselves a sort of equivalence': how, 'without training', the animal 'passes from a hundred frequencies in one register', that of visual stimuli, 'to a hundred frequencies in another', that of auditory stimuli.[175]

Lacan brings in this reference to Pavlov at the very end of the lesson. He is using it to illustrate something that he has been developing throughout it, about the concept of *aphanisis*. In the lesson, Lacan has been making a new rendition of the term *aphanisis*—which was first used by Ernest Jones to describe a disappearance of desire—that recasts it as a disappearance, or splitting, of the subject that occurs upon them entering the dialectic of desire with the Other. Lacan develops his notion of *aphanisis* as a redefinition of the '*Vorstellungsrepräsentanz*' that was first mentioned in Freud's 1915 article 'Repression'. Repression, as Freud conceives it there, has a direct, distorting effect on mental representations of reality: it 'turns [them] away and maintains them at a distance from consciousness'.[176] Freud hypothesises here the existence of 'a primal repression, a first phase of repression' lying at the core of mental representation, that would 'consis[t] in the psychical [or ideational] representative [*Vorstellungs-Repräsentanz*] of the drive being denied entrance into the conscious'.[177] What Lacan introduces in *Seminar XI* is an equation between Freud's notion of *Vorstellungsrepräsentanz*, and what he calls a 'binary signifier': the signifier that appears in the Other as a representative of the subject.[178] From the 'first signifying coupling', of subject and Other, he says, the

---

[174] Lacan, *Seminar XI*, p. 229.

[175] Lacan, *Seminar XI*, p. 228–229.

[176] Sigmund Freud, 'Repression', in *The Standard Edition of the Complete Psychological Works of Sigmund Freud, Vol. XIV (1914–1916): On the History of the Psycho-Analytic Movement, Papers on Metapsychology and Other Works*, trans. by J. Strachey (London: Hogarth Press, 1957), pp. 146–158 (p. 147).

[177] Freud, 'Repression', p. 148.

[178] Lacan redefines *Vorstellungrepräsentanz* as 'that which takes the place of the representation' ('le tenant-lieu de la représentation'). '5. Tuché and Automaton', in *Seminar XI: The Four Fundamental Concepts of Psychoanalysis* (1964–1965), ed. by Jacques-Alain Miller, trans. by Alan Sheridan (London: Norton, 1998), pp. 53–66 (p. 60).

subject appears in the Other for the first time 'in so far as the first signifier, the unary signifier, emerges in the field of the Other and represents the subject for another signifier'.[179] But, he says, this first signifier, which represents the subject only for another signifier, simultaneously brings about a division of the subject. This leads Lacan to the formula that 'when the subject appears somewhere as meaning, he is manifested elsewhere as "fading", as disappearance'.[180] A dialectic of desire is thus set in motion concurrently with *aphanisis*, because the desire of the subject emerges, after the appearance of the binary signifier, out of the point of lack in the Other.[181] Lacan, in summary, revises Freud's notion of a primal repression—or a fundamental warping—at the core of an individual's reality, and makes of it the symbolic co-ordinate at which the first signifier both divides the subject, and represents them in the field of the Other.

Lacan then performs an innovative critique of philosophical idealism on the basis of his reconceptualisation of *aphanisis*. It remains true, he says—in a view that would agree with idealism—that 'every representation requires a subject'.[182] The ethical vision correlative to this, however, of a proliferation of pure subjects, each of whom is propped up by their singular *Weltanschauung*, or worldview, leads, he says, down a path where—as 'a backward psychology or psycho-sociology is still showing us'—truth may only be ascertained through 'the inquiry, the totalization, the statistics of different *Weltanschauung*'.[183] Subjects who are, as these naïve psychologies assume, 'each entrusted with the task of representing certain conceptions of the world', cannot, he demonstrates, exist if the theory of the signifier is taken seriously. The 'essential flaw of philosophical idealism', Lacan asserts, is that 'there is no subject without, somewhere, *aphanisis* of the subject'—the effacement by the signifier that he has been describing—and 'it is in this alienation, in this fundamental division, that the dialectic of the subject is established'.[184] No subject,

[179] Lacan, Lesson of 3 June 1964, 'XVII. The Subject and the Other: Aphanisis', in *Seminar XI*, pp. 216–229 (p. 218).

[180] Lacan, *Seminar XI*, p. 218.

[181] Lacan, *Seminar XI*, pp. 218–219.

[182] Lacan, *Seminar XI*, p. 221.

[183] Lacan, *Seminar XI*, p. 221.

[184] Lacan, *Seminar XI*, p. 221.

then, however unique or numinous, without it also disappearing in the dialectic of desire.

Lacan also makes clear, however, that despite occurring in the context of this virtuosic critique of idealism, his theory of *aphanisis* is based on a reading—and in fact is a new rendition—of Hegel's dialectic of master and slave. There is, Lacan says, 'a matter of life and death between the unary signifier and the subject, qua binary signifier, [the] cause of his disappearance'.[185] Lacan is drawing out this tangent from the dialectic of master and slave in an attempt, as he puts it, to undermine the possibility of any idealism. If Hegel, however, is the origin of this dialectic, then he is definitively not, in any unequivocal sense, on the side of the idealism that is being overturned by Lacan here. Of course, for Lacan, neither can anyone else worth reading ever really, irredeemably be placed on the level of the 'philosophical idealism'—which, in any case, he adds, 'cannot be sustained and has never been radically sustained'—that he has in his sights.[186]

In an earlier lesson of *Seminar XI*, Lacan has already addressed the association that was routinely made between psychoanalysis and idealism.[187] Freud, as the present chapter has been describing, was frequently reproached for making an idealistic reduction—as Lacan ventriloquises it in the fifth lesson of the seminar—of a materialist explanation of 'the reasons for our deficiencies' by 'the hard supports of conflict, struggle, [or] the exploitation of man by man' to, in Lacan's words, 'an ontology of the tendencies', which Freud supposedly 'regards as primitive, internal, already given by the condition of the subject'.[188] Freud is routinely accused, Lacan reiterates, of apoliticism: of ignoring material struggle and social antagonism, and of instead proposing the Oedipus complex, and other ancient, supposedly necessary psychic conflicts, as explanations for all human discontent. Though accusations of this kind were made by Politzer, Vygotsky, and many others in the Soviet Union, Lacan is opposed to this view. As he argues in this lesson, psychoanalysis can clearly not be

[185] Lacan, *Seminar XI*, p. 218.
[186] Lacan, *Seminar XI*, p. 221.
[187] See Lacan, 'V. Tuché and Automaton', in *Seminar XI*, p. 53.
[188] Lacan, *Seminar XI*, p. 53.

reduced to a radical idealism that would support 'some such aphorism as "life is a dream"'.[189] On the contrary—and against the idea that Freud supposedly retreated from real struggle and exploitation, in favour of primitive, internal tendencies—for Lacan, no praxis is more oriented than psychoanalysis 'towards that which, at the heart of experience, is the kernel of the real'.[190] As Lacan presents psychoanalysis here, its opposition to idealism comes from the way it reveals something about the real that cannot be accounted for by a framework that would merely pit materialism and idealism against each other as two alternatives. Freud, as Lacan reads him in *Seminar XI*, was more committed to the real—in the sense of being against an idealist dream of reality—than Marx. Psychoanalysis, he posits here, is more materialist than any existing materialism, because it takes to a limit a critical interrogation of the threshold between idealism and materialism. This was a threshold that was being felt out—as the present and the previous chapter have demonstrated, in their discussions of Vygotsky, Politzer, Wallon, Koyré, Kojève, Hyppolite, and others—by a whole host of figures prior to Lacan.

It is, says Lacan, the real that is the essential object of Freud's concern.[191] This real lies, as he puts it, 'behind the automaton' of the pleasure principle, and it is encountered as a point that always 'eludes us'.[192] The claim Lacan is making here is that, 'however far it is developed', the reality principle—the principle of mental functioning that, in a Piagetian reading of Freud, would facilitate the subject's contact with the real, material world—'leaves an essential part of what belongs to the real a prisoner in the toils of the pleasure principle'.[193] The reality principle had always been, for Freud, merely a detour, or temporary suspension, of the

[189] Lacan, *Seminar XI*, p. 53.

[190] Lacan, *Seminar XI*, p. 53.

[191] Lacan, *Seminar XI*, pp. 53–54. As demonstrated by the Wolf Man case study, in which Freud applies himself with commitment approaching 'anguish' to the question of 'the first encounter, the real, that lies behind the phantasy'; and by his question in *Beyond the Pleasure Principle*, of how the dream as 'the bearer of the subject's desire' can 'produce that which makes the trauma emerge repeatedly' (*Seminar XI*, pp. 54–55).

[192] Lacan, *Seminar XI*, p. 53.

[193] Lacan, *Seminar XI*, p. 55.

original, more fundamental pleasure principle.[194] As Lacan expands it here, regardless of the extent to which the reality principle cleaves the subject to a material world, there is always a portion of the real that touches this subject only on the level of the pleasure principle, and that is accessed, not via perception, but only through representation. This is why, as Lacan illustrates in this lesson of *Seminar XI*, dreams can be understood by psychoanalysis as giving access to a privileged level of the real: psychoanalysis identifies another reality, concealed behind representation, that impresses itself onto the reality of the dream.[195]

Through these various assaults, not just on idealism, but also on reflexology, Lacan carves out a new position for psychoanalysis in the context of the debates in materialist psychology that have been outlined in this chapter. The interweaving Lacan describes here of dream and waking reality, around a kernel of the real that penetrates through both, definitively relegates a standard opposition between idealism and materialism, and proposes a much more complicated basis on which their relationship needs to be understood. What troubled, concerned, appalled, blindsided, and confused materialist psychologists in France and the Soviet Union about psychoanalysis with regards to its status on the threshold of idealism and materialism, Lacan takes full advantage of here. It is not, for Lacan, that Freud made a mistake, that he did not realise something, or that he got something wrong, but that psychoanalysis is leaning—in a way that, it is true, remained only partially articulated by Freud—towards an entirely different topology than that upon which the old debates around materialism and idealism had been based. In the lessons of

---

[194] See Freud, 'Formulations on the Two Principles of Mental Functioning' (1911), in *The Standard Edition of the Complete Psychological Works of Sigmund Freud, Vol. XII (1911–1913)*, trans. by J. Strachey (London: Vintage, 1957), pp. 213–226.

[195] More generally, this allows Lacan to formulate that 'the phantasy is never anything more than the screen that conceals something quite primary, something determinant in the function of repetition'. What wakes us from a dream is, then, 'the other reality hidden behind the lack of that which takes the place of representation'—which Freud identified as the *Trieb* (Lacan, *Seminar XI*, p. 58). In the same lesson of *Seminar XI*, after Lacan has made clear why psychoanalysis is not an idealism, he makes the only reference to Wallon in the entire Seminar. In *Seminar XI*, Wallon is cited as an ally in emphasising the reality of *aphanisis*, the fundamental splitting of the subject. Interestingly, Wallon is brought into play here against Freud, as offering an alternative interpretation of the *fort-da* game described in *Beyond the Pleasure Principle* than the one Freud gives there. The game symbolises the repetition, Lacan argues here, of 'the mother's departure as cause of a *Spaltung*', or splitting, in the subject (p. 62).

Seminar XI described above, Lacan makes a tactical revision of Pavlov's famous experiments in reflexology, which presents them as having revealed, in a unique way, the operativity of the dimension of the signifier. Clearly, however, the break to this perspective can only take place because something fundamental about Pavlov's own epistemological assumptions has been rejected by Lacan. Lacan does not invalidate Pavlov's experiments. He connects them to what he considers to be a more satisfactory and comprehensive theoretical framework, and then uses them to make clear that his own view of subjectivity, as a dialectic of desire with the Other, has radical consequences for the position of psychoanalysis with respect to science. As Lacan develops in his later, third reading of Pavlov, the theory of the reflex stands upon an unscientific faith in the nature of the material, which, as he will argue, betrays certain fundamental tenets of what the proponents of materialism had always considered it to be.

Pavlov III: Materialism Supposes Knowledge in the Real

Lacan makes a third reading of Pavlov in 1967, in the first lesson of *Seminar XV: The Psychoanalytic Act* (1967–68). This lesson is predominantly taken up by a discussion of Pavlov's experiments. In the lesson, Lacan makes a new critique of these experiments, as a means to outline the status of the 'psychoanalytic act', which is the theme of that year's seminar as a whole. The Pavlovian schema, as Lacan presents it here, effaces the kind of act that is central to psychoanalysis, because all motor functions of the body, 'once you insert [them] into the reflex arc', appear as mere passive effects, and as 'pure and simple response[s] to stimuli'.[196] It is 'precarious', Lacan says, even to designate reflex responses as 'actions', when these do not necessarily even amount to motor responses, but—as in Pavlov's experiment—can be merely secretory functions like salivation. Lacan continues here the line of argument he began a decade ago, in

[196] Lacan, Lesson 1, of 15 November 1967, in *Seminar XV: The Psychoanalytic Act* (1967–1968), unpublished. For an unofficial translation, see Gallagher, <http://www.lacaninireland.com/web/wp-content/uploads/2010/06/Book-15-The-Psychoanalytical-Act.pdf>, pp. 3–4.

Seminar V (1957–58), that Pavlov's experiment reveals the function of the signifier. He puts it more starkly and audaciously here in *Seminar XV*, however, by describing Pavlov not only as a 'structuralist ahead of time', but as a 'structuralist of the Lacanian observance', because his experiment demonstrates—in the way Lacan argued in *Seminar V* and *Seminar XI*—Lacan's formula that 'the signifier is what represents a subject for another signifier'.[197] In this first lesson of *Seminar XV*, Lacan also reads Pavlov's experiment as a neat demonstration of another of his classic formulae, that the speaking being 'receives his own message in an inverted form'.[198] After hooking the sound of the artificial stimulus onto the physiological sequence involving salivation, what the scientist receives, Lacan illustrates, 'is an inverse sequence in which the animal's reaction presents itself as attached to this sound'.[199] The Pavlovian scientist, as subject, observes a reverse version of the sequence that they themself have put into play.

What Lacan adds in *Seminar XV*, to the reading of Pavlov that he began in the early 1950s, is an interpretation of Pavlov's experiments as an allegory for the operation of modern science itself. Lacan uses this reading of the experiments to demonstrate the antagonistic position towards modern science that he understands psychoanalysis to occupy. Whilst Lacan's theory of the signifier does away with any idealistic, spiritual reference, it retains, he emphasises, a firm reference to the subject. This is made clear by the definition he gives the signifier from the early 1960s, as 'what represents a subject for another signifier'.[200] As he emphasises in *Seminar XV*, this means that 'there is no operation involving signifiers as such which does not imply the presence of the subject'.[201] The signifiers involved in the experiment can be understood, therefore, to represent a subject. This subject is obviously not implied to be present in the dog, because, as Lacan puts it, Pavlov 'constructs this experiment precisely to show that one can do very well without a hypothesis about

[197] Lacan, Lesson 1, *Seminar XV*. See Gallagher, p. 8.

[198] Lacan, 'Seminar on "The Purloined Letter"' (1955), in *Écrits*, pp. 6–48 (p. 10).

[199] Lacan, Lesson 1, in *Seminar XV*. See Gallagher, p. 10.

[200] Lacan, Lesson of 27 May 1964, 'XVI. The Subject and the Other: Alienation', *Seminar XI*, pp. 203–215 (p. 207).

[201] Lacan, Lesson 1, *Seminar XV*. See Gallagher, p. 9.

what the dog thinks'.[202] The subject whose existence is demonstrated can therefore, says Lacan, only be the same one who gives the demonstration: 'namely, Pavlov himself', who is in the position that Lacan also describes as that of the 'subject of science'.[203] This subject is represented in the experiment, according to Lacan's formula, 'for another signifier'. Lacan identifies this other signifier as the gastric secretion—which 'takes on its value [...] from the fact that it is not produced by the object that one would expect to produce it', and 'is an effect of deception', because in it 'the need in question is adulterated'.[204]

The experiment, Lacan points out, does not transform the dog into a different kind of animal. It does not, he says, even produce the kind of modification that took place in dogs historically in order to domesticate them. The experiment merely allows, in his reading of it, a demonstration of the effect that the signifier has on the 'living field'—an effect that it clearly does have on domesticated dogs, who can both respond to commands and recognise a master.[205] As a result of Lacan's reading of the experiment as proof, not of the reflex, but of the function of the signifier, its theoretical consequence is, as Lacan presents it here, that it pits the signifier—and not, as the traditional materialist physiology had viewed it, the organic substrate of the nervous system—against an idealistic spiritualism based on the mind, consciousness, or soul. Pavlov's experiment shows, says Lacan, that 'where there is language, there is no need to search for a reference in a spiritual entity'.[206] The classical materialist subversion of idealism, in which this experiment represented such a triumph, is reoriented by Lacan, away from the theoretical framework of reflexology, and onto his own theory of the operation of the signifier.

Presenting, as Lacan does here, the experiment's artificial stimulus as a signifier that represents a 'subject of science' has implications for Lacan's understanding of modern science much more generally. The second stage of Lacan's argument in this lesson is that Pavlovian materialism is in fact

[202] Lacan, Lesson 1, *Seminar XV*. See Gallagher, p. 9.

[203] Lacan, Lesson 1, *Seminar XV*. See Gallagher, p. 8.

[204] Lacan, Lesson 1, *Seminar XV*. See Gallagher, p. 9.

[205] As Lacan comments in *Seminar X*, p. 58.

[206] Lacan, Lesson 1, in *Seminar XV*. See Gallagher, p. 9.

on the side of precisely the spiritualism that it attempts to jettison, because it resurrects this in the form of a new spiritualism of science. Pavlov's experiment is based, Lacan argues, on a fundamental misrecognition of the very function of language that he also, as summarised above, used it to demonstrate. Lacan repeats the very same point made by Vygotsky in the 1920s, and then by Politzer in the 1940s: that existing materialist psychologies have collapsed into a renewed form of spiritualism that is in fact entirely palatable for an extreme metaphysical idealism.[207] Reflexology is, Lacan comments, 'very well accepted by spiritual authorities', and in fact leads to a form of 'ecumenism', through a 'reduction of the field of the divine' to a level acceptable to all—a gathering, as he jibes, of 'all the little fish [...] into the same big net'.[208] The new spiritualism that Lacan identifies in Pavlov resides, he says, in the way that reflexology supposes knowledge to be already there 'waiting for us', before it is discovered. As he expands:

> everything that is concealed in terms of foundations for belief, of hope for knowledge, of an ideology of progress in the Pavlovian functioning, if you look closely at it, resides only in the fact that the possibilities that the Pavlovian experimentation demonstrates, are supposed to be already there in the brain.[209]

What makes the Pavlovian framework ultimately only, for Lacan, a fallacious escape from spiritualism, is that it supposes that any and all knowledge discovered by Pavlov's experiments is already there in the organic material of the body, waiting to be known. What was supposed to be reflexology's ultimate strength as a materialist science—allowing

[207] See Vygotsky, 'The Methods of Reflexological and Psychological Investigation' (1926), p. 65; Politzer, *La Crise*, pp. 92–3; and Chap. 3, pp. 93–94 and p. 110. Not a single psychologist, says Vygotsky in 'The Methods', 'not even an extreme spiritualist and idealist, disclaimed the physiological materialism of reflexology', but '[o]n the contrary, all forms of idealism always invariably presupposed it' (p. 65). For Politzer, materialism, as it currently exists in psychology, merely 'tries to express the "spiritual"', by the 'classic means' of 'the nervous system; viscera; the glands with internal secretion', or 'the organism considered as a whole'. Medical, physiological, or biological materialism is, Politzer claims, 'still only a negative reaction against spiritualism', which is 'cast on the mould of spiritualism' (*La Crise*, pp. 92–3).

[208] Lacan, Lesson 1, in *Seminar XV*. See Gallagher, p. 11.

[209] Lacan, Lesson 1, in *Seminar XV*. See Gallagher, p. 12.

psychology to do away with any notion of either a soul or an isolated psychical entity—becomes, in Lacan's hands, its fundamental flaw.

Here, Lacan reiterates Vygotsky's critique from the 1920s and 1930s, of the proximity of reflexology to spiritualism. Where Vygotsky, however, was aiming his criticisms at specific, malformed elements in reflexology (introduced by Pavlov, Bekhterev, and others), he maintained faith that the science could ultimately be sharpened into its proper form. Lacan, on the other hand, in *Seminar XV*, is fundamentally disabling reflexology with respect to the position that it gives to knowledge. Lacan argues here that reflexology assumes knowledge to be something intermingled with the material of the body. He thereby unveils the reflex as a fetish, which conceals a deluded assumption that the body 'knows' how to respond to various stimuli. Instead of banishing the idealist ephemera of consciousness or subjectivity, Pavlov, Lacan alleges, merely flattened these into the material substrate of the nervous system, by converting them into a knowledge that is supposed, absurdly, to exist in the real. As a result, Lacan places materialism itself into profound question as an intellectual position. The 'reduction described as "materialist"', he alleges here, 'deserves to be taken as such for what it is, namely, symptomatic'.[210] Materialism is given a new designation here by Lacan, as the mark, or symptom, of a conflict in the nature of knowledge itself: of a failure by science to know something about knowledge.

Psychoanalysis is thereby given an entirely new position by Lacan in the debates described in this chapter. For both Vygotsky and Politzer, Freud was on the side of the idealism that they wrote so stridently against, whilst also having something in him—something they were unable to isolate or to articulate fully without encountering serious difficulties—that could open a vital path to a dialectical materialist psychology. Approaching psychoanalysis slightly differently, but still with ambivalence, Wallon made it a bridge from idealism to materialism in psychology, by appealing to a rehabilitated Freud whose theories could be given credence by empirical verification. Following these partial attempts to recruit Freud in the service of materialism, Lacan turns Freud around from the position that Vygotsky and Politzer had put him in. He makes

[210] Lacan, Lesson 1, in *Seminar XV*. See Gallagher, p. 11.

Freud, not an inadvertent idealist, but the key to an effective critique of idealism. The way Lacan reads Freud in the passages discussed above also suggests one reason for Vygotsky's and Politzer's common inability to deploy him in a similar way. Freud, Lacan demonstrates, could not be unleashed onto idealism without also destabilising the fundamental ground of *materialism*. With Lacan, Freud becomes an abrasive that eats away at the facades of both idealism and materialism, to reveal the very different foundations upon which they had both always stood.

Psychoanalytic Materialism

This chapter has been describing how psychoanalysis was treated with profound ambivalence by the partisans of a materialist psychology. As was eloquently articulated by Vygotksy, the pursuit of this materialist psychology had made clear that the theoretical basis of the science was beset by crises. Vygotsky proposed, as a result, the need for its total transformation, but he could not settle clearly on what function Freud would have in this renaissance. The spectre of the reformed psychology that Vygotsky imagined was then repeated in what Politzer envisaged as a 'concrete psychology', which was to take something from Freud—indeed, to base its entire 'dramatic' approach to subjectivity on the clinic of psychoanalysis—whilst also purging its theories of the dregs of idealism it was supposed to have preserved. Following Politzer, Wallon borrowed a Freudian logic to make the psychic interior a mirage generated by material, dialectical processes, and produced by exchanges between a body and its external environment. Lacan, who began his psychoanalytic career as a student of Wallon, took advantage of what had troubled and frustrated materialist psychologists about Freud in France and the Soviet Union for decades. He made a different approach to the problems they identified, by posing a new topology for the relationship between idealism and materialism. In the process, he both fulfilled and undermined the necessity that the other figures discussed in this chapter had attributed to this conflict. Freud is read by Lacan as having revealed, in a way that had been imperceptible until this point, a conflict, not between idealism and materialism, but *within* materialism itself.

One important implication of the history narrated in this chapter is the insufficiency of the idea that there was a successful trueness to Marxism achieved either in Soviet science, or in scientific theories by partisans of dialectical materialism in the West, that psychoanalysis would not be able to approach, or that it would necessarily require supplementation or modification by Marx in order to do so. As the chapter has demonstrated, Marxist psychologists—and Marxist thinkers in general—both in and out of the Soviet Union, very rarely lived up to the standards of intellectual sophistication that the most ambitious of them sought to. Secondly, as the chapter has also shown, psychoanalysis was clearly not one thing in this context: Freud's thinking contained so many points of contention that they couldn't be judged as anti-Marxist, because they did not settle into a straightforward final form without a sustained effort being made to produce it. One reason why Luria and Vygotsky's introduction to *Beyond the Pleasure Principle* is such an interesting document is that they are aware—as illustrated by their image of the 'difficult and prolonged' labour of rescuing the 'materialistic buds' from the 'bowels' of bourgeois science—both that Freud's work contains something immensely fruitful, but also that this fruit was yet to be extracted from it.[211]

There was a shared expectancy in the writings of the psychologists this chapter has summarised, that a different, more satisfactory way of articulating the conflict between idealism and materialism laid on the horizon. This is gestured to in the various spectres they conjure, of 'dialectical materialist psychology', 'concrete psychology', 'Marxist psychology', 'dialectics of psychology', or 'general psychology', which haunt their writings. These were promises of a future coherence that, ultimately, failed to emerge. One of the defining ways, however, in which Lacan has been received by contemporary theorists is as the messenger and the distiller of exactly this new position. He is, for example, in Alenka Zupančič's *What is Sex?* (2017), described as the herald of a new materialism that 'is not guaranteed by any matter', but grounded in 'the notion of conflict or contradiction', the 'primacy of a cut', and 'the "parallax of the Real"

---

[211] Lev Vygotsky and Alexander Luria, 'Introduction to the Russian translation of Freud's *Beyond the Pleasure Principle*' (1925), in *The Vygotsky Reader*, p. 17.

produced in it'.[212] The unconscious in Lacan becomes, for Zupančič, not 'a subjective distortion of the objective world', but a mark of a radical, mutant materialism that amounts 'first and foremost [to] an indication of a fundamental inconsistency of the objective world itself'.[213]

If Lacan produced this new materialism, he did so only by bringing to light an inconsistency within materialism itself as a theoretical position. As this chapter has demonstrated, Lacan shows how materialism, in its existing forms, ultimately defeats itself, because it amounts to a point that is not distinct from idealism. This is an argument that Vygotsky, Politzer, and Wallon had each been close, in their own way, to making before Lacan. They, however, made this accusation of what they considered to be botched materialist theories, whereas Lacan extends its scope to target materialism as a whole. He identifies materialism as, in his words, a symptom of a failure in the consistency of scientific knowledge. There remains, for Lacan, another break required in order to escape from this—one that had not yet been made by Marx and Engels, but that could be understood, as he sees it, to have been traced out by Freud.

Lacan, as the present chapter has demonstrated, responds to the question of the relationship between idealism and materialism by performing a broader analysis of the underlying epistemological co-ordinates of science. In *Seminar XV*, he describes psychoanalysis as a field that 'proves that it would not be futile, but frivolous, to think that [...] knowledge [*savoir*] is already there waiting for us before we make it emerge'.[214] It is a field, in other words, that defies the supposition of knowledge in the real that Lacan criticises in reflexology. Psychoanalysis, for him, is able to crystallise and to communicate something about the effect that modern science made on the nature of knowledge itself, in a way that had not been possible before Freud. For Lacan, this status of knowledge is something that Marx was ultimately unable to realise. This is why Lacan cannot—just as Freud could not, as Vygotsky, Politzer, and Wallon made so clear—be stitched into the framework of an existing Marxism. The supposition of knowledge in the real is identified by Lacan as an error that

[212] Alenka Zupančič, *What is Sex?* (London: MIT Press, 2017), p. 78.

[213] Zupančič, *Why Psychoanalysis? Three Interventions* (Aaarhus University Press, 2008), p. 16.

[214] Lacan, Lesson 1, in *Seminar XV*. See Gallagher, p. 13.

haunts, not just reflexology, but also materialism more generally. As the following chapter will discuss, despite Althusser's attempt to ascribe psychoanalysis a pivotal place in this history, this error can also be found in his own theories of the history of science. Althusser's work is often taken as a means of aligning Lacan with Marx. A close reading of his work, however, serves to demonstrate what it is in Marxist thought that Lacan criticises, and what in it he attempts to break away from.

4

The Symptom as a Principle of History: Althusser's Reading of Marx

So far, this book has made detailed discussion of two particular facets of the history of Marxism, in order to illustrate how Lacan's theories of the 1940s, 1950s, and 1960s have an important place in this history. Chapter 3 situated Lacan's reading of Hegel in the context of questions that dominated French Hegelianism in the 1920s and 1930s. It focused on concerns, first put forward by Kierkegaard, about the role of subjectivity in Hegel's dialectic that became central in this context, and showed how Lacan responded to these in his own strategy of reading Hegel. Chapter 3 followed this with an account of the history of materialist psychology as it was developed in the Soviet Union and France. It explored how a parallel question was encountered in this field to those that concerned the French Hegelians, when the attempt was made by psychologists to study the human mind without recourse to assumptions about subjectivity that went beyond the material. Vygotsky and Politzer, the chapter described, each criticised reflexology for unintentionally resorting to a new spiritualism in order to solve this problem.

The present chapter will discuss how Louis Althusser unites this question of subjectivity, which had presented obstacles both to reading Hegel and to the development of materialist psychology, with a corresponding

M. Maher, *Symptom Invented*, The Palgrave Lacan Series,
https://doi.org/10.1007/978-3-032-12267-4_4

question about history. The chapter will elaborate how the structuralist movement is haunted by an elision that would resurface in Althusser's version of the notion of the 'epistemological break'. For Althusser, following Bachelard, and in a theory of history building on structuralist ideas, the history of science is constituted not by the accumulation of knowledge, but by a series of convulsive ruptures, each of which propels a temporary structure of science into a new constellation. Again after Bachelard, Althusser describes these seismic shifts as 'epistemological breaks'. To this, however, Althusser adds the role played by the individual subject in producing these shifts. He asks how a radical shift away from any given conceptual framework, which pierces through that framework's points of inadequacy, is precipitated, on a psychological level, by the historical individual who first articulates it. In lieu of this problematic, one of Althusser's most influential theoretical innovations was to make the epistemological break not only a shift in the history of science, but also simultaneously, and inseparably, the mechanism of Marx's personal departure from Hegel. Althusser presents the epistemological break as operating on two levels—within the history of science, but also within an individual's biography—and as therefore requiring a psychological explanation, as well as a depersonalised, historical one.

The question then remains, for Althusser, of how to articulate a mechanism to act as the joint between these two levels of subject and history. As Chap. 3 summarised, one of Vygotsky's main concerns was how psychology could view its subjects materialistically, independently of any spiritual, subjective excess, and as constituted instead purely by stimuli and responses—but how it could also, at the same time, avoid pretending that there was no such thing as the mind. The present chapter will outline, in its opening section, how a structurally equivalent problem was encountered, without being approached as rigorously, by Lévi-Strauss. When he attempted to comprehend subjectivity as a grid of unconscious social practices, Lévi-Strauss would, as if not knowing how fully to give up the obscurantist residues associated with idealism, end up resorting to the 'brain' or the 'human spirit' as the material origin of this network of co-ordinates. This chapter will present Althusser's work from the 1960s as an attempt to solve these questions that had been posed both to Marxism and to structuralism, on the levels of subjectivity and history, through his introduction of a logic of the 'symptom'. The chapter summarises a series of problematic points in structuralist thought that are decisive for Althusser's work. It gives an abridged intellectual history of structuralism, that hones in on how the structuralist movement opened up the gap to think what would be named by Althusser and Lacan as a logic of the symptom—a logic that understands a rupture within a given order, not as a pathology of that order, but as its truth. Following this, the chapter reconstructs how Althusser operationalises the logic of the symptom as a principle for reading Marx, that he uses to make sense of the conflicts and tensions that exist within Marx's writings. It then discusses how Althusser expands this symptomatic reading of Marx into a model for the movement of the history of science, and points to the various obstacles that appear in his attempt to make this leap.

As the following, final chapter will develop in detail, Lacan's own way of understanding the history of science in the late 1960s and early 1970s is very different to Althusser's own. In his teaching of these years, Lacan makes a reading of *Capital* with reference to Althusser's extensive work on the text, which clearly takes much of its impetus from him. However, Lacan's understanding of history departs from Althusser's in the paradoxical historical position that Lacan, as discussed in detail in the following chapter, also gives to Marx. Lacan's much more ambivalent position towards Marx resulted from his involvement in a tradition of thought that was pressing the consequences of Marx's theories to surprising new ends. As a result, the present chapter will argue, Lacan's theories cannot be viewed, as they are by some, as a tool to complete or to correct something in Althusser's work.

Structuralism and History

In light of the historical detail laid out in the previous two chapters, it is possible to approach the structuralist movement with a new, slightly refined set of emphases. Structuralism is often understood to have originated as a reaction to, and a rejection of, currents of thinking that were hegemonic in French intellectual life prior to its eminence—above all, existentialism and phenomenology, two movements that Lacan also sought to depart from. One possible way to view the ascendance of Claude Lévi-Strauss and Roland Barthes in the 1950s, and Lacan and Foucault shortly after, is as a rise to prominence of an ideological movement amongst a new generation of intellectuals who were seeking an alternative to a phenomenologically-oriented existentialism that they saw as having been made 'defuct' and blunted by popularisation.[1] Structuralism is viewed, as a result, not only as an anti-phenomenology and an anti-existentialism, but also, as François Dosse puts it in his history of the movement, as an opponent of the Marxist politics that also characterised these groups—as an intellectual movement that 'took off where Marxism left off' in France.[2] Structuralism amounted, as Edith Kurzweil presents it, to a means for intellectuals 'to deradicalize themselves', by gaining distance from Marxism 'without abandoning their humanist convictions'.[3] Despite its theoretical complexity and occasional aura of the arcane, structuralism, as this perspective would have it, amounted to the expression of a new left-wing conservatism that absorbed and dissipated the political impact of revolutionary Marxist movements amongst the French intelligentsia.

On the other hand, it does not require much ingenuity to point out the ways in which structuralism was shaped by—and not simply a rejection of—classic hallmarks of Marxism; and even of Stalinism.[4] As summarised in the Introduction to this thesis, the heavy-handed extension of dialectical materialism to the natural and human sciences in the Soviet Union had resulted in the technocratic, biologist, evolutionist dogma of Stalinist 'diamat'.[5] Despite its excesses, there is a potential analogue to this Soviet thinking in the work of key players in twentieth-century

[1] John Sturrock, *Structuralism and Since* (Oxford: Oxford Paperbacks, 1980), p. 2.

[2] François Dosse, *History of Structuralism* (University of Minnesota Press, 1998), p. 158.

[3] Edith Kurzweil, *The Age of Structuralism* (London: Transaction Publishers, 1996), p. 4. The 'complexities of structuralist methods', she adds, 'obscured the fact that structuralism would become the new conservatism of the left'.

[4] For philosophers who sought to adhere to the texts of "orthodox" Marxism, there were, broadly speaking, three options: an evangelical scripturalism and corresponding science of history; an abstraction of Marx's dialectical logic and method; or the extension, following Engels, of dialectical materialism to the fields of natural and human science. See Ted Benton, *The Rise and Fall of Structural Marxism: Althusser and His Influence* (Macmillan, 1984), p. 4.

[5] See Introduction, p. 8.

French sociology. As Ted Benton points out, Comte and Durkheim, like Stalin, also opposed a 'subject-centred history' and 'subject-constituted knowledge' in favour of a model of individual consciousness 'made up of representations in which the imperatives of an external social order are internally inscribed', and into which a liberal subjectivity could be dissolved.[6] Lévi-Strauss's pursuit of a depersonalised 'unitary and universal "depth-grammar" of the mind' which was to encompass all cultural practices, is clearly also in sympathy with this anti-subjectivism. As this book has been attempting to demonstrate, more complex networks of connection exist behind currents of thought associated with Marxism than can be articulated by drawing lines of allegiance, which only ever stand precariously upon the historical complexities they attempt to partition. If the advocates of structuralism were seeking—in part—an alternative to Marxism, there were nevertheless manifest and significant continuities between these bodies of thought.[7]

This section of the present chapter will outline some of the ambiguities of this relationship in more detail, with particular attention to Althusser's criticism of the work of Lévi-Strauss. Chapter 3 narrated the historical difficulties encountered by psychologists committed to Marx when they attempted to enlist Freud to their various projects. It identified the tensions that are embodied in the Freudian unconscious' ambiguous position between idealism and materialism. The unconscious would also occupy a contested and complex position in structuralist thought, as a concept that was both theoretically appealing and, in its Freudian guise, not quite assimilable with its premises. An idea of the unconscious is central to the way Lévi-Strauss imagines the all-encompassing structures at the foundations of human culture. His structuralist anthropology owed a large debt to Freud, and one that he frequently acknowledged.[8]

[6] Benton, *The Rise and Fall of Structural Marxism*, p. 10.

[7] See Lacan's comment in 'Radiophonie', in *Autres écrits* (Paris: Seuil, 2001), pp. 403–448 (p. 408): 'Pas de raison pourtant de parquer les structuralistes, si ce n'est à se leurrer qu'ils prennent la relève de ce que l'existentialisme a si bien réussi: obtenir d'une génération qu'elle se couche dans le même lit dont elle est née' ('No reason however to enclose the structuralists, except to deceive oneself that they are taking up the baton where existentialism was so successful: getting a generation to get into the same bed from which it was born').

[8] Lévi-Strauss had discovered Freud in his schooldays, and 'read what had been translated of Freud until then' between 1925 and 1930, a formative encounter which, as he acknowledged, 'played a

Yet Lévi-Strauss's view of the unconscious, as laid out in his *Introduction to the Work of Marcel Mauss* (1950), also clearly operates according to the Maussian logic of exchange: his is a purely formal unconscious; a structure mediating between subjects, emptied of affect, and functioning as the absent cause of all social practices.[9] This in itself points to several of Lévi-Strauss's significant departures from a Freudian unconscious. Doing away, as Dosse points out, with the 'dynamic dimension' of the Freudian unconscious—the movements of conflict, reversal, and evolution that characterise the mechanisms of repression, condensation, displacement, and censorship—leads Lévi-Strauss to downplay the centrality of desire, in which he declared himself to be 'not in the least convinced'.[10]

Ultimately, Freud was of value to Lévi-Strauss as the architect of a mythological metastructure, whose underlying logic structural anthropology sought to distil in a purified form. As Althusser would criticise—in a letter to Lacan from 1963, and then later, in more detail, in a 1966 article 'On Lévi-Strauss'—one consequence of this untethering of the unconscious from individual subjectivity is the attribution of a functionalist subjectivism to this social unconscious. The notion of desire rejected by Lévi-Strauss reappears, Althusser criticises, in the displaced form of a 'will to survive' that he attributes to society itself.[11] For Lévi-Strauss, as Althusser reads him, the unconscious is therefore only a convenient conceptual intermediary between the individual and the social, and he allows it to fall away and lose its significance once problematic distinctions between these two points have been elided. Just as offensive to Althusser would be Lévi-Strauss's contradictory recourse to the 'brain' or 'human spirit' as potential origins of his unconscious structures. In this respect, as

very important role in shaping my thinking'. See Dosse, *History of Structuralism*, p. 112. Lévi-Straussian structuralism is allied with Freud in its attempts to extend reason to phenomena seemingly beyond it, and to strive to uncover a reality beneath ordinarily assumed appearances. For many, Lévi-Strauss's *Structural Anthropology* had a revolutionary impact comparable to *Capital* or *The Interpretation of Dreams* (See Dosse, *History of Structuralism*, p. 19), a grouping which points to its proximity to the 'hermeneutics of suspicion' that Ricoeur identified in the work of Marx, Freud, and Nietzsche.

[9] Dosse, *History of Structuralism*, p. 114.

[10] Dosse, *History of Structuralism*, p. 115.

[11] Althusser, letter to Lacan of 11 July 1966, in *Writings on Psychoanalysis* (Columbia University Press, 1999), pp. 170–171 (p. 171); and 'On Lévi-Strauss' (1966), in *The Humanist Controversy* (London: Verso, 2003), pp. 19–32 (p. 25).

Peter Dews observes, Lévi-Strauss repeats a Freudian, materialist "insurance policy" of supposing that 'statements about the "human mind" should ultimately be reducible to statements about the physical structure of the brain'.[12]

Lacan departs from Freud on this basis, by jettisoning any recourse to a neurological substrate of the unconscious. This also represents, therefore, a departure from those materialist suppositions that are preserved in Lévi-Strauss. This is true in spite of Lacan's famous enlistment of structural linguistics and anthropology in the return to Freud—as announced in the watershed of the 1953 'Rome Discourse', published in the *Écrits* as 'The Function and Field of Speech and Language in Psychoanalysis'. Language, the lecture argues, is the manifestation of an inescapable intersubjectivity, a forcefield of the Other in which the body is trapped, and the material in which the human encounters its own being. Lacan recasts the Oedipus complex in Lévi-Straussian mode, as an effect of the exchange of women in marriage bonds, which he understands at root as the exchange of a debt.[13] The unconscious is then neatly redefined by him as 'that part of concrete discourse *qua* transindividual, which is not at the subject's disposal in reestablishing the continuity of his conscious discourse'.[14] If this, in its externality and 'transindividuality', echoes the metaphysical ledger of Lévi-Strauss's unconscious, it also departs from it significantly. The unconscious in 'Function and Field' is also the 'chapter of my history that is marked by a blank or occupied by a lie: it is the censored chapter'.[15] Lacan allows the unconscious to remain an aporia, an absence, and an interruption, rather than becoming bureaucratically crystallised into an encyclopaedic monolith, or an architecture of

[12] Peter Dews, 'Structuralism and the French Epistemological Tradition', in *Althusser: A Critical Reader* (Wiley-Blackwell, 1994), pp. 104–141 (p. 110). Freud, too, had hypothesised, in the early 'Project for a Scientific Psychology' for example, the existence of a neurological network whose structure determined psychic activity. See Freud, 'Project for a Scientific Psychology' (1950 [1895]), in *The Standard Edition of the Complete Psychological Works of Sigmund Freud, Vol. 1 (1866–1899): Pre-Psycho-Analytic Publications and Unpublished Drafts*, trans. by James Strachey (London: Hogarth, 1966), pp. 281–391.

[13] Lacan, 'The Function and Field of Speech and Language in Psychoanalysis' (1953), in *Écrits*, trans. by B. Fink (London: Norton, 2006), pp. 197–268 (p. 231).

[14] Lacan, 'The Function and Field', p. 214.

[15] Lacan, 'The Function and Field', p. 215.

knowledge. Even at this point, Lacan's unconscious is structured like language only in perpetually exceeding structure: as he presents it, structure, like the secondary revision of a dream, is always a delayed attempt to register the unconscious, or the trace in which the unconscious is registered. This limit at which structure is 'holed' by an unstructurable excess would, as Chap. 5 will outline in detail, be decisive in the way that Lacan reads Marx in the late 1960s.

One rhetorical position of Lacan's work in the 1950s is that Lévi-Strauss, Jakobson, and even Saussure are, as he puts it in 'Function and Field', reconquering terrain already traversed by Freud. Indeed, Lacan's projection of metaphor and metonymy back onto the Freudian mechanisms of condensation and displacement in 'The Instance of the Letter in the Unconscious' (1957), has, as Dosse reads it, the effect of making Freud look like no less than the inventor of structuralism.[16] There is an irony here, in that, as described above, the notion of the unconscious to which Lévi-Strauss appeals is very different to that whose operation Lacan articulates according to structuralist linguistics. Lacan appeals to structuralism with a distinct air of opportunism: he is not particularly concerned with pointing out the limitations of its theoretical project, but with demonstrating how it allows something to emerge conceptually when it is approached in a particular way. In 'Function and Field' and 'The Instance of the Letter', Lacan finds that he can use what Saussure, Lévi-Strauss, and Jakobson deduced about structure as a hook, an opening, or a framework to articulate something about the unconscious. Unlike Althusser, who challenges Lévi-Strauss for his failure to pay due attention to the fundamentals of Marxist theory, Lacan does not—though he would have had just as much grounds to do so—reproach Lévi-Strauss for not being Freudian enough.

As mentioned above, Althusser was often fiercely critical of certain aspects of the general project of structuralism. There is a tension in his work, more explicit than in Lacan's, between an application and a criticism of structuralism. As Dosse describes, Althusser only 'adopt[ed] the structuralist orientation while maintaining a critical distance in the name

[16] Dosse, *History of Structuralism*, p. 106. See Lacan, 'The Instance of the Letter in the Unconscious, or Reason Since Freud', in *Écrits*, pp. 412–444.

of Marxism'.[17] Althusser, says Dosse, aimed to use the 'momentum, the propulsion, the scientistic side' of the 'rather optimistic linguistic positivism' of structuralism.[18] By this, Dosse refers to the structuralist hubris of declaring to 'interpret all reaches of knowledge with a total semiology, starting from a simple phonological model', whilst also remaining 'critical of those who believed themselves able to create such a metalanguage'.[19] In 1966, Althusser published a short, but precise and powerful, critique of Lévi-Strauss, which centres on the claim that his structuralist anthropology fundamentally misunderstands Marx. As Althusser points out here, Lévi-Strauss 'claims to draw his inspiration from Marx', declares several of his theses to be 'Marxist', and aims 'to produce a theory of ideologies', but he ultimately fails either to attain this objective, or to 'know' Marx truly. Lévi-Strauss's failure to grasp the ideological stems, for Althusser, partly from his omitting to question the foundations of 'ethnological ideology'.[20] His notion of a 'primitive society' preserves a myth of origin, says Althusser, despite the fact that Marx had decisively eliminated such a myth, and substituted for it the idea of a 'mode of production' responsible for the development of any legal-political and ideological superstructure.[21] Lévi-Strauss, Althusser alleges, directs no critical attention to the reasons for the structures of cultural substitution and variation that he maps out.[22] Vague appeals to an underlying structure of 'human spirit'; a cybernetic view of neurology; a 'functionalist' view of kinship structures (rules to govern marriage in primitive societies only exist, according to Lévi-Strauss, so that the societies can continue to survive); and the notion of a social unconscious, are wheeled out by Lévi-Strauss to plug this gap. Lévi-Strauss, Althusser remarks elsewhere, 'will not, *philosophically* speaking, play a role commensurate with the highly suspect success he has been accorded'; the 'keys to our future', as Althusser

[17] Dosse, *History of Structuralism*, p. 290.

[18] Dosse, *History of Structuralism*, p. 290.

[19] Dosse, *History of Structuralism*, p. 290.

[20] Althusser, 'On Lévi-Strauss' (1966), in *The Humanist Controversy*, pp. 22–23.

[21] Althusser, 'On Lévi-Strauss', pp. 22–24.

[22] Althusser, 'On Lévi-Strauss', p. 23.

sees them, lie in the less well-known figures of Bachelard, Canguilhem, and Lacan.[23]

Despite Althusser's attack, there is clearly a rapprochement with Marx of a certain kind at the core of structuralism. In his early years certainly, Lévi-Strauss was, as Dosse puts it, both '[l]oyal to Marx, and strictly orthodox in his Marxism', citing Marx in *Tristes Tropiques* (1955) as one of his 'three mistresses', along with Freud and geology.[24] Lévi-Strauss's announcements of allegiance to Marx are widespread in this period of his work: Marx, says Lévi-Strauss elsewhere in *Tristes Tropiques*, 'established that social science is no more founded on the basis of events than physics is founded on sense-data'.[25] Reading the ahistoricity of their structures generously, Saussure and Jakobson enabled, as Dosse puts it, a better understanding of 'something that evolved not as a function of class or of social change, but outside of conscious will'.[26] Combined with Lévi-Straussian anthropology, this meant, on a political level, that 'other visions of the world and other systems of representation could be considered'.[27] This was a departure, then, from some of the classic hallmarks of Marxism, but one that indirectly opened up possibilities for Marxism's broader political project. In taking up the baton of lines of thinking about society and history previously dominated by Marxism, structuralism was, in Dosse's estimation, the 'real beneficiary' of the crisis of loyalty to the Soviet Union that began among western, left-wing intellectuals in 1956, following Khrushchev's denunciation of Stalin's purges in the Secret Speech, and the USSR's repression of the Hungarian Revolution.[28] Structuralism, from this perspective, took the place of Stalinist dogma by giving 'scientificity' and 'operationality' to disciplines 'by preserving the goal of universality that prior forms of commitment had held to, without making this one part of the desire to transform the

---

[23] Althusser, 'The Philosophical Conjuncture and Marxist Theoretical Research', in *The Humanist Controversy*, pp. 1–18 (p. 9).

[24] Dosse, *History of Structuralism*, p. 14. Marx might even be included alongside Lévi-Strauss's other, more obvious, intellectual forebears, Comte, Durkheim, and Mauss.

[25] Claude Lévi-Strauss, *Tristes tropiques* (Pengiun Classics, 2011), p. 57.

[26] Dosse, *History of Structuralism*, p. 164.

[27] Dosse, *History of Structuralism*, p. 164.

[28] Dosse, *History of Structuralism*, p. 164.

world'.[29] The movement also, for Dosse, represented a limited attempt 'to better understand the world by integrating alterity and the unconscious into it'.[30] Structuralism certainly shared with Marxism this combination of a striving towards totality, and a method of levelling illusions to discover the scaffolding behind them. It was accepted by many in France as a heuristic that could take Marxism's place.

As Althusser makes clear, however, Lévi-Strauss's reverence towards Marx makes it no easier to say whether or not structuralist anthropology represents a true conceptual heir of Marxism. One self-evident way that structuralism, in its Saussurian–Lévi-Straussian form, departs from Marx, is by seeming to elide an understanding of history as a process of change. Saussure, as the linguist André Martinet criticises, overlooks the question of how and why phonetic changes happen so regularly in the history of language.[31] This phenomenon requires structure to be studied diachronically (as changing through time) rather than synchronically (without this historical dimension).[32] Saussure, Martinet alleges, escaped from linguistic evolutionism only by sleight-of-hand, by depicting the history of language as a series of synchronic, self-contained slides arranged one after the other, and by merely ignoring the question of what mechanism allowed for the transition between them.[33] Lévi-Strauss takes a similarly ahistorical position in his critique, in *La pensée sauvage* (1962), of Sartre's view of history as a convergence towards a single universal ideal. Lévi-Strauss's dismissal of this progressive idea of history means he is able to preserve the value of past societies and cultures, which are seemingly diminished by the Sartrean theory to primitive steps towards a superior future civilisation. Lévi-Strauss's wholesale rejection of this Sartrean logic of history results, however, in his reduction of historical changes to effects of mere contingency and accident that, for him, cannot be scientifically studied.[34] As Dews puts it, by disqualifying the possibility that history could be an object of rigorous knowledge, history exists for Lévi-Strauss

[29] Dosse, *History of Structuralism*, p. 164.
[30] Dosse, *History of Structuralism*, p. 164.
[31] Interview with François Dosse, cited in *History of Structuralism*, p. 47.
[32] Dosse, *History of Structuralism*, p. 47.
[33] Dosse, *History of Structuralism*, p. 48.
[34] Dews, 'Structuralism and the French Epistemological Tradition', pp. 106–7.

'as a reservoir of facts to be absorbed and ordered by synchronic analysis'.[35] Lévi-Strauss affirms that history should be relegated to subjectivity because it consists of 'a method with no distinct object corresponding to it'.[36] As Dews also points out, however, it is difficult to see why anthropology is any less impaired, as a scientific field, by a preferential and arbitrary organising of information of the kind that Lévi-Strauss finds in history.

Saussure and Lévi-Strauss were, it seems, attempting to rethink history so radically that they might appear to have repressed or ignored its existence to an unacceptable extent. But it is also true that their work enabled a definitively structuralist view of history, which developed out of the Lévi-Straussian revolution. Canguilhem, following Bachelard, would shape a theory of history around precisely the gaps and contingencies that Saussure and Lévi-Strauss had left in it.[37] Transforming history from the Sartrean model of an ascending narrative whereby truth and knowledge were progressively unveiled, Bachelard and Canguilhem move towards a view of history, not as a white noise of disordered information, but as a series of errors and breaks that precipitated dramatic transformation. It is Bachelard's theory of the epistemological break that forms the basis for Althusser's view of history, and for his positioning of Marx and Freud in the history of science. However, as the following section will discuss, history continues to pose problems for Althusser when he makes it the object of a structuralist theory. When Althusser comes to apply structuralist ideas to a reading of Marx, the central question remains of what mechanism could be invoked to understand the production of an epistemological break.

[35] Dews, 'Structuralism and the French Epistemological Tradition', p. 108.

[36] Dews, 'Structuralism and the French Epistemological Tradition', p. 110, n. 16.

[37] See Gaston Bachelard, *La formation de l'esprit scientifique: Contribution à une psychanalyse de la connaissance objective* (Paris: Vrin, 1938); Georges Canguilhem, *La connaissance de la vie* (Paris: Vrin, 1952); and Canguilhem, *La formation du concept de réflexe aux XVIIe et XVIII siècles* (Paris: Vrin, 1955).

Reading Symptomatically

For Althusser, following Bachelard, the history of science is constituted not by a linear accumulation of knowledge—as a naïve, liberal positivism would have it—but by a series of convulsive ruptures that propel each temporary structure of science into a new constellation. Again after Bachelard, Althusser describes these seismic shifts as 'epistemological breaks'.[38] His breaks are precipitated when a disruptive, repressed, or 'invisible' element of a science, as it is constituted in a given historical moment, is made 'visible' in a way that signals precisely that element's absence from the previous field. An epistemological break occurs when this new element forces the reorganisation of the field as it existed prior to this point. This process is not smooth, like a mechanical changing of gears, or the Hegelian dialectic's elegant, inevitable choreography of spirit; it happens not in a dimension of 'ideas', or as dictated by an irrepressible, meta-historical logic, but through the same human struggle and conflict, and beset by the same convulsions, friction, and confusion, that characterise Marx's own account of history. Despite Althusser's clear debt to Bachelard, Canguilhem, and to some extent Foucault, for his understanding of the epistemological break, it is not, for him, exclusively a model for history. One of Althusser's foremost innovations was to make the epistemological break simultaneously, and inseparably, a framework for the interpretation of texts. Althusser applies the notion of the epistemological break as a tool for identifying structural boundaries within Marx's oeuvre. It becomes his main conceptual weapon in establishing once and for all the relationship that Marx's writings, and the thinking they perform, can be understood to have with Hegel.

The parameters of the epistemological break as a principle for reading are laid out in Althusser's 1961 essay 'On the Young Marx'. This text represents Althusser's definitive intervention on the status of Marx's early work, whose Hegelian and Feuerbachian influences had troubled interpreters of Marx for decades. Althusser relegates it as blunt insufficiency merely to 'set up Marx against his own youth' by jettisoning this early

[38] Bachelard first uses the term 'epistemological break' in *La formation de l'esprit scientifique: Contribution à une psychanalyse de la connaissance objective* (Paris: Vrin, 1938).

work.[39] Equally unsatisfactory, though, for him, is the opposite position, that would reconcile Marx with his youth, 'rounding him up' so that '*Capital* is no longer read as *On the Jewish Question*, *On The Jewish Question* is read as *Capital*' and 'the shadow of the young Marx is no longer projected on to Marx, but that of Marx on to the young Marx'.[40] Such an inadequate principle of reading can only be justified by erecting 'a pseudo-theory of the history of philosophy in the "*future anterior*"'—or future perfect, the tense characterised by what 'will have' happened—an assumption, in other words, of a future that was always destined to occur. Althusser identifies this as an unexamined logic which is 'quite simply Hegelian' in its teleology. What he deems vitally necessary instead, in order to escape this spectre of Hegelianism, is a general rethinking of how to read Marx. 'It is not possible', Althusser affirms, 'to commit oneself to a Marxist study of Marx's *Early Works* (and of the problems they pose) without rejecting the spontaneous or reflected temptations of an analytico-teleological method which is always more or less haunted by *Hegelian principles*'.[41] This method's presuppositions must be broken away from, in favour of applying 'the Marxist principles of a theory of ideological development'.[42] In order to break from such an unsatisfactory method of reading, Althusser poses the notion of the 'problematic', a term he uses to describe the ideological unity of a text, and the presence in it of inherited terms beyond its 'conscious', explicit references to other figures, other concepts, or other bodies of work.[43]

Althusser makes clear in the essay than the central target in his sights is a teleological view of Marx's biography, which would smuggle Hegelianism into a reading of Marx undetected. If he wants, understandably, to do away with this unfounded reliance on progression, more problematic is the question of what then comes to replace this as a logic that could guide the reading of inconsistencies in Marx's oeuvre. This means that Althusser can neither merely side-step the problem of diachronic,

[39] Althusser, 'On the Young Marx' (1961), *For Marx* (London: Verso, 2005), pp. 49–86 (p. 54).

[40] Althusser, 'On the Young Marx', p. 54.

[41] Althusser, 'On the Young Marx', p. 62.

[42] Althusser, 'On the Young Marx', p. 62.

[43] Althusser, 'On the Young Marx', p. 66.

historical change, as Saussure was alleged to have done, nor fall back onto a weak, Lévi-Straussian idea of history's pure, unintelligible contingency. Althusser rejects a model of bibliographic 'supersession'—an 'innocent but sly concept' which, he claims, sustains the spirit of a Hegelian *Aufhebung*, and which amounts merely to 'the empty anticipation of its end in the illusion of an immanence of truth'.[44] In its place, he prescribes a '*logic of actual experience and real emergence*', a 'logic of *the irruption of real history in ideology itself*', which would 'put an end to the illusions of *ideological immanence*'.[45] Althusser appeals to history, as a 'logic of actual experience' and a 'real emergence', as a levelling force able to correct the falsity of Hegelian presuppositions. In Althusser's hands, the 'irruption of real history' provides exactly the unstructurable force required to puncture ideological mystification.

Althusser draws here on the part played by Marx's subjective personhood in shaping his work. Althusser's logic of experience and of the history-in-ideology would, he claims, 'give some real meaning to the *personal style* of Marx's experience, to the extraordinary sensitivity to the concrete which gave such force of conviction and revelation to each of his encounters with reality', and to a 'dramatic genesis of Marx's thought'.[46] At the point, however, immediately following his valorisation of this attention to Marx as a living person, Althusser immediately steps back from this dimension, allowing it to remain a somewhat vague and mysterious solution to the problem he sets himself. Althusser declines to

> give a chronology or a dialectic of the *actual experience* of history which united in that remarkable individual the Young Marx one man's particular psychology and world history so as to produce in him the *discoveries* which are still our nourishment today.[47]

What Althusser is attempting here is to make a link, on the most fundamental level, between individual subjectivity—a mysterious and unshared 'experience', as he puts it—and an overarching, collective

[44] Althusser, 'On the Young Marx', p. 82.
[45] Althusser, 'On the Young Marx', p. 82.
[46] Althusser, 'On the Young Marx', p. 82.
[47] Althusser, 'On the Young Marx', p. 83.

movement which *can* be conceptually metabolised, in this case as 'history'. At its root, this is a problematic case that was central both to French Hegelianism and to materialist psychology in the early twentieth century. As Chap. 3 discussed, the question of the relationship between the subjective irresolution of unhappy consciousness and the conclusiveness of absolute knowledge led French readers of Hegel to identify the necessary limits of the Hegelian dialectic. Chapter 3 followed this by identifying how the problem of resolving subjective experience into a stable, logical grid also laid behind the difficulty posed to reflexology by the mind. Althusser stops here, however, at this point in the essay, on the pretext that such details about Marx's psychology are available in Auguste Cornu's biographical study of Marx's early work, to which Althusser gives high praise.[48] There is, he says, 'no access to the Young Marx except by way of this real'—i.e., biographical—'history'.[49] We must appreciate, he proclaims, the '*contingent beginnings* (in respect to his birth) that he had to start from', the '*gigantic layer of illusions he had to break through before he could even see it*', his 'prodigious break with his origins', his 'heroic struggle against the illusions he had inherited from the Germany in which he was born', and his 'acute attention to the realities concealed by these illusions'.[50] If, adds Althusser,

> "Marx's path" is an example to us, it is not because of his origins and circumstances but because of his ferocious insistence on freeing himself from the myths which presented themselves to him as the *truth*, and because of the role of the experience of real history which elbowed these myths aside.[51]

Like Lévi-Strauss, Althusser seeks to do away with the notion of historical progression. Unlike Lévi-Strauss, though, he does not want to elevate 'primitivity' or 'earliness' to a status equal to that of historically later moments of development. Reading for structural contradiction and friction as Althusser does leads him simply to break off Marx's early work

[48] Auguste Cornu, *Karl Marx: L'Homme et l'œuvre. De l'Hégelianisme au matérialisme historique (1818–1845)* (Paris: Librairie Félix Alcan, 1934).

[49] Althusser, 'On the Young Marx', p. 83.

[50] Althusser, 'On the Young Marx', p. 83.

[51] Althusser, 'On the Young Marx', p. 83.

as fundamentally irreconcilable with the later, true Marxism which it produced. A notion of a 'logic of experience', and an elevation of Marx's character are introduced by him here instead. The problem remains, though, of defining the mechanism that produced this break, beyond Althusser's references—still considerably vague in the passages quoted above—either to Marx's genius or to the peculiarity of his circumstances.

Althusser's efforts responded to a pressing need amongst readers of Marx, at a time of deep uncertainty about the achievements of communism, to curate a valid form of Marxism out of a body of work that contained evident, significant discrepancies. His notion of Marx's epistemological break was an attempt, as Ted Benton puts it, 'to establish a series of discontinuities, differences, dislocations within and between texts' and 'on the basis of these discriminations to establish a principle of selection (*this* is acceptable, authentic, validated—*that* is not)'.[52] The ground on which Althusser bases such a filtering process—or the ground on which he *explains* discrepancy, and the meta-narrative that gives the body of work coherence in its incoherence—is Marx himself, as a living human being. There is more than a touch of the psychobiographical here: in order for the epistemological break to function as a principle of discrimination and selection, it has simultaneously to be an element of biography—and more (or less) than this, an element (if such a thing could be isolated) of human experience. For an epistemological break to occur, Marx himself had to have made an epistemological break in his own thinking—in his own life—and a break that was an enlightening step towards truth in an objective sense.

One explicit intention of Althusser's method of reading Marx is to reconceive of how the relationship between Marx and Hegel, and the traces of Hegel that exist in Marx, could be understood. In his 1962 essay 'Contradiction and Overdetermination', Althusser refers to Marx's distinction between the 'mystified form' of the Hegelian dialectic, and the 'rational figure' of Marx's own dialectic.[53] He reads this as an indication that the 'mystical shell' is not a detachable aspect of the Hegelian dialectic,

[52] Benton, *The Rise and Fall of Structural Marxism*, p. 21.

[53] Althusser, 'Contradiction and Overdetermination' (1962), in *For Marx*, pp. 87–128 (p. 92).

but rather a 'mystified form', an 'internal element' that is 'consubstantial' with it.[54] The operation performed by Marx on Hegelian thought is therefore much more complex and extensive than a mechanical portioning-off of mystified Hegelian dregs. We are given by Althusser a Marx who entirely dismantled the Hegelian dialectic, and who gave it an entirely new basis in the way that he made it approach the real, rather than merely amputating its diseased parts, or adjusting its mechanism slightly. The relationship between Hegel and Marx can no longer, then, be thought of in the uncomplicated but reductive terms of an 'inversion'. But there is a paradoxical element to the transition that Althusser names the epistemological break: it may rapturously redeem one system of thought, precisely by having seeded a new one, but—in a contradiction Althusser does not address—it must, as it did Marx's break from Hegel, have been produced *from* that very pre-existing system. If Althusser wishes, according to his structuralist approach, to make the process of history composed entirely of impersonal, inhuman structures—of discourses relating to one another independently—this leaves no mechanism for the emergence of *new* configurations. He is left having either to fall back on some quasi-teleological logic of history, whereby discourses give birth to each other by necessity, or to valorise the individual in their ineffable, vaguely fetishised heroism—to an extent that even Sartre did not.

Althusser seeks to articulate a way of reading Marx that would solve several problems at once. He attempts to relegate humanism, Hegelianism, and other unwanted foreign objects from Marx in one decisive movement, whilst also preserving everything that he thinks is still of clear value in Marx's work. Yet there are undercurrents of Althusser's argument here that simultaneously undermine these intentions. Althusser wants seemingly to have things both ways: to be rigorously scientific, yet also acutely attentive to Marx's individual subjectivity.

The lyrical passage below from 'On the Young Marx' draws together much of what Althusser has so far articulated about his prescribed method of reading, but also returns to several of its underlying problems:

[54] Althusser, 'Contradiction and Overdetermination', p. 92.

> Of course, we now know that the Young Marx *did* become Marx, but we should not want to live faster than he did, we should not want to live in his place, reject for him or discover for him. We shall not be waiting for him at the end of the course to throw round him as round a runner the mantle of repose, for at last it is over, he has arrived. [...] We *scan* [*scandons*] the necessity [*nécessité*] of [authors'] lives in our understanding of its nodal points, its reversals and its mutations. In this area there is perhaps no greater joy than to be able to witness in an emerging life, once the Gods of Origins and Goals have been dethroned, the birth of necessity.[55]

In place, here, of teleologically reducing Marx to his final form—a reduction that Althusser casts as patronising, presumptuous, and hubristically impatient—he unveils the idea of 'necessity'. Something emerged in Marx's life, Althusser proposes, on the level of his lived experience, that necessitated a response in the form of changes of direction in his work. The analysis Althusser offers here appears as something of a bibliographical prosody—amounting, in the way he describes it above, to a purely formal, even metrical, portioning of a life.

There is a repressed psychoanalytic basis for the idea of 'scanning' Marx's life for its 'nodal points', shifts, and reorientations. In their introduction to the English translation of Althusser's 1964 article 'Freud and Lacan', Oliver Corpet and François Matheron print the following note from an early draft of 'On the Young Marx', which Althusser had made in the above passage after the word '*scan*' ('*scandons*' in his original French). He writes: 'I borrow this term from Jacques Lacan. Among those disciplines attentive to events and major advents, there are no doubt correspondences and affinities that a single word is capable of freeing from the rest'.[56] Lacan uses the word '*scande*' fairly regularly in the *Écrits*, particularly up to the mid-1960s. It is the verb form of what translates to the English word 'scansion', the prosodic technique of determining the metrical pattern of a line of verse, whose infinitive, *scander*, is usually translated as 'to scan' or 'scanning'. In his English translation of the *Écrits*, Bruce Fink introduces the neologism 'scand' as a translation of *scande*, to

[55] Althusser, 'On the Young Marx', pp. 70–71.

[56] Oliver Corpet and François Matheron, 'Introduction to "Freud and Lacan"', in *Writings on Psychoanalysis*, pp. 7–12 (pp. 7–8).

distinguish it from the ordinary, colloquial uses of 'scan' in English ('looking over rapidly, quickly running through a list, taking ultra-thin pictures of the body with a scanner, or "feeding" text and images in digital form into a computer').[57] As Fink glosses it, Lacan uses the word *scande* to refer, more specifically, to 'cutting, punctuating, or interrupting something', usually 'the analysand's discourse'.[58] The word, as Lacan uses it, also has the more specific connotation of a dialectical transition, through which something shifts on the level of a subject's identifications, to produce a transformation or irruption in knowledge. Examples of Lacanian 'scansions' given in the *Écrits* are: the renunciations 'scanding' the history of psychic development, whose pattern is expressed in the '*fort-da*' game Freud observes in *Beyond the Pleasure Principle* (1920); the 'dialectical reversals' in Dora's case history; the time intervals in 'Logical Time and the Assertion of Anticipated Certainty', which reorient the knowledge of the subjects in the group described in the article's sophism (1945); and the punctuation made by the end of an analytic session.[59]

Althusser's use of the word *scande* in 'On the Young Marx' is intended to highlight 'correspondences and affinities' between Marxism and psychoanalysis. It is invoked by Althusser to signal an appreciation of the structural turning-points in Marx's life, and to make any claim about the superiority of Marx's later work rest on the idea that the virtues of this mature work emerged only through his immersion in a structural nexus external to him that precipitated his break from Hegel—a structural nexus that, as far as Althusser understands it, was described in Lacan's early theories. Closer attention to one of Lacan's examples of scansions in the *Écrits*, however, highlights some of the distance between Lacan's and Althusser's usages of the term. Here is how Lacan, in his 'Presentation on Transference' (1951), describes the way that Freud lays out the case of Dora in *Fragment of an Analysis of a Case of Hysteria* (1905). Freud structures the case, says Lacan, as a 'series of dialectical reversals'. This, he says,

---

[57] Bruce Fink, 'Translator's Endnotes', in *Écrits*, pp. 759–849 (p. 842).

[58] Fink, 'Translator's Endnotes', p. 842.

[59] Lacan, 'Presentation on Psychical Causality' (1946), in *Écrits*, pp. 123–160 (p. 152); 'Presentation on Transference' (1951), in *Écrits*, pp. 176–188 (p. 178); 'Logical Time and the Assertion of Anticipated Certainty' (1945), in *Écrits*, pp. 161–175; and 'Function and Field', p. 209.

'as Freud clearly states here', is no 'mere contrivance for presenting material whose emergence is left up to the patient'.[60] Rather,

> What is involved is a scansion of structures in which truth is transmuted for the subject, structures that affect not only her comprehension of things, but her very position as a subject, her "objects" being a function of that position. This means that the conception of the case history is *identical to* the progress of the subject, that is, to the reality of the treatment.[61]

The rhythms of transition and transformation that scand the process of Dora's analysis are always, as Lacan reads the case here, both changes on the level of her knowledge, *and* changes in her position as a subject with respect to certain objects. The case history that narrates these transitions can therefore be, as Lacan stresses here, 'identical to' Dora's own progress, because these transitions amount to her position in the structures that the case history describes. Later in the presentation, Lacan will articulate transference—which Freud understood to have been the obstacle to Dora's treatment—as a subject's fixation on a congealed moment in the dialectic of knowledge. As Chap. 2 described, Lacan made this fixation an integral component *of* knowledge, based on his reading of Hegel. An analyst's interpretation of transference amounts, therefore, for him, to '[n]othing but [filling] the emptiness of this standstill with a lure', whose function is to push beyond the stagnant fixation to which the transference amounts.[62]

As Chap. 2 of this book described, the object of transference is designated by Lacan as the 'subject supposed to know'; the 'nothing' of knowledge that functions as a prosthetic site for absolute knowledge.[63] In an obvious irony, it is a Hegelian logic that Lacan is deploying in his redesignation of the mechanics of transference. It is through this Hegelian logic of transference that, as Lacan's 1951 reading of the Dora case study is just one example, he articulates the notion of 'scansion' that Althusser then uses to make a Marxist ambush of Hegel. Beyond this

[60] Lacan, 'Presentation on Transference', p. 178.

[61] Lacan, 'Presentation on Transference', p. 178.

[62] Lacan, 'Presentation on Transference', p. 184.

[63] See Chap. 2, pp. 68–73.

unintentionally inherited Hegelianism, though, there is more to the distance between Lacan and Althusser that is made visible here. In 'On the Young Marx', Althusser is trying to use psychoanalysis as a way out of the problem posed by diachronicity to ahistorical structural cross-sections. This problem, as the first section of this chapter summarised, itself manifested a crisis in a structuralist approach to history and subjectivity. Some other entity—some impulse to facilitate transitions and interactions between these two levels—was clearly required, but Althusser is only able loosely to propose 'necessity' as such a mediator. He still lacks a means to unite the two levels of history and individual subjectivity. In the attempt to find it, he encounters the same problem as Vygotsky had pointed out several decades earlier. Materialist psychology should not be allowed, Vygotsky argued persuasively, to reduce people to reflexological machines—but nor should it, on the other hand, allow subjectivity to manifest as some unobservable excess of the soul. In seeking to banish, whether from history as a whole or from the biography of an individual, the notions of purpose and destination—as reflexology had on the level of psychology—Althusser repeats the same situation criticised by Vygotsky. He is forced to generate a vaguely spiritualistic account of subjectivity, relying on an untouchable excess to explain the precipitation of epistemological breaks.

There is nothing of the 'necessary' in the Lacanian scansion. Lacan was equally opposed to the kind of latent spiritualism that Vygotsky criticised, and it was on this basis that he made the extended critique of Pavlov summarised at the end of Chap. 3. Pavlovian reflexology amounts, for Lacan, to a new scientific spiritualism, because in supposing the mechanism of the reflex to be 'already there in the brain', Pavlov inscribed knowledge into the real, as some mysterious entity that exists there 'already waiting for us' to be discovered.[64] If teleological predestination is put off the table for Althusser, 'necessity', in the way Althusser unwillingly falls back onto it in 'On the Young Marx', preserves the same assumptions for which Lacan criticised Pavlov. This is far from what

[64] Lacan, Lesson 1,15 November 1967, in *Seminar XV: The Psychoanalytic Act* (1967–1968), unpublished. For an unofficial translation, see Gallagher, <http://www.lacaninireland.com/web/wp-content/uploads/2010/06/Book-15-The-Psychoanalytical-Act.pdf>, p. 12.

Lacan is deploying in his notion of scansion. Althusser inscribes a set of motivations in a zone of the real that is untouchable and imperceivable, and transforms them thereby into what Lacan critically identified as 'knowledge in the real'.

Inversion and Symptom

Another target of Althusser's project in the 1960s is the notion that there exists a relation of 'inversion' between Marx and Hegel. The theme of Marx's so-called inversion of Hegel was an object of obsessive concern amongst communists in the mid-twentieth century.[65] The famous spatial metaphor, of setting the dialectic 'right side up again' after it had been 'standing on its head' in Hegel, had first been articulated in the second German edition of *Capital* in 1873, near the end of the Afterword.[66] This passage had been reductively interpreted, Althusser alleges in 'On the Young Marx' (1961), to imply that the ideas Marx inherited from Hegel in the mid-1800s contained a truth that Marx merely needed to extract from them by a simple geometric manoeuvre; by a little twist, or sleight of hand. To this, Althusser responds, with biting simplicity, and taking seriously the topology implied in Marx's metaphor, that 'to turn an object right round changes neither its nature nor its content by virtue merely of a rotation'.[67] It is not enough, then, merely to 'invert' the idealist abstraction—which understands concrete objects as products of general concepts—into a materialist abstraction, which would reverse this to understand abstract concepts instead as the products of concrete objects.[68]

[65] See, for example, Maurice Godelier, *Rationalité et Irrationalité en Economie* (Paris: Éd. Maspéro, 1966); Lucio Colletti, *Il Marxismo e Hegel* (Laterza, 1969); and Trần Đức Thảo, 'Le "noyau rationnel" dans la dialectique hégélienne', in *La Pensée* (Jan–Feb 1965), 4–5.

[66] Marx, 'Afterword to the Second German Edition' (1873), in *Capital: A Critique of Political Economy*, trans. by Samuel Moore and Edward Aveling (London: Lawrence and Wishart, 1974), pp. 12–22 (p. 19). 'The mystification which dialectic suffers in Hegel's hands, by no means prevents him from being the first to present its general form of working in a comprehensive and conscious manner. With him it is standing on its head. It must be turned right side up again, if you would discover the rational kernel within the mystical shell.'

[67] Althusser, 'On the Young Marx', p. 73.

[68] Althusser, 'On the Materialist Dialectic', in *For Marx*, pp. 161–218 (p. 189).

The belief that all that was required to obtain Marx from Hegel was to turn upside-down the relation Hegel gives to the concept and the real is, Althusser warns, a trap that results in a merely illusory materialism. Worse, Althusser argues, this reductive schema in fact delivers supposed Marxists into the throes of a new idealism. Althusser denounces, in an article 'On the Materialist Dialectic' (1963) a few years later, not only the 'idealism of consciousness', but also a '"mechanistic" materialism' of the reductive kind that he has in mind here, as equally compromised types of thinking. Each merely assimilates 'the structured unity of a complex whole to the simple unity of a totality'.[69] They both take 'the complex whole [...] as purely and simply the development of one *single* essence or original and simple substance', and they do so in a way that 'slide[s] back from Marx to Hegel, at worst, from Marx to Haeckel'.[70]

The argument Althusser makes here—that a clumsy, naïve materialism in fact results in a new idealism—is very close to that made by both Vygotsky and Politzer decades earlier in the context of psychology. As summarised in Chap. 3, part of Vygotsky's critique of reflexology was his identification of its unintentional proximity to a spiritualistic idealism. The attempt of naïve reflexologists to 'build a psychology without a mind', Vygotsky argues in 1926, amounted to 'the dualism of subjective psychology turned inside out'—it preserved this dualism between mind and behaviour, because it allowed them to remain 'not one but two'.[71] Psychologists who sequestered the mind from the possibility of study, Vygotsky alleges, produced an 'idealism of the highest order', and 'a dualism that might more correctly be called an idealism turned upside down'.[72] What Vygotsky makes clear is that the kind of botched materialism he identifies in reflexology has the capacity to ruin the science of psychology, because it precludes the possibility of developing either a proper method for the science, or an effective theoretical technology to purge it of its limitations. It had allowed the science instead to languish in idealism with diminishing hope of escape. Politzer makes the very

69 Althusser, 'On the Materialist Dialectic', p. 202.

70 Althusser, 'On the Materialist Dialectic', p. 202.

71 Vygotsky, 'The Methods of Reflexological and Psychological Investigation' (1926), in *The Collected Works of L.S. Vygotsky, Vol. 3*, pp. 35–50 (p. 65).

72 Vygotsky, 'The Methods', p. 46.

similar claim, in the 1940s, that supposedly 'materialist' psychological theories were still fundamentally idealist. The science remained, for him, 'cast on the mold of spiritualism', because it still tried 'to express the "spiritual"', but by the means of 'the nervous system; viscera; the glands with internal secretion', or 'the organism considered as a whole'.[73] In the 1960s, Althusser is arguing that to believe turning Hegel's dialectic upside-down would solve its problems is to remain within idealism. In both cases—materialist psychology, and readings of Marx—Vygotsky, Politzer, and Althusser find idealism to be a spectre that can persist even when it is assumed to have been exorcised.

Althusser's treatment of the relationship between Marx and Hegel was one of a host of others being made in France at the time. This was a problem that had troubled Marxist philosophers for decades—but it was, in part, the treatment of this relationship as a puzzle to be solved that had made it such a stumbling block for Althusser's contemporaries. The comprehensive history in Michael Kelly's book *Modern French Marxism* (1982) gives detailed descriptions of the most significant of the responses made in France to this problem. Those who published on the question of this relationship included Maurice Godelier, Lucio Colletti, Trần Đức Thảo, Roger Garaudy, and Jean Hyppolite. Though their reiterations or dismissals of the question of the 'inverted' dialectic had elements in common with Althusser's in some cases, none posed such radical notions as a consequence. Althusser hones in on the vital importance of something that remains totally unaccounted for by a model of an inverted dialectic.

One result of this rejection of the model of inversion is the privileged position Althusser gives to the notion of 'symptom', which becomes a structural principle in his thinking, with clear connections to both Freud and Spinoza. In *Reading Capital* (1965), Althusser describes Marx's second reading of Hegel as '*symptomatic*' (*symptomale*), for the way that it draws out, not something present in Hegel, but something precisely absent from him. Marx's symptomatic reading of Hegel, says Althusser, 'divulges the undivulged event in the text it reads', and 'in the same movement relates it *to a different text*, present as a necessary absence in the

[73] Politzer, *La Crise de la Psychologie Contemporaine* (Paris: Éditions Sociales, 1947), pp. 92–93.

first'.[74] Althusser elaborates the effect this has in Marx's own writing through a theatrical metaphor: if, he illustrates, Marx "plays" with Hegelian formulae, it is to constitute from them '*the action of a real drama*, in which old concepts desperately play the part of something absent *which is nameless*, in order to call it onto the stage in person'.[75] Yet the concepts placed 'onto the stage' by Marx produce, he says, the presence of the nameless thing only 'in their failures, in the dislocation between the characters and their roles'.[76] Though Marx was unable to discover, in his own historical context, a concept adequate to think the nameless entity that he summoned, Althusser names this entity as '*the concept of the effectivity of a structure on its elements*'.[77] What Althusser has in mind is a historical deficiency: what Marx could not say was that which was beyond the limits of the sayable, due to the configuration of Marx's world. Therein lies the value of structuralism, for Althusser, in providing concepts to express, or at least to hone in on, what remained only a pre-emptive phantom—a ghost from the future—in Marx.

But were Marx and his world really waiting for a messianic 'concept of the effectivity of a structure on its elements'? Following Althusser's own reflections elsewhere, it seems that precisely this was provided amply, and powerfully, by Spinoza in the 1600s. In a series of lectures from 1963, on 'Psychoanalysis and the Human Sciences', Althusser spends some time framing Spinoza's philosophy as an alternative to Cartesian epistemology. Central to Descartes's philosophy, as Althusser reads it, is a division between truth and error, which results in error being seen 'simply as the exterior of a truth, as exclusion from a truth'.[78] The psychological subject, says Althusser, is made possible by Descartes in order to act as a battle-ground for these two principles, with all the pathologies of the psychological subject—'memory, attention, haste, prejudice, imagination,

[74] Althusser, 'From *Capital* to Marx's Philosophy', in *Reading Capital*, trans. by Ben Brewster and David Fernbach (London: Verso, 2016), pp. 11–70 (p. 28).

[75] Althusser, *Reading Capital*, p. 29.

[76] Althusser, *Reading Capital*, p. 29.

[77] Althusser, *Reading Capital*, p. 29.

[78] Althusser, 'Psychoanalysis and Psychology', in *Psychoanalysis and the Human Sciences*, pp. 45–88 (p. 81).

feeling'—being defined by him negatively, as being exterior to the truth.[79] This makes the psychological subject's pathologies the other side of Descartes's subject of objectivity.[80] But Descartes, as Althusser criticises him, did not attempt to conceive of or to criticise the objective social structure in which he lived. On this basis, Spinoza's idea of the 'imaginary' opens an entirely different, more expansive framework. Spinoza conceives of the imaginary not, with Descartes, 'as a psychological category', but 'as the category through which a world is conceived'—not as a function of the psyche, but as something more like a Hegelian 'element': 'a totality into which the psychological functions are integrated and on the basis of which they are constituted'.[81] The imaginary, for Spinoza, is not 'a faculty of the mind', or of the psychological subject; instead, 'the imagination is a world', one example of which is the world-forming category of 'historical existence', as described in his *Tractatus Theologico-Politicus* (1677). For Spinoza, the imagination is not a function of the psychological subject, but there is a profound reversal, and an evident critique of the *cogito*; psychological subjects are instead taken by him to be constituted as functions of the world that is the imaginary. The role of the Cartesian subject of objectivity as an arbiter for the production of new knowledge in history is thereby radically destabilised. Spinoza, as Althusser reads him, critiques the constitution of this supposedly sovereign subject, as having merely been imposed by the structure of the imaginary, because the imaginary amounts to 'a social structure that necessarily produces this subject in order to be able to subsist'.[82] The Spinozan imaginary is a structure, then, that produces an element—the Cartesian subject—that denies its own status as an element in this structure.

As has been remarked by several commentators on his work, Althusser's enthusiasm for Spinoza is central to much of his thinking. Of all the philosophers in France in the 1960s, says Warren Montag, 'none is more closely associated with Spinoza than Althusser'.[83] Indeed, Montag adds,

[79] Althusser, 'Psychoanalysis and Psychology', p. 78.

[80] Althusser, 'Psychoanalysis and Psychology', p. 78.

[81] Althusser, 'Psychoanalysis and Psychology', p. 79.

[82] Althusser, 'Psychoanalysis and Psychology', p. 80.

[83] Warren Montag, 'Spinoza and Althusser Against Hermeneutics: Interpretation or Invention?', in *The Althusserian Legacy*, pp. 51–58 (p. 51).

although '[t]o speak of the influence of Spinoza on Althusser is already to grant a conceptual regime that both thinkers refused', Althusser's work constitutes 'a theoretical project profoundly internal to the conceptual space delimited by Spinoza's works'.[84] Althusser also personally identified, like Lacan, with Spinoza's apostatism, and experienced the theoretical climate of 1960s France as a repetition of the forces that framed Spinoza's persecution in the seventeenth century. It is the Spinozist notion that matter exists in different modalities that allows Althusser to postulate, famously, that ideology has a material existence, and that it can be understood according to a Marxist logic of production.[85]

Althusser's introduction of Spinoza into the debates that raged in French Marxism in the 1960s, even if it was a covert introduction, reframed them irreversibly.[86] One seeming contradiction borne out by this work on Spinoza, however, is that, whilst *Reading Capital* makes '*the concept of the effectivity of a structure on its elements*' the concept that is *missing* from Marx (and also, perplexingly given Spinoza lived two centuries earlier, a concept that was missing from Marx's world in general), Althusser also clearly wants to understand the relationship between Marx and Hegel on exactly this basis. This is borne out in the non-linear structure he attempts to give to Marx's biography: if the end of Marx must not be allowed, in Hegelian fashion, to subsume his beginning, the *whole* of Marx can bring out elements in his texts that are absent from any one of those texts in isolation. What is being implicitly attempted here is the development of a functioning, subtle, structuralist theory of history from a Spinozist logic of causation. Yet, still, Althusser writes as if Marx was *applying* precisely this method of reading. Marx, for Althusser, conducts a "symptomatic" reading of Hegel—in which the missing piece is diagnosed from the whole—yet Marx also *lacks* a *concept* of the symptom.

The question is, then: on what level is the knowledge of structural causality, which allows a theory of the symptom, present for Marx, if it is also true that he was unable to articulate this theory as such? Althusser

---

[84] Montag, 'Spinoza and Althusser', p. 51.

[85] See Althusser, 'Ideology and Ideological State Apparatuses', in *On the Reproduction of Capitalism: Ideology and Ideological State Apparatuses* (London: Verso, 2014), pp. 232–272.

[86] He would later distance himself from this work, in his 1972 essay 'Elements in Self-Criticism'. See Althusser, *Essays in Self-Criticism*, trans. by Grahame Lock (London: New Left Books, 1976).

falls back here into appeals to Marx's 'unconscious' knowledge; to something that presses through as a trace in Marx, but that Marx was not fully able to articulate. However, he thereby merely defers the question. Then there are Althusser's appeals to Marx's psychobiography, his heroic subjectivity, and the enigmas of 'necessity' and the 'force of history'; but none of these notions are developed sufficiently to answer this question. The problem is usefully parsed out in Paul Ricoeur's critique of Althusser, which puts significant pressure on his account of the epistemological break. In general, what Ricoeur's reading of Althusser highlights is how difficult it becomes, if we follow Althusser's account of ideology, to imagine how any break from an ideological formation could ever be possible. Because ideology, for Althusser, is tied 'to the mirror stage of the imagination', as an imaginary grounding for subjectivity, it is unclear to Ricoeur 'from where we could borrow the forces to resist the [state] apparatus if not from the depths of a subject having claims that are not infected by this supposed submissive constitution', or how anyone could 'produce a break in the seemingly closed shell of ideology'.[87] Precisely by raising the enemy's power to its maximum, Althusser loses any ground for the revolutionary impetus he needs in order to resist it. As an extension to this point, Ricoeur poses a similar query to the notion that Marx experienced his own epistemological break. Is, he asks, 'a complete break understandable without some kind of intellectual miracle, a sense of someone emerging from the dark?'.[88] Ricoeur gestures here not only to the problem of the unfeasibility of the epistemological break—the fact that it seems to require some kind of deus ex machina to take place, given the impossible odds stacked against its occurrence—but also the vague romanticism that it retains. How, he asks, can the break be conceived of in its very implausibility, except as a divine revelation?[89]

[87] Ricoeur, 'Althusser's Theory of Ideology', in *Althusser: A Critical Reader*, ed. by Gregory Elliot, pp. 44–72 (p. 65).

[88] Ricoeur, 'Althusser's Theory of Ideology', p. 67.

[89] Ricoeur's further dispute with Althusser is that his representation of the epistemological break 'does great damage not only to the theory of ideology but to the reading of Marx', as it 'causes us to place the break at a different point from where it should be' ('Althusser's Theory of Ideology', p. 67). A more significant change 'at the philosophical level' comes, for Ricoeur, earlier than where Althusser locates it: 'not after *The German Ideology* but between the *Manuscripts of 1844* and *The German Ideology*, that is to say, in the emergence of the concept of the real human being, real *praxis*,

Ricoeur's criticisms of Althusser stem partly from his own reluctance to consider how a structural theory of causality transforms any notion of motivation, and indeed an existentialist understanding of subjectivity more broadly, when the latter traditionally put so much weight on the centrality of freedom of choice. Ricoeur's criticisms are still helpful, however, in clarifying certain places of porousness within Althusser's theory of the epistemological break. A large part of the problem remains in Althusser's need for the epistemological break to operate in a way that would cut across two levels: the level of Marx as an individual, in terms of his biography, and the level of history, understood as a series of theoretical developments that can be abstracted from the work of several individual figures. Althusser does not offer a mechanism to join together these two levels of the epistemological break, and he instead falls back on an appeal to Marx's supposedly remarkable ability to tap into and express a certain 'historical' pressure. But how did the force of history emerge into Marx's life in a way that moved him to conduct the epistemological break? How does an individual obtain a glimpse of the invisible object on which an ideological framework is based? Althusser's idea of 'necessity' is just as suspect in this respect as Lévi-Strauss's appeals to a 'social unconscious' and to 'human spirit', or the Freudian 'insurance policy' of a neurological substrate of the unconscious. The way Marx's symptomatic reading of Hegel operates, as Althusser presents it, is by using inadequate concepts to mime the adequate ones that did not exist yet. This framework preserves, however, the ghostly presence of a divine truth that pierces through epistemological frameworks and makes them break, without explaining either how this truth does so, what it is, or where it comes from.

individuals acting in certain given conditions' (pp. 67–68). Althusser's division of Marx puts forward a conflation, says Ricoeur, under the single heading of 'anthropological ideology', of an 'ideology of consciousness', with which Marx and Freud 'rightly' broke away, and 'the ideology of real, concrete, human being, a being composed of drives, labour, and so on'. The latter should not be confused with idealism, Ricoeur asserts, favouring the development of a 'non-idealistic anthropology'. Marx's breakthrough, far from abandoning a 'deep-rooted interest in the plenitude of individual existence', must, Ricoeur argues, make sense at this level.

History and the Symptom

Against the reductive schema of inversion that Althusser attacks in the early 1960s, which he accuses of being a return to idealism, he pits perhaps his best-known concept, that of 'overdetermination'. The notion of overdetermination is offered by Althusser as a defence both against, on the one hand, slipping back from materialism into a vulgar idealism, and on the other, against a Hegelian view of totality as an incessant movement towards ultimate, intrinsic identity. Hegel, Althusser observes, 'in one movement, rejects both the structured complex whole and its conditions of existence by his prior assumption of a pure, simple interiority'; he impatiently rejects, in other words, whatever might exist in excess of an elegant symmetry.[90] By contrast, the kind of structure that Althusser refers to as 'overdetermined' consists of an irresolvable complexity containing manifold layers of contradiction, within which there is one dominant structural component.

As Althusser outlines in his article 'Contradiction and Overdetermination' (1962), when applied to history, the concept of overdetermination removes the imperative for a revolutionary transformation to occur with purity. Althusser uses the concept to describe how pre-revolutionary elements inevitably remain after revolutions, 'overdetermining' the new structure of post-revolutionary society. This in itself is, once more, Althusser's intended means of departing from a Hegelian view of history. Althusser accuses Hegel of subjectifying history by attributing to it the psychological function of memory. In Hegel, as Althusser reads him, 'the survival of the past as the "*superseded*" (*aufgehoben*) is simply reduced to the modality of a *memory*, which, furthermore, is merely the inverse of (that is, the same things as) an *anticipation*'.[91] This is why, for Hegel, 'the present can feed on the shades of its past, or even project them before it, just as the great effigies of Roman Virtue opened up the road to Revolution and Terror for the Jacobins'.[92] The past of this present 'is never anything more than itself and only recalls to it that law

[90] Althusser, 'On the Materialist Dialectic', p. 208.

[91] Althusser, 'On the Materialist Dialectic', p. 115.

[92] Althusser, 'On the Materialist Dialectic', p. 115.

of interiority which is the destiny of the whole Future of Humanity'.[93] Althusser dismisses what he finds in the way Hegel treats history, which he takes to amount, for Hegel, to a memory that is inscribed in the present. The way Marx receives the concept of 'supersession' does away completely, as Althusser reads him, with 'this dialectic of historical comfort'.[94] For Marx, the past is not an abstract, ideal realm containing forms that can be reconfigured along the axis of time; the past is, as Althusser puts it, 'no shade, not even an "objective" shade—it is a terribly positive and active structured reality, just as cold, hunger and the night are for his poor worker'.[95] It is precisely because history is not, for Marx, a shadow falling coolly on the present, but a sharp, material reality, that its structures can, for him, be definitively broken away from.

Yet the material realism that Marx attributes to history also means we can accept, Althusser argues, that no break is complete, immediate, or, in a word, ideal. Overdetermination means both that 'a revolution in the *structure* does not *ipso facto* modify the existing superstructures and particularly the *ideologies* at one blow' and 'that the new society produced by the Revolution may itself *ensure the survival, that is, the reactivation of older elements*'.[96] The view of history Althusser takes from Marx is one of complex, delayed, superimposed, and uneven development; a process that is improvised and scrambling, without the encircling, propulsive logic of the world spirit.

One of Althusser's particular aims in *Reading Capital* is to develop a theory of the history of science. He attempts this by extending his account of the relationship between Marx and Hegel to a general principle for the structure of this history. After acknowledging his debt to Lacan, Bachelard, Cavaillès, Canguilhem, and Foucault, Althusser describes, once more, but with particular precision, the break that he understands Marx to have made with what he describes as 'the Hegelian conception of the whole as a "spiritual" [...] *expressive* totality'.[97] Implicit once more here is Althusser's

[93] Althusser, 'On the Materialist Dialectic', p. 115.
[94] Althusser, 'On the Materialist Dialectic', p. 115.
[95] Althusser, 'On the Materialist Dialectic', p. 115.
[96] Althusser, 'On the Materialist Dialectic', pp. 115–116.
[97] Althusser, 'From *Capital* to Marx's Philosophy', in *Reading Capital*, p. 17.

distinction between Hegel's 'expressive' logic, and Spinoza's 'structural' logic of causation.

Althusser articulates the distinction between these two logics further through an analysis of Marx's critique of fetishism. In *Capital*, Althusser summarises, Marx 'measures a distance and an internal dislocation (*decalage*) in the real, inscribed in its structure'.[98] There is something, as Althusser reads Marx here, that is fundamentally broken about reality as a result of class conflict. Social antagonism does not exist, in this reading, on another level to the real, because all human experience of reality is structured *around* this social antagonism—the real itself, therefore, has these dislocations inscribed into it. However, this 'dislocation' that Marx measures in the real, as Althusser reads him, also makes its own effects 'illegible', so that the 'ultimate apex' of these effects is 'the illusion of an immediate reading of them'.[99] The antagonisms of capitalism are inscribed onto reality, then—but the most important effect of this, says Althusser, is exactly the illusion that this dislocation could be comprehended directly. The effect of the dislocated real is, in other words, that it projects a substitute for itself that appears to consciousness to be easily and totality comprehendible. Belief in this illusion—the illusion that dislocation in the real can be simply and immediately understood—is itself, for Althusser, the act of fetishism. If Hegel says that the real may bear its secrets legibly, then Marx responds that the real is ruptured beyond comprehension, and he labels the assumption of its legibility as a fetish. Hegel is therefore the fetishist *par excellence*, because his logic of 'expressive totality' leads to this fetishistic belief in a legible real. Spinoza's 'structural' logic, Althusser is arguing, led Marx to generate a precise critique of this logic in his analysis of fetishism.

The way Marx thereby punctures to the very heart of Hegel's theoretical framework is exemplary, Althusser expands, for the pattern of all true scientific development. The production, he says, 'of a new problem endowed with this *critical* character (critical in the sense of a critical situation)', like the problem that Marx articulates in his concept of fetishism, 'is the unstable index of the possible production of a new theoretical

[98] Althusser, 'From *Capital* to Marx's Philosophy', p. 17.

[99] Althusser, 'From *Capital* to Marx's Philosophy', p. 17.

problematic, of which this problem is only one symptomatic mode'.[100] This transition comes down, says Althusser, to a distinction between what is 'visible' and what is 'invisible' within a given theoretical framework. Any object or problem, 'situated on the terrain and within the horizon, i.e., in the definite structured field of the theoretical problematic of a given theoretical discipline, is visible'.[101] In the 'shadowy obverse' of the visible, however, are the objects 'defined [as] excluded, *excluded* from the field of visibility and *defined* as excluded by the existence and peculiar structure of the field of the problematic; as what forbids and represses the reflection of the field on its object'.[102] These objects are 'invisible' in the field of the existing theory, 'because they are *forbidden* by it', 'rejected in principle, repressed from the field of the visible'.[103] If 'their fleeting presence in the field [...] does occur (in very peculiar and symptomatic circumstances)', it '*goes unperceived*, and becomes literally an undivulgeable absence—since the whole function of the field is not to see them, to forbid any sighting of them'.[104] These blind spots, common to all epistemological fields, conceal that which is unthinkable within any given one of them.

The privileged example Althusser gives of the invisible-object-made-visible is surplus value. He understands Marx to have produced this object from the inferences that existed before him, tangentially, in political economy.[105] The idea of the 'value of labour' in political economy contains inside itself, says Althusser, 'an internal lack' that points to 'a real but absent question outside itself', and which therefore serves as a model of 'the *absence of a concept behind a word*'.[106] The term 'value of labour'

[100] Althusser, *Reading Capital*, p. 25.
[101] Althusser, *Reading Capital*, p. 25.
[102] Althusser, *Reading Capital*, p. 26.
[103] Althusser, *Reading Capital*, p. 25.
[104] Althusser, *Reading Capital*, p. 25.
[105] Marx did not invent the term 'surplus-value', and it was already used routinely in classical political economy. But Marx radically transformed its meaning, and it is the consequences of this transformation that Althusser is developing here. Political economy saw surplus value as the product of labour that exceeds the amount paid to the labourer. Marx's key innovation was to recognise the distinction between surplus *labour*—the daily labour in excess of the worker's daily wage—that is enforced by capital, and the surplus value that 'expresses' this surplus labour.
[106] Althusser, *Reading Capital*, p. 33.

served, for political economy, to veil this absent concept of surplus-value. This, says Althusser, is because surplus-value—which is the facilitating principle of capitalism, because it turns value into capital by allowing value to increase itself—is made possible because of an internal dislocation *within* the value of labour. Althusser then extends the structure of Marx's discovery of surplus value to a general theory of the history of science. He illustrates this process of making-visible with the example of oxygen with regards to the earlier, dominant 'phlogistic' theory of chemistry.[107] According to this seventeenth-century theory, a fire-like element that it named phlogiston is contained in combustible elements, and is released when these objects are burnt. Lavoisier overturned this model of chemistry by naming a previously 'invisible' element—*oxygen*—and then articulating the role of this element in combustion. After this point, the entire structure of the theoretical framework of chemistry was transformed around the now 'visible' object of oxygen. Althusser emphasises how this is structurally similar to the break Marx makes from political economy.

As Althusser quotes Engels, before Marx, the words 'value' or 'worth' were applied, reductively, as '*literally* directly to the useful things themselves'.[108] Engels clarifies this in a colourful analogy. This idea that value and worth are inherent properties of objects, as Althusser quotes Engels, 'has as much to do with the *scientific definition* of commodity "value" as the fact that the word salt was first applied to cooking salt by the ancient world, and that therefore since Pliny *sugar*, etc., have figured as *kinds of salt*, etc.'.[109] Because 'salt' was originally the name used for all cooking salts, this meant that sugar and other ingredients used to be called 'salts'. Finding value to be *literally in* useful objects is, Engels is illustrating, similarly arbitrary and flawed. The way that political economy understood value is made by Engels to appear hopelessly backward, and as having preserved an outmoded and erroneous framework, which is incapable of articulating, and therefore of thinking, its own concepts.

[107] Althusser, *Reading Capital*, p. 25.
[108] Althusser, *Reading Capital*, p. 146–7.
[109] Althusser, *Reading Capital*, p. 147.

Althusser quotes another particularly penetrating culinary-chemical example given by Engels as an analogue to the state of political economy before the discovery of surplus value:

> [It] is reminiscent of the old chemists before chemistry was a science: because edible butter, which in ordinary life was just called butter (according to nordic custom), has a soft consistency, they called chlorides butter of zinc, butter of antimony, etc., or butyrous humours.[110]

Being a chloride was not, unlike the softness attributed to butter, something that could have been observed empirically by chemists. In the cases of chlorides or salts, the invisible object cannot be 'seen' by any degree of empirical scrutiny. Similarly, an economist can no more 'see' the form of exploitation named by surplus value in the measurable economic facts of 'prices, exchanges, wages, profits, rents, etc.' than he can 'see' the 'law of attraction in falling bodies, or the pre-Lavoisierian chemist could "see" oxygen in "dephlogisticated" air'.[111] Just as bodies could be seen to fall before Newton, exploitation was 'seen' before Marx. But the economic 'forms' of that exploitation, the 'economic existence of the relations of production', and their structural domination of political economy, 'did not then have any theoretical existence'.[112] Smith and Ricardo, says Althusser, may have 'produced' the 'fact' of surplus value, in the 'fact' of rent and profit, but they could not 'think it in its concept, nor draw from it its theoretical consequences', because they did not realise what they had 'produced'. Neither they nor the culture of their time imagined that a 'fact' like surplus value might be the existence of a '*relation* [...] consubstantial with the entire mode of production', and one dominating the fate of that mode of production.[113]

As Althusser presents them, every given epistemological framework has at its centre an 'invisible' object that is unthinkable and forbidden within that framework. The emergence of this object onto the field, when

---

110 Althusser, 'The Epistemological Propositions of *Capital* (Marx, Engels)', in *Reading Capital*, pp. 145–157 (p. 147).

111 Althusser, 'Marx's Critique', in *Reading Capital*, pp. 165–181, (p. 181).

112 Althusser, 'Marx's Critique', p. 181.

113 Althusser, *Reading Capital*, pp. 150–151.

it does occur, precipitates the reorientation of that field, and it has a kind of purifying effect, resolving tensions that had appeared to be irresolvable within the previous constellation. Althusser, as described above, is here explicitly using his analysis of the relationship between Hegel and Marx as a framework or model for all epistemological development. Althusserian epistemological breaks are enabled, in general, in the same way as Marx made his own: by reorganising conceptual elements taken up from older frameworks, in order to allow the 'invisible objects' to come into view; by using old concepts, as Althusser depicted in his metaphor, to 'play the part of something absent *which is nameless*, in order to call it onto the stage in person'.[114]

Because of this, Althusser adds, a later shift brought about by another figure may be necessary in order to complete an epistemological break. Based on this framework, Althusser illustrates how not only Marx, but also Freud, fit into the history of science. He draws several parallels between Marx and Freud in this process. In his lecture on 'The Place of Psychoanalysis in the Human Sciences'—part of a series delivered in 1963—Althusser describes how Freud was forced to set forth his theory using 'imported concepts' from the sciences of biology, thermodynamics, and political economy. This, he says, necessarily produced an 'inadequation between the concepts that Freud uses in his texts and the content that these concepts are intended to grasp'.[115] As Althusser remarks in a preliminary note to his article 'Freud and Lacan' (1964), in this respect Freud was like Marx, who was 'constrained to think through his discovery in certain Hegelian terms'.[116] Lacan's role was, according to Althusser, to complete the scientific shift that had been begun by Freud. Lacan, he says, extends Freud's 'theoretical reflection' into a 'theoretical transformation' and converts Freud's 'imported concepts into domestic concepts'.[117]

The great scientific achievement of psychoanalysis was, for Althusser, to have performed a fusion between biology, on the one hand, and sociology on the other. This fusion was, he says, completed by Lacan's

[114] Althusser, *Reading Capital*, p. 29.

[115] Althusser, 'The Place of Psychoanalysis in the Human Sciences', in *Psychoanalysis and the Human Sciences*, pp. 1–44 (p. 5).

[116] Althusser, 'The Place of Psychoanalysis', p. 14.

[117] Althusser, 'The Place of Psychoanalysis', p. 6.

importation of structuralist concepts to Freud's theories.[118] Althusser describes Freud as having found what he metaphorically refers to as the "pineal gland" between biology and society—their precise intersection, or 'infinitesimal point of encounter'—in the bourgeois, patriarchal family.[119] But Freud only found it in this place, Althusser adds, because of the cultural context in which psychoanalysis originated. Since other societies will have 'a pineal gland different from our own'—that is, a different fulcrum between the biological and the social—it would be possible, Althusser speculates, to develop a 'theory of other pineal glands', and even a 'general theory of the possibility as such of forms of concrete variations on the Western pineal gland'.[120] Hence, for Althusser, the significance of Bronisław Malinowski's research into alternative familial structures, and Lévi-Strauss's relativising comparison between psychoanalytic treatment and shamanism. Lévi-Strauss, Althusser says, 'is becoming an expert in generalizing the pineal gland, because it is itself his object'.[121] The redesignation Althusser gives to psychoanalysis here is impressive: in this lecture, just as in the work by Malinowski and Lévi-Strauss that he champions here, any understanding of psychoanalysis as the science of some fetishised realm of subjectivity is definitively deflated. Psychoanalysis is instead presented by him purely in terms of its position in the history of science, relative to other sciences, and specifically as a unification of the two fields of biology and sociology.

When it comes to the relationship between psychoanalysis and the human sciences, Althusser determines two 'Archimedean points' that have created bridges between them. The first of these he identifies as 'the problematic inaugurated by Marx', and the second he finds in the 'consistent, rigorous, valid, theoretical definition of psychoanalysis' made possible by Lacan.[122] According to Althusser, Lacan's break was achieved by rearticulating what Althusser describes as the 'becoming-human' of a child: Lacan, he says, moves away from the traditional view of this

[118] Althusser, 'The Place of Psychoanalysis', p. 26.
[119] Althusser, 'The Place of Psychoanalysis', pp. 26, 30.
[120] Althusser, 'The Place of Psychoanalysis', pp. 30.
[121] Althusser, 'The Place of Psychoanalysis', pp. 31.
[122] Althusser, 'The Place of Psychoanalysis', p. 40.

movement as a linear, causal development that progresses from the biological to the cultural, and instead offers a view of the cultural as actually having an effect on the biological. As Althusser understands him, for Lacan, culture is 'constantly preced[ing] itself,' and 'absorbing the being that is to become a human subject'.[123] Althusser identifies Lacan's achievement, in light of this, as the full extension of the Saussurian break that was made by structural linguistics. Lacan, he says, draws out this earlier Saussurean break into one that achieves a full generalisation of psychoanalysis, by uniting it with the human sciences. As Althusser sees it here, Lacan's reading of structuralism allows him to invert the supposed relation between biology and culture, to make culture (or in Lacanian terms, the signifier) the agent that acts on and integrates a biological human body. Lacan's work therefore makes psychoanalysis able to function as this previously unthinkable fulcrum between biology and culture. In this lecture, Althusser uses his understanding of Marx's position in the history of science—which he describes fully in *Reading Capital*—as a template to understand the positions of Freud and Lacan in this history. Freud, as Althusser presents him, demonstrated that a 'pineal gland' could be found between the cultural and the biological. Lacan then completed this revolution, by generalising this theory of how those two dimensions intersect.

Whilst doing away with a teleological view of history in either its Hegelian or Sartrean forms, what Althusser's insertion of Lacan and Freud into this historical sequence of epistemological breaks demonstrates is that his historical schema clearly has its own satisfyingly neat, interlaced structure. Even if epistemological breaks are not preordained, they appear according to a choreography that he takes to be ubiquitous, and that he imagines as tending towards unification and synthesis. This chapter has been pointing out some of the limitations of this view of history, and comparing these limitations to the points of crisis encountered, as summarised in Chaps. 1 and 2, in French Hegelianism and Marxist psychology. For all the elegance of Althusser's rendition of the epistemological break, it relies on the supposition of a succession of 'objects' that manifest as 'blind spots' in any given framework. It therefore makes the history of science into a procession of constantly emerging 'pineal glands',

[123] Althusser, 'The Place of Psychoanalysis', p. 59.

which gravitates towards both revelation, and the integration of different fields. As suggested above, there is a rendition here of what Lacan criticised in Pavlov as belief in a 'knowledge in the real', because Althusser assumes that there is a 'necessary' impingement of knowledge on the movement of history.

Althusser, as described earlier in this chapter, harshly criticises Lévi-Strauss for the obscurantist residues remaining in his work. Whilst he deems it a useful and ambitious attempt to map out ideological frameworks and their cultural effects, he also argues, in his 1966 critique, that structural anthropology represents a regressive step away from Marx's theory of ideology, because it detached these frameworks from the historically dependent modes of production that Marx located at the source of ideologies. Lévi-Strauss, as a result, resorts to unsatisfactory appeals to the 'brain' or 'human spirit' as material origins of the unconscious structures whose logic he traces out. Althusser's reading of Spinoza allows him to facilitate a reconciliation between structuralism and the Marxist theory of ideology, through the notion of structural causality—the idea that structural wholes act on the individual elements they contain. Viewing the subject of ideology as an *effect* of ideology—as a body bequeathed subjectivity through the action of culture—removes the need for any appeal to Lévi-Strauss's suspect materialist substrates. At the same time, though, raising ideology to this degree of pervasiveness leaves the question, posed by Ricoeur, of how these structures are ever to be escaped or transformed—of what, in other words, there is remaining in subjectivity to resist ideology. Althusser follows Bachelard here in putting forward the idea of the epistemological break as a mechanism for such a transformation on the level of scientific development. He goes further than Bachelard, however, by also indexing the epistemological break onto the level of individual biography, and by making the epistemological break the mechanism for an individual's personal break with an ideological framework. This allows Althusser to tackle in an original way the problem of how to mark the division between Hegel and Marx.

As this chapter has been pointing out, however, when Althusser isolates the symptomatic points and structural contradictions within Marx—and when he attempts to use the passage of Marx's own biography to illustrate how an epistemological break is precipitated in an individual's life—what is missing, in the last instance, is another mechanism to explain the epistemological break, beyond either a reliance on Marx's subjective personhood, an appeal to Marx's psychobiography, or the idea of the 'experience of history'. The questions remain in Althusser of how Marx could say what he, by very definition, could not say—and of how the veil of ideology can be understood as all-pervasive, whilst also preserving the possibility of breaking through it to the truth.

Butters of Enjoyment

Lacan has his own, different way of articulating the relationship between Marx and Hegel. Like Althusser, though, he also does so with reference to the dimension of the symptom. The first time Lacan describes this relationship is in the chapter of the *Écrits* 'On the Subject Who Is Finally in Question'. The text was written in 1966, just one year after the publication of *Reading Capital*, and is clearly responding to the ideas Althusser put forward there in 1965. The view of the symptom Lacan articulates in 'On the Subject' gives a distinct reorientation to the idea of the epistemological break. In the text, Lacan gives a brief outline of the pre-history of the Freudian logic of the symptom. The pre-psychoanalytic 'dimension' of the symptom, says Lacan, represented what he describes as 'the return of truth as such into the gap of a certain knowledge'.[124] It is a logic that identifies truth at the point of failure of knowledge. A logic of the symptom, says Lacan, allows this gap in knowledge to be viewed not as 'a failure of representation' but as 'a truth of another reference than the one [...] whose fine order it manages to disturb'.[125] This is so far in line with Althusser's view of transitions between epistemological fields. To see a hole or void in a system—what Althusser calls an invisible object with respect to scientific fields—as a symptom is, for Lacan too, to see it as part of another, as-yet imperceptible, order of truth. In this sense, Lacan identifies Marx's role in the development of this logic as follows:

[124] Lacan, 'On the Subject Who Is Finally in Question', in *Écrits*, pp. 189–196 (p. 194).
[125] Lacan, 'On the Subject', p. 194.

> one can say that this dimension is highly differentiated in Marx's critique, even if it is not made explicit there. And one can say that a part of the reversal of Hegel that he carries out is constituted by the return (which is a materialist return, precisely insofar as it gives it figure and body) of the question of truth. The latter actually forces itself upon us, I would go so far as to say, not by taking up the thread of the ruse of reason, a subtle form with which Hegel sends it packing, but by upsetting these ruses (read Marx's political writings) which are merely dressed up with reason[.][126]

The 'question of truth', as Lacan presents it here, is warded off by Hegel's account of the way spirit manipulates individual historical actors. But this 'question of truth' comes returning in full force when Hegel's logic is punctured, in this case by truth being 'given figure and body' by Marx. Truth is given this 'figure and body' by him, because he finds it in the material reality that interrupts knowledge, rather than in knowledge's own neat choreography. Lacan is in sympathy here with the Althusserian idea of Marx's 'symptomatisation' of Hegel. Marx's critique of Hegel, says Lacan, facilitates the return of truth as a 'gap' in knowledge, by upsetting Hegel's ruses of reason, and marking them as deficient. As Althusser also outlines, Marx brings to the fore something that Hegel cannot articulate, but something that is also immanent to Hegel in a certain, unregistered form. Marx is presented by Lacan here in the same way that he is by Althusser: as making a break away from Hegel, and into a new framework of thought that Marx structured around something that is missing from Hegel.

Lacan continues 'On the Subject', however, by giving Freud a position in this drama, and in relation to Marx's introduction of the logic of the symptom. As Lacan mentions in the passage quoted above, the 'dimension' of the symptom is 'not made explicit' by Marx. In this context, Freud, he says, makes a radical leap. Freud fully realises the dimension of the symptom, for Lacan, because the Freudian symptom is not a 'representation' of truth; the Freudian symptom *is* truth. Freud, says Lacan:

> sets himself apart from the rest by clearly linking the status of the symptom to the status of his own operation, for the Freudian operation is the

[126] Lacan, 'On the Subject', p. 194.

> symptom's proper operation, in the two senses of the term. Unlike a sign—or smoke which is never found in the absence of fire, a fire that smoke indicates with the possible call to put it out—a symptom can only be interpreted in the signifying order. A signifier has meaning only through its relation to another signifier. The truth of symptoms resides in this articulation. Symptoms remained somewhat vague when they were understood as representing some irruption of truth. In fact they are truth, being made of the same wood from which truth is made, if we posit materialistically that truth is what is instated on the basis of the signifying chain.[127]

Because Lacan understands a Freudian symptom as a signifier, he positions symptoms here not as pointing to a truth of another order, but as existing, as all signifiers do, only in relation to other co-ordinates of the symbolic field of signifiers. The central example of this would be Freud's classical method of interpreting hysterical symptoms. For Freud, the hysteric's paralysed limb or incurable cough does not point to another order, of the neurological or the spiritual, but has a position only in a symbolic network, and is only treatable on this basis. Lacan makes Freud the architect of a flattened epistemology: for him, there is no dimension of truth to be pointed to or distinguished on its own terms; truth is 'instated' by the signifying chain, and the symptom is but one element in this signifying chain.

There is a subtle but significant gap between what Lacan is saying here, and how Althusser presents the positions of Hegel, Marx, and Freud in the history of science. In the way that Lacan presents this relationship, there is no sense, as there is in Althusser, of Marx struggling to articulate something post-Hegelian via concepts that are ill-equipped to perform this articulation. Marx's break amounts, for Lacan, to a shift in perspective, away from understanding the obstacles to a given order as failures of this order's truth, that instead sees these obstacles *as* its truth. Marx is taken by Lacan to be responsible, in this way, for a new order of thought, which breaks through the ruses of reason to find truth in the gaps in this facade.[128]

---

[127] Lacan, 'On the Subject', p. 194–195.

[128] Lacan later describes this as Marx's departure from the order of the 'semblance'. See Lacan, Lesson of 16 June 1971, 'X. Du mythe que Freud a forgé', in *Le Séminaire, Livre XVIII, D'un dis-*

Like Althusser, Lacan identifies in Freud a recuperation or continuation of Marx. For Althusser, both Freud and Marx were instrumental in synthesising the sciences of the biological and the social. In the passages from 'On the Subject' quoted above, Lacan also presents Marx as having made a materialist turn, and Freud as having repeated this in the position his theories gave to the symptom. Freud is not taken by Lacan, however, to have synthesised fields, or to have joined together regimes of knowledge. Lacan does not retain the idea, latent in Althusser, of pieces of science being put together in the correct way, or of secret truths being revealed by them. What Lacan also departs from here is the idea that a privileged object—which Althusser had identified in surplus value—was produced by Marx. As this chapter has been suggesting, the sequence of invisible objects that, for Althusser, form the motor for the history of science, preserves something of the 'irruption of truth' that Lacan, in the passage above, understands the dimension of the symptom to have broken *away* from. The endpoint of Lacan's historical vignette here is not an 'object', but rather Freud's approach to the symptom, as the appearance of the signifier in the body.

Despite the fact that, in the passage above, Lacan clearly privileges Freud as the true herald of the symptom, Lacan in many ways makes clearer there than it is made by Althusser what Marx really mobilised epistemologically. The question, for example, that this chapter has identified as still remaining in Althusser, of whether or not Marx stumbled independently on a Spinozist logic, is not an important one for Lacan, because he is not attempting to use Spinoza to defeat Hegel. This means that he does not have to pretend that this logic came to Marx independently of Hegel. Lacan, unlike Althusser, sees Marx as having been able to articulate the dimension of the symptom *because* he was responding to Hegel—and not because he simply stumbled, as he appears to have in Althusser's account, on something Spinozist, in the Hegelian tea leaves that he then discarded. Lacan seems here, rather, to think of Marx as reading Hegel—at least on the level, where he sees Marx as being most successful, of his differentiation of the symptom—in the same way that

cours qui ne serait pas du semblant (1971), ed. by Jacques-Alain Miller (Paris: Seuil, 2007), pp. 163–178 (pp. 164)

Lacan himself reads Hegel. As discussed in Chap. 2, Lacan's understanding of absolute knowledge led him to think of neither himself nor of anyone else as going 'beyond' Hegel. To repeat the words he used to describe Kierkegaard, Lacan takes Marx to have realised the 'truth of the Hegelian formula'—a truth that would overturn this formula through a strategy of pure, limitless assent. In Lacan's article 'On the Subject Who Is Finally in Question', Marx is not described as breaking from Hegel, but as doing quite the opposite: like Kierkegaard, he gets right to the heart of Hegel, and realises one full version of the truth of his philosophy.

The aim of the present chapter of this book is not only to stage a comparison between Althusser and Lacan. Beyond cataloguing the differences between the way each understands Marx's part in the history of the symptom, it also seeks to emphasise the consequences these differences held for the way Lacan has, much more recently, been positioned in relation to Marx. One result of Althusser's inability, which this chapter has highlighted, to unite the levels of subjectivity and history, is the position given to *jouissance* in Žižek's theory of ideology. As discussed earlier in the chapter, the trouble with finding ideology everywhere in subjectivity, as Althusser does in his famous essay on 'Ideology and Ideological State Apparatuses' (1970), is that everything in subjectivity then *becomes* ideology.[129] Althusser therefore has to argue that all constitution of subjectivity is a distortion, because he claims that a subject is only formed by being interpellated by an ideological structure. But what, then, of the significance that Althusser gives to the epistemological break? How can breaking through to the truth from any ideological formation be possible for a subject, if subjectivity is permeated by misrecognition to the very core? What point, as Ricoeur asks, 'would there be in a critique of miscognition if it were not for the sake of a more faithful recognition?'.[130] This uninhibited recognition is made impossible if there is no gap between the subject and the structures of ideology for the subject to escape through. Yet the possibility of 'true recognition' beyond the veil of

[129] Althusser, 'Ideology and Ideological State Apparatuses', in *On the Reproduction of Capitalism: Ideology and Ideological State Apparatuses* (London: Verso, 2014), pp. 232–272.

[130] Ricoeur, 'Althusser's Theory of Ideology', p. 65.

ideology is, as Ricoeur argues, something Althusser wants to rescue—and he reserves the epistemological break as a mechanism for its realisation.

Lacan, from one perspective, might appear to step in to solve this problem for Althusser. This is one way to read a certain thread that recurs frequently in Žižek's work; an explicit aspect of which, particularly in his earlier writings, is the use of the Lacanian elements of *jouissance* and the object *a* to elaborate how a subject is 'hooked' into ideology. The object *a* was originally introduced by Lacan in the late 1950s, in an explicit departure from the British object relations school of psychoanalysis, to articulate the object of desire sought by the subject in the other. As will be described in detail in Chap. 5, the significance Lacan gives to the object *a* later undergoes a distinct shift, in *Seminar XVI: From an Other to the other* (1968–69), where Lacan positions the object *a* as the fulcrum between formless *jouissance* and the structure of the symbolic order. The position Lacan gives to the object *a* as a mediator between these levels allows Žižek to appeal to the object *a* as a supplement to Althusser's theory of ideology. The concept of the object *a* is used by Žižek for the combined purposes of providing a mechanism for the subject's ideological interpellation and, simultaneously, of propping up the gap, which disappears in Althusser except in a vague, ill-defined form, between the subject and ideology. Žižek positions the object *a* as the 'sublime object of ideology'—the 'fantasmatic support of ideological propositions'.[131] Dovetailing Lacan's theory of fantasy and Althusser's theory of ideology, Žižek makes the object *a* the event horizon of ideological frameworks, that invests them with the subjective enjoyment of *jouissance*, and enables them to hold sway over their subjects.

Žižek also gives the account, which was missing in Althusser, of how the 'traversal of the fantasy'—the fantasy to which, for Žižek, an ideological framework amounts—is possible. The grasp of ideology can be escaped if I am able to perceive my *jouissance* for what it truly is in this context: if, says Žižek, I '"unhook" my *jouissance* from its fantasmatic frame, and acknowledge it as that which is properly undecidable, as an indivisible remainder that is neither an inherently "reactionary" support for historical inertia, nor a liberating force enabling us to undermine the constraints

[131] Žižek, *The Parallax View* (Cambridge, Massachusetts: MIT Press, 2006), p. 40.

of the existing order'.[132] Žižek's quite open intention here is to position *jouissance* as the missing substance of Althusser's theory of ideology. *Jouissance* becomes a magic bullet—the ultimate pineal gland—able to replace all of Althusser's remaining reliance on unconscious impulses or historical necessity. Instead, it is this core of senselessness at the heart of the subject's connection with the symbolic that makes sense of the epistemological break. Two problems that were immanent to structuralism—of the material connection of structure to individuals, and of how structures shift and change—appear thereby to have been resolved.

In this way, Žižek makes Lacan the missing piece of Althusser's theories of ideology and history. However, something is ignored when Lacan is used in this way. This is the idea—which Lacan introduces in the mid-1960s—that the knowledge of the unconscious made possible by psychoanalysis enables a much more fundamental departure from any kind of knowledge that came before. Chapter 3 summarised part of the first lesson of *Seminar XV: The Psychoanalytic Act* (1967–68), delivered in 1967, for the critique Lacan carries out there of Pavlov's experiments in reflexology. In the midst of the lesson's reading of Pavlov, there is a brief discussion of how the emergence of psychoanalysis subverts idealism. Lacan is clear here that there exists a firm connection between the 'question of the act' in psychoanalysis—the topic of that year's seminar—with the 'question of the act of the *birth* of psychoanalysis'; the question of its appearance historically.[133] 'Did this field', Lacan asks, that psychoanalysis 'organises, over which it reigns in more or less governing it, did this field exist before?'.[134] The question Lacan is asking is whether the field of the unconscious can be understood to have existed before psychoanalysis. Obviously, as he points out, what Freud would name the unconscious made its effects felt before the act of the birth of psychoanalysis: it was through these effects that Freud was first able to study it. But the intervention Lacan makes here is to point out the effect that the origin of psychoanalysis, and the knowledge of the unconscious that it produced,

132 Žižek, *The Parallax View*, p. 687.

133 Lacan, Lesson 1, of 15 November 1957, in *Seminar XV: The Psychoanalytic Act*, unpublished. Available in an unofficial English translation by Cormac Gallagher, at <http://www.lacaninireland.com/web/wp-content/uploads/2010/06/Book-15-The-Psychoanalytical-Act.pdf>, p. 5. My italics.

134 Lacan, Lesson 1, in *Seminar XV*. See Gallagher, p. 5.

had on the level of scientific knowledge as a whole. The question of 'who knew' that this field of the unconscious existed is, he says, 'perhaps not without import here'.[135] Therein lies Lacan's strict delineation of the break psychoanalysis makes from any idealism. This centres on his distinction between *connaissance* and *savoir*, the two words for 'knowledge' in French:

> In effect, does this question have any other import than the *Epoché*,[136] the idealist suspension, that which is founded on the idea, taken as radical, of representation, as founding all knowing [*connaissance*], and which therefore asks: outside of this representation where is reality? It is absolutely certain that the question which I am raising in the form of "who knew [*savait*] this field of psychoanalysis?" has absolutely nothing to do with the fallacious antinomy on which idealism is founded, it is clear that there is no question of contesting that reality is prior to knowing [*connaissance*]. Reality, yes! But know*ledge* [*savoir*]?[137]

The argument of this passage can be broken down into three points. Firstly, that idealism makes a subsumption of reality under representation. As Lacan points out, this is based on what he calls a 'fallacious antinomy', between representation and reality. Chapter 3 discussed in detail Lacan's concern in the mid-1960s with demonstrating how ineffectual this dichotomy truly is. There is, as he argues in *Seminar XI*, a more acute form of traumatic reality encountered in the psychic representations of dreams.[138] It is incontestable, he clarifies in the above passage from *Seminar XV*, that reality exists prior to '*connaissance*'—which can be translated into English as 'knowing'. The idealism he criticises

---

[135] Lacan, Lesson 1, in *Seminar XV*. See Gallagher, p. 5.

[136] Or 'bracketing' in English, the phenomenological tool of setting aside assumptions and beliefs developed by Husserl in *Ideas* (1931).

[137] 'En effet, cette question n'a-t-elle pas d'autre portée que l'époché, la suspension idéaliste, celle qui se fonde sur l'idée, prise comme radicale, de la représentation, comme fondant toute connaissance et qui dès lors demande hors de cette représentation où est la réalité. Il est absolument certain que la question que je lève sous la forme du qui le savait? ce champ de la psychanalyse n'a absolument rien à faire avec l'antinomie fallacieuse où se fonde l'idéalisme, il est clair qu'il n'est pas question de contester que la réalité est antérieure à la connaissance. La réalité, oui! mais le savoir?' (Lesson 1, *Seminar XV*, unpublished manuscript)

[138] See Lacan, Lesson of 12 February 1964, 'V. 'Tuché and Automaton', in *Seminar XI: The Four Fundamental Concepts of Psychoanalysis* (1964–1965), ed. by Jacques-Alain Miller, trans. by Alan Sheridan (London: Norton, 1998), pp. 53–66.

here is concerned with this level of 'knowing'. Lacan is making a distinction here between '*connaissance*', or 'know*ing*', and '*savoir*', or '*knowledge*'. Reality may be prior to *connaissance*, but not, he posits here, to *savoir*.

Secondly, the passage above identifies two opponents to the epistemological intervention Lacan understands psychoanalysis to have made. The first opponent is the level of *connaissance*, privileged by idealism; which wrongly—for reasons discussed in detail in Chap. 3—pits representation against the real, and which, as a result, raises the false problem of whether reality can be found outside of representation. As also described in Chap. 3, Lacan criticises Pavlov in this lesson of *Seminar XV*, for propagating the second opponent of psychoanalysis that he identifies here: the materialist belief that knowledge—*savoir*—is there in the real waiting for the scientist to make it emerge. Lacan identifies this belief, in the following passage of the lesson, with the spiritualism usually associated with the mystifications of idealism:

> What it is all about when it comes to the divine dimension and generally that of the spirit revolves entirely around this: what do we assume to be already there before we find it? If over a whole field it turns out that it would not be futile, but trivial, to think that this knowledge [*savoir*] is already there waiting for us before we bring it up, this could be of a nature to make us carry out a much more profound questioning.[139]

In the passage above, he is determining the stakes of psychoanalysis in this question of what is 'already there' before a scientific discovery. Because psychoanalysis abandons the belief—which Lacan accuses of Pavlov of cultivating—that knowledge waits to be discovered in the real, psychoanalysis also departs from what Lacan characterises here as a 'divine dimension' of the 'spirit'. It is in the rejection of both these positions—of the dichotomy between representation and real; and the belief in

---

[139] Lacan, Lesson 1, in *Seminar XV*. 'Ce dont il s'agit quand il s'agit de la dimension divine et généralement de celle de l'esprit, tourne tout entier autour de ceci: qu'est-ce que nous supposons être déjà là avant que nous en fassions la trouvaille? Si sur tout un champ il s'avère qu'il serait non pas futile, mais léger, de penser que ce savoir est déjà là à nous attendre avant que nous le fassions surgir, ceci pourrait être de nature à nous faire faire une tellement plus profonde remise en question'.

knowledge in the real—that psychoanalysis, as Lacan presents it here, amounts to a definitive departure from idealism and the spiritualism associated with it. Lacan can be read as operating here with the same logical clarity that Althusser displays in his account of Marx's position in the history of science; but as extending this account, with precision, to a question raised to it by Freud. Oxygen, according to Althusser, was not an object before Lavoisier, and surplus value was not an object before Marx. But what, asks Lacan here, was the status of the unconscious before Freud, if the unconscious *is* knowledge that is not known? Freud cannot be subsumed into the Althusserian co-ordinates for mapping the history of science, if the epistemological consequences of psychoanalysis are expressed as Lacan does so here.

Thirdly, this passage from *Seminar XV* gives the epistemological consequences of psychoanalysis a level of *historical* significance. As this book as a whole has been arguing, a different, more precise, and more subtle relationship can be understood to exist between Marx and Lacan than that put forward in contemporary scholarship, when this relationship is read in the context of developments in Marxist thought. The book will continue, in the following chapter, by focusing on Lacan's own concern with the position of psychoanalysis in history. One purpose of the extended discussion of Althusser's philosophy in the present chapter has been to introduce how these same questions were approached by him. This chapter has been identifying the ways in which Althusser's work of the 1960s repeats the crises described in Chaps. 1 and 2 of the thesis: firstly, the question of how to think about breaks in a philosopher's oeuvre in terms of shifts in their biography, which preoccupied the French Hegelians struggling to reconcile an existential subject with Hegel's work; and secondly, the problem of how to respond to the limits that were encountered when reflexology was used as a means of understanding, geometrising, and giving structure to subjectivity.

For Althusser, capitalism is a veil covering all human experience. In his theory of ideology, it becomes a kind of original sin which fundamentally wounds reality, in a way that bars human perception from accessing this reality. It is not clear how this condition could be escaped, because, for Althusser, belief in unhindered access to this reality would be the biggest illusion of all. A logic of the symptom, as he operationalises it, is able at least to appreciate this trap for what it is. In certain respects, this Althusserian position towards capitalism and ideology is taken even further by Lacan. However, as the following chapter will illustrate, whilst maximising the idea of the ensnaring nature of capitalism, Lacan does away with any notion remaining in Althusser of an escape from its logic. His own reading of Hegel leads him to understand capitalism in a very different way. Lacan does not think that Marx made a break from anything: he instead emphasises Marx's ultimate *continuity* with a subterranean logic that had existed before him, and that was manifested in capitalism. Lacan even argues that Marx unleashes the potential of this logic more fully than anyone else.

The theoretical impasses Althusser encounters are obstacles to the translation of his theories into a practical politics. This chapter has shown how Lacan has been used by Žižek to supress these impasses. Lacan, however, does not solve the problems in Althusser' theories, but only makes them more apparent. Something else has to be appreciated about Lacan that does not sit so easily with a set of Marxist assumptions, but that holds a no less important position in the history of Marxism this book has been depicting. The present chapter has discussed the limits of Althusser's theory of a history of science guided by the logic of the symptom. The following chapter will develop further how Lacan's own way of understanding the history of science in the late 1960s and early 1970s responds to, and departs from, both Althusser, and structuralism more generally. For Lacan, as the chapter will show through close readings of *Seminar XVI*, *Seminar XVII*, and 'Radiophonie', Marx invented the logic of the symptom only by misrecognising the change that he also brought about on the level of knowledge in history—a change that Lacan describes as the 'founding of capitalism'.

5

Capitalism and the Symptom: Marx's Two Inventions

This book has been articulating how Lacan's work responded to pressing questions encountered in the history of Marxism. It has been demonstrating that, when Lacan is situated in the historical context of Marxist thought, and of traditions of thought closely associated with it, different facets to this relationship can be identified to those that have been registered in existing literature. The book has not been laying out a cache of correspondences between Marx and Lacan. An increasing number of their readers have already taken something more like this approach, and have mapped these out thoroughly, and in some cases elegantly.[1] This book is arguing that, as a direct result of contemporary enthusiasm about that set of correspondences, the subtleties of Lacan's position in the history of Marxism have been neglected. The previous three chapters have

[1] See, for example, Pietro Bianchi, 'The Discourse and the Capitalist. Lacan, Marx, and the Question of the Surplus', *Filosofski vestnik*, 31, no. 2 (2010), 123–137; Ceren Özselçuk and Yahya M. Madra, 'Enjoyment as an Economic Factor: Reading Marx with Lacan', *Subjectivity*, 3 (2010), 323–347; Roger A. Salerno, 'Imagining Marx Imagining Lacan', *Critical Sociology*, 44, no. 2 (2018), 259–266; David Pavón-Cuéllar, 'Lacanianizing Marxism: The Effects of Lacan in Readings of Marx and Marxist Thinkers', *Critique*, 6, no. 1 (May 2019), 262–289; and Samo Tomšič, 'Homology: Marx and Lacan', in *Journal of the Jan van Eyck Circle for Lacanian Ideology Critique*, 5 (2012), pp. 98–112 (pp. 110–111); Slavoj Žižek, *The Sublime Object of Ideology* (London: Verso, 1989); and Alenka Zupančič, *What is Sex?* (London: MIT Press, 2017).

M. Maher, *Symptom Invented*, The Palgrave Lacan Series,
https://doi.org/10.1007/978-3-032-12267-4_5

attempted to restore these subtleties through discussions of French Hegelianism, the pursuit of a materialist psychology, and Althusser's theories of the history of science. Each chapter has described how Lacan identified questions in these milieux of thought, and attempted, with important results, to position psychoanalysis as an opening onto different ways to approach these questions. This chapter will move on to discuss in detail the extended response to Marx made by Lacan in the late 1960s and early 1970s.

This episode amounts in part to Lacan's distancing of himself from the structuralist project. It is also an explicit response to Althusser's work, which contains Lacan's own full, revised elaboration of the relationship that Althusser imagined to exist between Marx and psychoanalysis. As the chapter will discuss at length, in 1968, in *Seminar XVI: From an Other to the other* (1968–69), Lacan announces that a 'homology' exists between his and Marx's theories—that they have a continuous logic. He then develops a theory of the signifier and *jouissance* that adapts the theory of value laid out in Marx's critique of political economy. The theoretical detail of this episode has been reconstructed assiduously by several philosophers and psychoanalysts.[2] This chapter breaks from them, however, by emphasising the moments where Lacan announces a *departure* from Marx—where he outlines a fundamental break between psychoanalytic theory and either the theory or politics of Marxism.[3]

As the present chapter will discuss, there was a clear reformulation of Lacan's theories at this point in the late 1960s. This was a reformulation in which Marx's critique of political economy played an important role.

---

[2] See Jacques-Alain Miller, 'A Reading of the Seminar *From an Other to the other*, Part I', trans. by Barbara P. Fulks, *lacanian ink*, 29, pp. 8–61; Samo Tomšič, *The Capitalist Unconscious: Marx and Lacan* (London: Verso, 2013); Alenka Zupančič, '3. Contradictions that Matter', in *What is Sex?* (London: MIT Press, 2017), pp. 35–72.

[3] For summaries of Lacan's references to Marx, see Mauricio Cardoso and Vinicius Darriba, 'A Referência a Marx no Ensino de Lacan', *Psicologia; Teoria e Pesquisa* 32, no. 1 (January–March 2016); and Pierre Bruno, *Lacan and Marx: The Invention of the Symptom*, trans. by John Holland (London: Routledge, 2019). For other more specific accounts of Lacan's reading of Marx, see Sidi Askofaré, 'Le symptôme sociale' (1989), in *Marx et Lénine, Freud et Lacan, Actes de 2e Colloque de La Découverte Freudienne*, ed., by A. Soueix (Toulouse, Mirail, 1992); David Pavon-Cuellar, *Lacan, lecteur de Marx* (Rouen: Universite de Rouen, 2013); François Regnault, 'Le Marx de Lacan', *La Lettre Mensuelle de l'ECF*, 242 (2005), 4–6; and Fabio Vighi, Capitalist Bulimia: Lacan on Marx and Crisis, *Crisis and Critique*, 3 (2016), 414–432.

It did not, however, amount to a 'Marxification' of his earlier theories, or, as has been suggested, to a 'second return to Freud' that supplemented Lacan's earlier reference to structural linguistics with Marx's critique of political economy.[4] From the late 1960s onwards, Lacan emphasises very clearly both what it is crucial to learn from Marx, and what he considers to be the limits of Marx's theories. Lacan claims at this point that Marx does not represent an antidote to capitalism, but that his theories, when they are understood by way of Lacan's theory of discourse, actually unwittingly played a central role in the operation of capitalist logic. Lacan delineates, in this way, what he considers to be Marx's paradoxical status. This chapter will interpret Lacan's reading of Marx as an important context for the position he gives to psychoanalysis in the history of science, and for the function he understands psychoanalysis to have in civilisation. Lacan argues that there is a point of fundamental contradiction framed by Marx, and that this—rather than a political or theoretical programme—is the most significant element to be taken from Marx's work. Psychoanalysis, the chapter will show, is positioned by Lacan as a science that inherits, and that only exists because of, this point of flux.

These aspects of Lacan's thinking about Marx have not been fully appreciated in existing analyses of their relationship. The idea that a 'homology' exists between the two has too often been used as grounds to turn Lacan into something of a supplement to Marx, as if the logic of Marx's critique of political economy is extended by Lacan into a complete theory of ideology and subjectivity. The previous chapters of this book have shown how conflicts in the history of Marxist thought make this approach redundant, because Lacan was deliberately responding to *gaps* and *crises* that had been encountered by Marxist thinkers. The present chapter follows by making it clear how Lacan understands his own relationship to Marx. After outlining the homology presented by Lacan in *Seminar XVI*, and challenging the reading of it made by Samo Tomšič, this chapter goes on to summarise the critique of Marx made by Lacan in *Seminar XVII* and his 1970 radio interview, published later that year as 'Radiophonie'. The chapter will present Lacan's interpretation of Marx as a historical event, and as a significant moment in the history of Marxism.

[4] See Samo Tomšič, *The Capitalist Unconscious: Marx and Lacan* (London: Verso, 2013), p. 2.

It will articulate the subtleties of this reading, and point out how it took up the radical shifts in reading Marx that, as described in earlier chapters, had been precipitated by Lacan's contemporaries.

The Scissors' Cut: Inaugurating a Homology

The seminar Lacan gave in the years 1968–69, *Seminar XVI: From an Other to the other*, is the text where he gives his most sustained attention to Marx. Its very first lesson opens with a direct discussion of Marx. In this and its following two lessons, Lacan makes a detailed, theoretically dense response to Marx's critique of political economy. As this section of the present chapter will emphasise, Lacan is not, here, transposing Marx's discoveries from the plane of economics and onto that of psychic structure, in an operation whose paradigm would be the Freudo-Marxism of Reich or Marcuse, or the 'monstrous combinations' formed by the awkward stewing of Marxist philosophy and Freudian metapsychology that Vygotsky had ridiculed in the work of Luria and Fridman.[5] Lacan's work is instead much more like the kind of thorough reading of Marx that Vygotsky had in mind when he wrote 'The Meaning of the Historical Crisis in Psychology'. What Lacan begins in *Seminar XVI* is an attempted intervention in the trajectory of existing Marxist thought, and in existing readings of Marx.

Seminar XVI also carries out a shift in Lacan's theory of the signifier. This shift is directly and explicitly connected to Lacan's reading of Marx at this point. Lacan's earlier theoretical paradigm, as articulated most fully in 'The Subversion of the Subject and the Dialectic of Desire in the Freudian Unconscious' (1960), takes *jouissance* to be off-limits for the subject of the signifier. *Jouissance*, at this point, is presented by Lacan to be 'prohibited to whoever speaks', and the Oedipal subject, who is founded on 'that very prohibition', is understood to have no access to

[5] See Chapter 3, p. 97, n. 55; and L.S Vygotsky, 'The Meaning of the Historical Crisis in Psychology', in *The Collected Works of L.S. Vygotsky, Vol. 3: Problems of the Theory and History of Psychology*, trans. by René van der Veer (New York: Springer, 1997), pp. 233–244.

jouissance.[6] According to that earlier paradigm, there is an effect of 'pure loss' on the speaking being as a result of the very presence of the signifier, and their subjection to the signifier makes it fundamentally impossible for them to attain *jouissance*.[7] The shift Lacan makes in *Seminar XVI* is to understand the signifier not as a barrier to *jouissance*, but instead as productive of—or, in other words, as the *cause* of—*jouissance* in a certain form. The name Lacan gives to his new theoretical invention, of what is produced by the loss of *jouissance*, is '*plus-de-jouir*'. This roughly translates as 'surplus-enjoyment' in English.[8]

To put it another way, what Lacan engineers from the late 1960s is a perspectival shift on his previous work, after which he treats loss as having a positive manifestation, on a structural level, as an excess, or a surplus. Loss of *jouissance* is understood by Lacan, after this shift, not as the absence of *jouissance*, but as a new modality of *jouissance*. As the opening lessons of *Seminar XVI* describe, the logic of Marx's critique of political economy, and in particular his theory of the production of surplus value, is the model for this later theoretical paradigm.[9] The same recognition—that loss can be made to register as *surplus*—is made by Marx in *Capital*: according to Marx, what political economy failed to comprehend was how capitalism deploys this perspectival shift on the level of economics, in order to generate capital. As the current section will outline in detail, Lacan theorises from 1968 onwards that, just as capital produces surplus value, the signifier produces *plus-de-jouir*. At this point in the late 1960s, Lacan uses Marx's critique of political economy as an index for the structure of subjectivity.

---

[6] Lacan, 'The Subversion of the Subject and the Dialectic of Desire', in *Écrits*, trans. by Bruce Fink (London: Norton, 2006), pp. 671–702 (p. 696).

[7] Alenka Zupančič, *What is Sex?* (London: MIT Press, 2017), p. 46. As Zupančič puts it, in the later paradigm this 'pure loss' now appears 'on the side of the signifier, which no longer has, or relates to, another side (pure organic need on which it would perform its inaugural operation); what it has is a reverse side (*l'envers*)'.

[8] Because the word *jouissance* is usually used left untranslated in English, I have chosen to keep the word *plus-de-jouir* in French here as well. Other writers discussed in this chapter use 'surplus-enjoyment' or 'surplus *jouissance*' as a translation of *plus-de-jouir*. Where they do so in passages cited below, I have amended their translation to the original French '*plus-de-jouir*'. I have also italicised their uses of the word *jouissance*, in line with this book's typography.

[9] Though not the latest—this represents a transitional episode, after which Lacan moves to his final phase, which attempts to think the unstructurable through topology and knots.

Lacan begins *Seminar XVI* by placing emphasis on his concept of 'discourse', and by distancing himself from the structuralist movement with which he had been associated, and had associated himself, since the 1950s. Before the start of the first lesson, Lacan has written the following phrase on the blackboard: 'The essence of psychoanalytic theory is a discourse without speech [*parole*]'.[10] This formula acts as a summation of the place Lacan is giving structuralism within psychoanalysis. As Lacan articulates it in the opening of this lesson, what structuralism takes seriously is 'knowledge [*savoir*] *qua* cause': the idea that *knowledge* (*savoir*) itself produces effects in the world.[11] Lacan reiterates his description of the status of the unconscious in these terms. The unconscious, he says, is a network of signifiers; a knowledge (*savoir*) that does not appear in words, but that nevertheless functions as a cause for all human phenomena. The psychoanalyst, he adds, occupies a position from which they are able to show where a discourse 'breaks down [*défaillance*]', into the holes that, for Lacan, always exist in its structure.[12] At this point in the first lesson of *Seminar XVI*, Lacan begins his reference to Marx. He points out how the integration of Marx into his theories had been long anticipated, and how Marx 'certainly has his place' in them.[13] He also makes an oblique reference to Althusser's work on the 'object of *Capital*' in the 1965 lectures that had been published the same year in *Reading Capital* (*Lire le Capital*).[14]

In this opening lesson, Lacan takes up the question of the 'object' of a science into the register of psychoanalysis. As outlined in the previous chapter, this idea was central to Althusser's account of the history of science. Althusser argues that surplus value was both the object of Marx's economics, and its key discovery, and that this object was structurally unthinkable within the context of the theory of political economy that he overturned. Sciences in general, as articulated by the Bachelardian schema

---

[10] Jacques Lacan, Lesson of 13 November 1968, 'I. From Surplus Value to Surplus Jouissance', in *Seminar XVI: From an Other to the other*, ed. by Jacques-Alain Miller, trans. by Bruce Fink (London: Polity, 2024), pp. 3–16 (p. 3).

[11] Lacan, *Seminar XVI*, p. 6.

[12] Lacan, *Seminar XVI*, p. 7.

[13] Lacan, *Seminar XVI*, p. 8.

[14] Louis Althusser, *Lire le Capital* (Paris: Maspero, 1965).

Althusser builds on, transform, or emerge in the first place, by introducing rogue objects to existing epistemological fields, that, since these objects cannot be comprehended by those fields, necessitate their transformation. In *Seminar XVI*, Lacan reformulates the status of the object *a* in light of this. Before this point, he had presented the object *a* more as a zone of the body—as a 'corporeal specimen', as Miller puts it.[15] In *Seminar XVI*, however, Lacan makes the object *a* the 'object' of psychoanalysis, in the Althusserian sense. Lacan makes it the object that, before him, had been as vaguely realised as surplus value had been by political economy.[16]

In this opening lesson of *Seminar XVI*, Lacan develops his classical formulation that 'the unconscious is the Other's discourse', by describing the field of the Other as a 'market'.[17] He rearticulates the Other in these economic terms, as having the structure, now, of a marketplace, so that he can posit the Other as the site of exchanges of *plus-de-jouir*.[18] Through this economic metaphor, Lacan establishes an identity between *plus-de-jouir* and the object *a*:

> *Plus-de-jouir* arises from the renunciation of *jouissance* owing to the effect of discourse. It is what gives object *a* its place. Insofar as the market defines any object whatsoever of human labour as a commodity, this object bears within itself some element of surplus value. *Plus-de-jouir* is thus what allows us to isolate the function of the object *a*.[19]

---

[15] As Jacques-Alain Miller glosses, in *Seminar X: Anxiety* (1962–63) the object *a* was 'understood through the signifier, but as a corporeal specimen', whereas in *Seminar XVI: From an Other to the other*, 'we see the object *a* understood as a pure logical function'. See Miller, 'A Reading of the Seminar *From an Other to the other*, Part I', trans. by Barbara P. Fulks, *lacanian ink*, 29, pp. 8–61 (p. 17).

[16] See Jacques Lacan, *Seminar XVI*, p. 32–3. 'We can't say that object *a* had never been broached before my own discourse did so, of course, but it was broached in a frankly inadequate way, as inadequate as was the definition of surplus value before Marx's discourse rigorously highlighted it'.

[17] Lacan, *Seminar XVI*, p. 9. For the classical formulation of the Other, see Jacques Lacan, 'Seminar on "The Purloined Letter"' (1955), in *Écrits* (London: Verso, 2006), pp. 6–48 (p. 10).

[18] For a precise account of the transformations in the meaning of Lacan's references to the Other, see Jacques-Alain Miller, 'A Reading of the Seminar *From an Other to the other*, Part IV', trans. by Barbara P. Fulks, *lacanian ink*, 29, 6–59 (pp. 21–24).

[19] Lacan, *Seminar XVI*, p. 10–11.

The object *a* is now defined in terms of *plus-de-jouir*. As formulated by Marx, in a capitalist economy, objects invested with surplus value by human labour are established as commodities. In Lacan's 'market of the Other', those objects that are invested with *plus-de-jouir* are established as *objets a*.

Lacan further develops the concept of *plus-de-jouir*, and its homology with Marx's critique of political economy, in relation to his formula defining the signifier. In the mid-1960s, he laid out the famous formula that 'the signifier is what represents the subject for another signifier'.[20] As he elaborates in the first lesson of *Seminar XVI*, one implication of this formula is that a subject is never represented to another subject, but only ever to another signifier.[21] The subject, then, is effaced—'stifled', as he puts it here—at the very moment of their appearance as represented by a signifier.[22] This is the division in the subject that, as Chap. 3 described, Lacan referred to in *Seminar XI* (1964–65) as *aphanisis*.[23] It means that the subject can only appear in the symbolic order as what they are not.[24] This idea is clarified if the formula is read, by a slight inversion, as a definition of the subject: 'the subject is what is represented by a signifier for another signifier'. This formula emphasises that there is a loss of identity inherent to subjectivity. Lacan presents this loss of identity as an elegant way of locating the object *a*:

> In whatever form the subject arises in its presence, he cannot reunite with his signifying representative without a loss occurring in the identity that is known, strictly speaking, as object *a*.[25]

Lacan does not hesitate to point out the parallel here with the gap, that is identified by Marx, between 'use value' and 'exchange value'. Just as the

---

[20] See Lacan, Lesson of 27 May 1964, 'XVI. The Subject and the Other: Alienation', in *Seminar XI*, pp. 203–215 (p. 207).

[21] Lacan, *Seminar XVI*, p. 12. Another consequence of this formula, as he adds, is that a signifier cannot represent itself: representation, by necessity, requires at least two signifiers.

[22] Lacan, *Seminar XVI*, p. 12.

[23] See Lacan, Lesson of 3 June 1964, 'XVII. The Subject and the Other: Aphanisis', in *Seminar XI*, pp. 216–229; and Chapter 2, pp. 139–141.

[24] Lacan, *Seminar XVI*, p. 12.

[25] Lacan, *Seminar XVI*, p. 12.

subject, as defined by Lacan, is what is represented by a signifier for another signifier, for Marx, use value is only ever represented as exchange value—and exchange value can only be co-ordinated as one value within a network of values. Use value is, in words aligning it with Lacan's formula for the subject, what is 'represented by an exchange value for another exchange value'. It is in this gap that surplus value falls, as what Marx describes as 'congealed' labour.[26] This labour reappears as a value after something immeasurable is lost from the gap between abstract (quantitative) labour and concrete (qualitative) labour. It is a structurally identical loss that produces *plus-de-jouir* from the subject whose identity is effaced by the signifier.[27]

In the second lesson of *Seminar XVI*, Lacan extends the scope of these formulations with a reference to energetics and thermodynamics. He uses this to develop the consequences that his theory of discourse holds for the natural sciences. As he states in this second lesson, one of his intentions in this seminar as a whole is to replace the classic Freudian reference to energetics with a new reference to political economy.[28] Lacan's means of doing so, however, is to subsume thermodynamics itself under the aegis of discourse, to the point of showing that energetics is 'only conceivable as a consequence of discourse'.[29] A reference to energy is only possible, he says, in relation to the thermodynamic hypothesis of a closed system. This hypothesis amounts, as he sums it up, to 'plot[ting] with signifiers the ranges and levels with respect to which the initial function of work, as understood in physics, can be assessed' to be involved in the system.[30] Here, Lacan is making the quite simple (and Althusserian) point that energy only exists because of a thermodynamic calculation—a calculation that, as he puts it here, amounts to the network of signifiers that forms a discourse. If this situation is taken seriously, Lacan puts forward, then energy can only be considered to have existed once this discursive

[26] Marx, *Capital: A Critique of Political Economy, Volume 1*, trans. by Ben Fowkes (London: Penguin, 1976), p. 141.

[27] Lacan, *Seminar XVI*, p. 13–14.

[28] Lacan, Lesson of 20 November 1968, 'II. The Knowledge Market and Truth (on) Strike', in *Seminar XVI*, pp. 19–31 (pp. 21–22).

[29] Lacan, *Seminar XVI*, p. 22.

[30] Lacan, *Seminar XVI*, p. 22.

framework was laid onto reality, and a historical origin of energy as an object can therefore be identified. After the elaboration of this discourse, energy exists in the world with very tangible effects. The 'consequences' of the establishment of this discourse are, Lacan emphasises, no less than the construction of an entire reality corresponding to the calculations of physics.[31]

Lacan is subsuming both political economy and the thermodynamics upon which Freud based the libido theory under the aegis of his theory of discourse. The holes in discourse that produce *plus-de-jouir* are a part of the discursive logic that he is hewing out. The parallels with Althusser here are clear—not just with respect to Althusser's theory of the history of science, but also to his theory of ideology. Lacanian discourse, like ideology for Althusser, penetrates subjectivity all the way down, because it is the cause of subjectivity. Lacan, however, does not encounter the same problems that Althusser does when he hypothesises, with reference to Marx's epistemological break, the role played by individual subjectivity in producing these shifts. Lacan's reading of Freud provides him with an anchor onto the kind of rigorous theory of subjectivity that Althusser was missing. This means that Lacan does not need to appeal even implicitly to some ephemeral but vaguely defined excess of discursive structures, or to the possibility of 'breaking' from these discursive structures, in the way Althusser does. As previous chapters have been describing, Lacan used Freud to try to solve the problems that subjectivity had posed to readings of Hegel, and to materialist psychology. This means that, when Lacan comes to approach the same questions as Althusser had, he is equipped with what he at least intends to be a materialist theory of the subject of the unconscious.

Science is understood by Lacan not, in what would be a more phenomenological way, as an epistemic 'framework' or paradigm, but as a means of simultaneously formulating, taming, and putting to use something of the fundamental nature of discourse. Modern science, by his account, is a refined deployment of discourse, and a means of intervening in discourse. This was possible because modern science introduced a shift in the very nature of knowledge, that occurred, for Lacan, co-extensively

[31] Lacan, *Seminar XVI*, p. 22.

with modern science's appearance in history. Just as it was for Althusser, surplus value remains the privileged reference point for Lacan here, because surplus value allows him to articulate what there is in common between the introduction of the capitalist marketplace, on the one hand, and the development of the discursive frameworks of science, on the other. He draws, once more, in this second lesson, a parallel between a 'discourse' and a 'market'. In structurally the same way as energy is made to appear by the calculations of physics, surplus value, says Lacan, is made to appear by the conversion, in Marx's terms, of 'concrete labour' into 'abstract labour', through what Lacan calls the capitalist 'absolutisation of the market' to include labour as a commodity. This shift was, in Marx's critique of political economy, what historically enabled the production of surplus value. Surplus value, as Lacan situates it here, 'is thus the fruit *of the means of articulation that constitute capitalist discourse*'.[32] This shift, says Lacan, 'is difficult to separate from the development of certain linguistic effects, which is why I introduced "*plus-de-jouir*"'.[33] What Lacan is putting emphasis on here is the underlying logic that maps out the operations of capitalism, and what this logic has in common with that underpinning modern science. This logic is what he isolates as a 'language effect' or 'discourse', and it is this connection that leads him to argue that science and capitalism hold consequences for the *jouissance* of subjects, dependent as it is, in the Lacanian schema, on language.

The 'Capitalist Unconscious'

From the conjunction with Marx with which Lacan begins *Seminar XVI*, it would be possible to view the object *a* as a powerfully unifying function: as a point extending the logic of surplus value to the structure of subjectivity, via the unconscious. A version of the object *a*, understood in this way, is central to the general project of the philosophers of the Ljubljana School, and it represents possibly the most important single concept for their work as a whole. The idea introduced by Lacan at this

[32] Lacan, *Seminar XVI*, p. 26. My italics.

[33] Lacan, *Seminar XVI*, p. 26.

point, that there exists a 'homology' between Marx and psychoanalysis, has been taken the furthest by Samo Tomšič, who has elaborated its consequences extensively over several publications. The longest of these is the book *The Capitalist Unconscious* (2013), where Tomšič argues that at this point in the late 1960s, Lacan staged a 'second return to Freud' by supplementing his earlier reference to structural linguistics with a reference to Marx's critique of political economy.[34] The book attempts to elaborate at length the network of ways in which Lacan and Marx tesselate. *The Capitalist Unconscious* includes a reading of Freud that outlines his 'labour theory of the unconscious', a theory that centres 'on the role of labour (*Arbeit*) in the satisfaction of the unconscious tendency (desire or drive)' and which uncovers 'the productive dimension of the unconscious'.[35] In the concept of *jouissance*, says Tomšič, Lacan unites Freudian libido with the notion of unconscious labour. This, Tomšič argues, required a theory of production, which is what motivated Lacan's shift from Saussurean structuralism to Marx's critique of political economy.

Lacan uses a particular metaphor to articulate the way in which his and Marx's theories are 'homologous'. When articulating what he means by a 'homology' in *Seminar XVI*, Lacan introduces the idea of a '*trait de ciseau*'—or 'scissors' cut'—in discourse.[36] This image of a 'scissors' cut' is used by Lacan to represent an intervention that can be made in a structure, that cuts through it, and dramatically reorients its topology:

> Owing to the way in which the scissors cut into structure, the latter is revealed for what it is. If the scissors cut one way, relationships change, such that what couldn't be seen beforehand can be seen afterward. Although saying that it is not a metaphor, I illustrated this cut using a Möbius strip; I cut it in such a way that it turned into a strip that was nothing like what it had been before. The next step we need to take is to realise, on the basis of this transformation, that the whole of the Möbius strip resides in the cut.[37]

[34] Samo Tomšič, *The Capitalist Unconscious* (London: Verso, 2013), p. 2.

[35] Tomšič, *The Capitalist Unconscious*, p. 11.

[36] Lacan, *Le Séminaire de Jacques Lacan, Livre XVI, D'un Autre à l'autre (1968–1969)*, ed. Jacques-Alain Miller (Paris: Seuil, 2006), p. 31.

[37] Lacan, *Seminar XVI*, p. 21.

Tomšič identifies this metaphor as an allusion to the first chapter of *Capital.* Here, Marx uses the example of tailoring to demonstrate the logic of commodity exchange, and the double character of labour.[38] In this first step of his critique of political economy, Marx illustrates how the labour of the weaver, which produces linen, and the labour of the tailor which produces a coat, are different forms of 'concrete labour'. Qualitatively they are not equivalent, and they produce a different use value: either linen, on the one hand, or a coat, on the other. As commodities, however, they can be expressed in equivalent exchange values, by forming the equation '20 yards of linen = 1 coat'.[39] The exchange value of the commodity then becomes another way to express the labour that formed it. This labour can be treated as 'abstract labour', and articulated in terms of the amount of exchange value that this labour adds to a commodity. In this way, Marx demonstrates how the double character of the commodity—its simultaneous 'concrete' and 'abstract' nature—is the foundation for the gap between 'concrete' and 'abstract' labour. As a result, Tomšič glosses, no labour 'is merely concrete labour; rather, it is part of a broader discursive logic that supports the capitalist organisation of labour'.[40] The cut of the tailor's scissors is, in a capitalist economy, *never* merely a 'concrete' form of labour. Each cut is already immediately and inevitably enmeshed in a discursive social network that is mapped out by exchange values. Because the cut of the tailor's scissors is productive of exchange value, its own 'abstract' nature is revealed by its being situated in this network of value.

Tomšič observes that there is a gesture to Marx's theory of the double character of labour in Lacan's notion of the 'scissors' cut' in discourse. Like Lacan's 'scissors' cut' in discourse, the tailor's labour 'is revealed for what it is' by the way that it 'cut[s] into structure'.[41] Its mark also makes 'relationships change, such that what couldn't be seen beforehand can be seen afterward', in the realm of commodity exchange.[42] The tailor's labour

[38] See Marx, 'The Value-Form or Exchange-Value', in 'Chapter 1. The Commodity', in *Capital*, pp. 138–153.

[39] Marx, *Capital*, pp. 139–140.

[40] Tomšič, *The Capitalist Unconscious*, p. 50.

[41] Lacan, *Seminar XVI*, p. 21.

[42] Lacan, *Seminar XVI*, p. 21.

changes the nature of the commodity it works on, and it reveals, in doing so, something of its own nature. More than just an inscription or an addition to a structure, though, both cuts—like the cut that can entirely transform the structure of a Möbius strip—radically and absolutely transform a structure from what it was previously. The tailor's cut transforms a commodity's (exchange) value, because it also operates on this abstract level, and a discursive cut produces a topological transformation of discourse, whilst making itself a part of this structure.

Does this really account, though, for what Lacan is saying about discourse, and for the act that he is claiming to make on the level of discourse? What would it mean to make a 'scissors' cut' *in* the discourse of Marx? Tomšič reads Lacan's assertion of a homological relationship between Marx and psychoanalysis as being pitched against a weaker, 'analogical' relationship between the two, like that posited by the Freudo-Marxists. To make such an analogy, he explains, 'would mean to see in surplus value a metaphor of *plus-de-jouir*, and the other way around; and we would be dealing with a parallel: what is surplus value in the capitalist social bond is *plus-de-jouir* in psychic life'.[43] However, because Lacan says that 'surplus value *is plus-de-jouir*', this, as Tomšič puts it, 'redirect[s] the debate on the logical articulation of the subjective and the social, and thereby also de-substantialis[es] the notion of *jouissance*'.[44] Lacan precludes, as a result, a vitalistic, Reichian understanding of libido.[45] The error of the Freudo-Marxist analogy was, by Tomšič's account, to have found in psychic life a representation of the economy in which the subject lives and, simultaneously, to have identified this economy as a representation of the pathologies of the psyche. Freudo-Marxism, in other words, made Freud and Marx the respective truths of each others' theories: Freud becomes the missing piece that completes Marx, and Marx becomes the missing piece that completes Freud. Lacan, however, is engineering a far more subversive perspectival shift. He instead identifies a

[43] Samo Tomšič, 'Homology: Marx and Lacan', *Journal of the Jan van Eyck Circle for Lacanian Ideology Critique*, 5 (2012), 98–112 (p. 104).

[44] Tomšič, 'Homology', p. 105.

[45] Tomšič, 'Homology', pp. 104–5.

mutually operative logic, that can be derived at the vanishing point between Freud's theories and Marx's.

Tomšič's reading of this discursive operation champions the levelling quality of discourse on which the claim to a homology is based. Despite this, it presents Marx's critique of political economy as being distinctly unaffected by this claim. Tomšič argues, for example, that Lacan's theory of discourse, whilst at first being 'synonymous to speech', later 'quite openly *translated* Marx's "mode of production"' as 'an attempt to formalise the inexistence of social relation and its material consequences'.[46] Tomšič is referring by this to *Seminar XVII: The Other Side of Psychoanalysis* (1969–70), where Lacan introduces formulas for four basic discourses, and attributes a 'product' to each of them. Moments such as this suggest that, whilst rejecting such a manoeuvre on the part of the Freudo-Marxists, Tomšič does silently position Marx's work as an original text that Lacan's own serves to represent, or 'translate'. Tomšič's reading of Lacan acknowledges that Lacan made adaptations to his own theories after reading Marx. This included, for Tomšič, no less than Lacan's second return to Freud, which Tomšič understands to have taken place as a redressal of structural linguistics inspired by a reading of Marx. Throughout Tomšič's writings, however, Marx emerges from this encounter just as unchanged as the catalyst of a chemical reaction.

Whilst Tomšič argues that Lacan radicalises aspects of Marx's analysis of capitalism, he does so in terms of a quasi-psychosocial mechanism. Psychoanalysis should, Tomšič argues, 'be considered in logical continuity with Marx's project of a critique of political economy' because psychoanalysis demonstrates how 'the capitalist mode of *jouissance* […] makes us all reproduce capitalism in the unconscious', and because psychoanalysis 'consists in modifying the subjective relation to *jouissance*'.[47] By this account, the 'mode of *jouissance*' characteristic of capitalism is imprinted onto the unconscious, and the political function of psychoanalysis is to recognise and formalise this situation, and then attempt to modify it. Something of Lacan's thinking is lost, however, in conceiving of psychoanalysis in this way, and in understanding the capitalist mode of *jouissance*

[46] Tomšič, *The Capitalist Unconscious*, p. 203. My italics.

[47] Tomšič, 'Homology', p. 111.

to 'reproduce' capitalism in the unconscious. In *Seminar XVI*, Lacan is finding a framework in Marx's critique of political economy for the operation of the signifier in general. Lacan is not, as Reich and Marcuse did, articulating pathologies of the psyche that appear because of capitalism—as if there would be a new kind of proletarian signifier under communism that would enable the redistribution of *jouissance*. At the same time, however, Lacan is also taking great pains to emphasise that he is *not* postulating something ahistorical. He is not suggesting that there is something that has been left untouched by, and that is independent of the existence of capitalism. Tomšič's argument cannot appreciate this fully, because it omits close attention to the particular view of history that is the ground for Lacan's reading of Marx.

A double standard emerges here as a result. There is, on one side of Tomšič's argument, an attempt to outline with precision the logical continuity between Marx and psychoanalysis. On the other hand, there is also an implicit view of capitalism as contingent; as an accident of history that has reproduced an equally accidental and contingent 'mode of *jouissance*' in the unconscious of capitalist subjects. The trace can be detected in Tomšič's argument of a view of the unconscious as a psychic interior into which the discourse of capitalism is projected, and within which it is reproduced. With it, there is an echo of the Freudo-Marxist problematic, which attempted to use Freudian theory as a psychology onto which the social manifestations of capitalism could be understood to be mapped out. In significant ways, Tomšič remains on the side of those he criticises, who treat the homology as a mere analogical substitution between Lacan and Marx.

Tomšič's reading of Lacan is one that is undeniably generous to Marx. The unspoken assumption of his work, and that of the Ljubljana School in general, is that discoveries of salvific revolutionary significance can be uncovered by following the contours of Lacan's engagements with Marxism and German idealism. It is usually openly acknowledged by them that the aim thereby is to produce salvaged, sharpened versions of the main players in these traditions—Kant, Hegel, Schelling, Kierkegaard, Heidegger—by hooking them up to the fortifying tincture of psychoanalysis. However, the key point that Lacan is making through the metaphor of the 'scissors' cut', partly in an ironic displacement of Marx, is that the homology also emphatically transforms the discourse in which it intervenes. This means, as Lacan puts it, 'what couldn't be seen beforehand can be seen afterward'.[48] Despite the comprehensiveness and accomplished theoretical edge of Tomšič's work, there is something not articulated by him of the shift that Lacan attempts to engender through his theory of discourse. Lacan is offering a new perspective on language and structure, which makes a radical detour through Marx, but which leaves in its wake no stable theoretical ground to fall back upon. Lacan understands homologies and metaphors as acts that fundamentally transform the topology of discourse, and not as nudges that realign them with some other privileged co-ordinate; Marxist or otherwise. The radical, unsettling transformation that Marx articulates in his theory of labour also applies when Lacan uses Marx's tailor's cut as a metaphor. Just as the tailor's labour transforms the nature of the linen he works on, Lacan's scissors' cut, according to him, transforms not just his own discourse, as Tomšič would have it, but also Marx's.

The Historical Dimension of *Plus-de-Jouir*

In *Seminar XVI*, Lacan is claiming that a logical identity exists between Marx's critique of political economy and psychoanalysis. Alongside this, he is also arguing that psychoanalysis inherited something of the Marxist discovery. He is saying, in other words, that something was transmitted, on the level of logic, from Marx to Freud.[49] This should not be confused with the argument that there is a 'homology' between Marx and psychoanalysis. It is important to understand this in order to appreciate the simultaneous, and equally stark, proximity and difference that Lacan is claiming to exist between Marx and psychoanalysis. For all the ways Lacan follows the path of their convergence, this path can, according to him, be taken only up to a certain limiting point. In many respects, the logical calculus in *Seminar XVI* is performed primarily in order to emphasise this limit. Beyond it, the gap between Marx and psychoanalysis could

[48] Lacan, *Seminar XVI*, p. 21.

[49] This is closer, then, to the other, biological definition of 'homology', which refers to a similarity of anatomical structures between different biological taxa, resulting from a shared ancestry.

not be more significant. The homology Lacan makes between surplus value and *plus-de-jouir* hinges, as described above, on his parallel between an 'absolutisation of the market' under capitalism, and the 'unification of science'. He identifies a historical shift underlying both, that produced a transformative effect on the nature of knowledge. This shift, he argues, triggered a set of consequences whose endpoint ultimately manifested in psychoanalysis.

Lacan's view of the histories of science, capitalism, and psychoanalysis rests on the idea, articulated in the second lesson of the seminar, that the discourses of capitalism and science have effects that are intertwined in significant ways. In this lesson, he describes the discourse of science as having reduced knowledge to what he calls a 'single market', and as having produced a different kind of knowledge as a result. Science made possible, Lacan says here, a kind of knowledge that can be entirely inscribed as a set of symbolic co-ordinates. He refers to this form of knowledge with the French word *savoir*. What he calls *savoir* is knowledge reduced to the level of the signifier, and alienated from the ego—distinct therefore from *connaissance*, the knowledge he associates with the imaginary register. Because *savoir* amounts to a network of differential points, it can be understood as knowledge that exists as a set of values that can be operationalised; as co-ordinates that only have meaning with respect to one another. Lacan is postulating a continuity between the two levels of scientific knowledge and economic value, via a third, unifying level of language as a field of signifiers.

The Saussurean signifier that Lacan adopted in the early 1950s thereby becomes the bridge between his understanding of modern science, his theory of *jouissance*, and Marx's critique of political economy. If *savoir* is knowledge on the level of the signifier, then it can be understood as being involved in the same economics of *jouissance* as the signifier. A subject can then be understood to 'know' (*savoir*) through the same process by which they become a subject of the signifier: through the labour of losing *jouissance*—which, in *Seminar XVI*, is now viewed by him as the labour of *producing plus-de-jouir*. Lacan formulates, in summary, that *savoir* is therefore the 'price paid for renouncing *jouissance*'.[50] He is claiming that

[50] Lacan, *Seminar XVI*, p. 28.

the homogenising absolutisation of knowledge by science establishes a 'market of *jouissance*':

> Owing to *savoir*, we finally perceive that *jouissance* is organised and can be established as sought after and perverse. This is not new, but it is only revealed on the basis of the homogenisation of fields of *savoir* on the open market.[51]

If, Lacan is posing here, the nature of the signifier is taken seriously, then the shift in civilisation that was instigated by the operations of modern science must be understood to have produced effects on the level of knowledge and *jouissance* that were structurally identical, or homologous, to those that were produced by the absolutisation of the market under capitalism.

The following, third lesson of *Seminar XVI* clarifies this vision of a historical shift in knowledge. Here, Lacan presents this shift as a pre-history—a kind of logical genealogy—of psychoanalysis. In the lesson, he gives what amounts to a description of the historical conditions that made possible the origin of psychoanalysis. All the while that Lacan is presenting *plus-de-jouir*, and its correlate the object *a*, as the product of the renunciation of *jouissance* under the signifier, he is also making clear that the object *a* is an 'effect of discourse'—that it is the effect of analytic discourse, in the same way that surplus value is an effect of Marxist discourse.[52] As Chap. 4 argued, the object *a* can be understood to represent a limit point in Althusser's theory of science. As Althusser formulates it in *Reading Capital*, each epistemic field of a science is overturned when a certain unthinkable object, whose invisibility is required in order for the field to function, is made visible. According to the schema Lacan is putting forward in *Seminar XVI*, the inclusion of an object into the epistemic field of a science would amount to this object's inscription as *savoir*. The object *a* clearly, then, holds a privileged limit-position with respect to Althusser's theoretical schema. The object *a* is the inscription as *savoir* of the object that is, by definition, the product, excess, and loss of the very

---

[51] Lacan, *Seminar XVI*, p. 29. Translation modified.

[52] Lacan, Lesson of 27 November 1968, 'III. Topology of the Other', in *Seminar XVI*, pp. 32–47 (p. 33).

inscription in the symbolic that creates *savoir*. The object *a* is the inscription as *savoir* of the object whose very nature is that it *escapes* exactly this signifying metabolisation. The object *a* is the category itself under which the holes in discourse—the unthinkable, invisible objects per se—are themselves subsumed.

The object *a* is recast in *Seminar XVII* as a strategic short-circuiting of the development of science as it is mapped out by Althusser. In *Seminar XVI*, Lacan presents the object *a* as the object of psychoanalysis. He thereby positions psychoanalysis as the science of an object that is *structurally unknowable*.[53] For this reason, Lacan is very clear that the object *a*, despite being the effect of analytic discourse, cannot be relegated to the status of an 'artifice'. The object *a* is articulable by psychoanalysis, and it began to be articulated by Freud, says Lacan, because the subjective position of the psychoanalyst appeared in history as a 'symptom', in his words, of that transformation in the relationship of knowledge to *jouissance* that Lacan, as described above, pins down and formulates as having been brought about by science. This 'question of artifice'—the question of whether the object *a* is merely a fictional invention generated by psychoanalysis—is, says Lacan in a dense but clarifying passage:

> modified, held in abeyance, and mediated by the fact that what was discovered in an effect of discourse already appeared as the effect of discourse in history.
>
> In other words, psychoanalysis only appeared qua symptom because a turning point regarding knowledge in history—I am not saying in the history of knowledge—or regarding the impact of knowledge in [the course of] history, was reached. That turning point distilled out, as it were, the function defined by object *a* in order to offer it up to us, in order to place it within our grasp.[54]

The object *a* is not merely the fanciful dream of psychoanalysis. It is Lacan's attempt to hone in on the historical shift that occurred in knowledge before the existence of psychoanalysis, of which psychoanalysis is but the symptom.

---

[53] But with the distinction, unregistrable in English, of un-*savoir*-able.

[54] Lacan, *Seminar XVI*, p. 33.

Lacan's formulation of the historical emergence of psychoanalysis in these lessons of *Seminar XVI* departs significantly from Tomšič's own understanding of psychoanalysis. There is, as suggested above, the ghost in Tomšič's 'capitalist unconscious' of an interior psyche into which the logic of capitalism could be understood to be projected. His name can therefore be listed as one more amongst those materialists, to whose ranks so many were condemned—by Vygotsky, Politzer, Althusser, and others—who ultimately failed to escape the clutches of idealism. In attempting to unite psychoanalysis with Marx, Tomšič sneaks in the implication of a rudimentary subjective interiority. The history described in Chap. 3, of the pursuit of a dialectical materialist psychology, is informative for understanding why Lacan is positing something different in the object *a*. Chapter 3 showed how Lacan positions the signifier as a refined substitute for the physiological reflex, that escapes the spiritualistic belief in knowledge in the real that he identifies in Pavlov's theories. Vygotsky, that chapter described, had asked in the 1920s how reflexology could give a satisfactory account of the mind without abstracting it metaphysically. In his writings, he criticises the attempt to build a psychology *without* the mind as amounting to 'the dualism of subjective psychology turned inside out', because, for this psychology, mind and behaviour remain 'not one but two'.[55] He claims that the psychologies that perform an isolation of the mind from empirical study actually backfire, and amount to 'a dualism that might more correctly be called an idealism turned upside down'.[56]

The object *a* can be understood as a dialectical response to these impasses of materialist psychology that were identified and criticised by Vygotsky. In *Seminar XVI*, Lacan formulates the object *a* as the hole in the supposed completeness of the field of signifiers, which appears as the *excess* of that field. Vygotsky berates the way in which the reflex did nothing to diminish the appeal of reflexology to spiritualistic idealists: because the reflex prohibited the plenitude of subjectivity, he points out, it actually preserved it in a more mystified, unscientific form.[57] The object *a* is

[55] Vygotsky, 'Consciousness as a Problem for the Psychology of Behaviour' (1925), in *The Collected Works of L.S. Vygotsky, Vol. 3*, pp. 63–80.

[56] Vygotsky, 'The Methods of Reflexological and Psychological Investigation' (1926), in *The Collected Works of L.S. Vygotsky, Vol. 3*, pp. 35–50.

[57] See Chapter 3, pp. 93–94.

an excess that is not walled-off, in the way that scientific psychology walled-off the mind and other subjective phenomena, but an excess that is *produced* by the signifier. In the object *a*, Lacan can be understood to position the structural excesses of subjectivity as the *product* of the signifier; a product that is *dependent* on the signifier, and that only registers *as* a component of the symbolic field. This object of psychoanalysis can be read, then, to defeat the idealistic sequestering of subjectivity that occurs when the subject is treated as something missing from the material, and which, as Vygotsky argued, had been the unintentional result of reflexology.

In *Seminar XVI*, however, the object *a* is also an explicitly historical object. For Lacan, the human mind is clearly by no means an eternal, ahistorical entity into which the structures of historically contingent economies are momentarily projected, in a way that would preserve the interiorised subjectivity of idealism. Even in the classical Marxist approach to psychology that understood the psyche as having been formed dialectically through its interaction with tools, the form of labour it engages in, and various economic forces, there was still *something* being shaped, and a mechanism, with responses that could be predicted and understood, was still believed to exist in the real.[58] Part of the significance of Lacan's theory of discourse is that it makes subjectivity entirely the product of a discursive structure, and not something that is shaped by it. This discursive structure is also, for Lacan, all that can be traced of subjectivity. This means that he eliminates all vestiges of the secret, interiorised remainder that had inhibited the pursuit of a materialist psychology.

By understanding science and capitalism as discourses in the way Lacan does in *Seminar XVI*—as structures with effects, but without words—he attributes to both science and capitalism a great and an inevitable impact on subjectivity. Science and capitalism are not, in Lacan, beasts that beset human life at the city gates of the psyche, or a plague that has infiltrated it, which could be defeated by a sufficiently powerful dialectical assault. For Lacan, science and capitalism are discourses with a history, and with a moment of origin. But they constitute, for him, the

[58] See Vygotsky, 'The Instrumental Method in Psychology' (1930), in *The Concept of Activity in Soviet Psychology*, ed. by J.V. Wertsch (New York: Armonk, 1981), pp. 134–143 (p. 137).

entire material of a world—a world that includes the deepest recesses of subjectivity that an idealism would have cloistered away. Even Althusser, as Chap. 4 argued, preserves this privileged realm, in the last instance, because he offers no means to account for the involvement of individual subjectivity in epistemological breaks. If Lacan is charting and explaining a homology in this seminar, he is also attempting a subsumption of Marx into a more general framework than that which can be found in Marx's writings; one that could deal satisfactorily with this question of subjectivity. Vygotsky is once more a vital reference point here, because of the scorn he always expressed towards attempts to catalogue parallels between Freud and Marx. What he instead prescribed in 'The Meaning of the Historical Crisis in Psychology' was no less than the formation of a new, general science—of which Marx, in his economic theories, had provided only one dimension. In this general science, all sciences other than economics would also be given an entirely new position, and they would be entirely transformed by it. There would be nothing 'Marxist' at all about this new general field of science: the name of Marx would be attributed merely to the economic theories and philosophical writings that took the first, halting, desperately incomplete steps towards what might be possible if it were realised. The following section will describe how Lacan, in the years when he makes his sustained reading of Marx, moves towards something in sympathy with this vision. Lacan stages a critique of Marx, in the interest of taking further what he finds to be the logic underlying Marx's theories.

How Did Marx Invent Capitalism?

There is a level on which Lacan is explicitly critical of Marx, which requires his relationship to anything named 'Marxism' to be understood with great subtlety. The title of this section is a reference to the first chapter of Slavoj Žižek's book *The Sublime Object of Ideology* (1989), which is called 'How Did Marx Invent the Symptom?'. This in turn is a reference to the claim that Lacan makes, firstly in *Seminar XVIII: On a Discourse that Might not Be a Semblance* (1971), and then several times in later years, that the logic of the symptom, as formulated by Freud, was first introduced by Marx. The reading Žižek gives of Lacan's claim is, briefly, as follows: Marx invented the symptom by identifying the proletariat as a point of inconsistency and rupture within bourgeois universalism, and by taking this point not, as it is seen from within that universalist framework, as the failure of this system to be fully manifested, but instead as the 'constitutive moment' on which the system depends. Marx, says Žižek, showed that the phenomena that appear to everyday bourgeois consciousness as contingent deviations, deformations, and degenerations of the '"normal" functioning of society'—including economic crises, wars, exploitation, and the existence of the proletariat—are instead 'necessary products of the system itself: the points at which the "truth", the immanent antagonistic character of the system, erupts'.[59] Marx's invention of the symptom lies, then, in this shift in perspective, which turns a lapse in a system into its truth.[60]

The foundation for the claim that Marx invented the symptom was laid by Lacan in the mid-1960s. In the chapter of the *Écrits* 'On the Subject Who is Finally in Question' (1966), in the passage discussed in Chap. 4, Lacan identifies the dimension of the symptom as having first been 'differentiated' in Marx's notorious 'reversal' of Hegel.[61] The stronger version of the 'invention of the symptom' claim, and the one Žižek directly quotes in *The Sublime Object of Ideology*, is made by Lacan in the final session of *Seminar XVIII*. In this seminar, Lacan repeats the argument that he made in 1966, but in terms of some of the concepts he develops in his later teaching, particularly that of the 'semblance'. In this final lesson of *Seminar XVIII*, Lacan outlines how Marx subverted a tradition of thought that was rooted in *connaissance*—knowledge in the imaginary register, which is based on mirages of illusory completeness, wholeness, and unity. Lacan broadly associates this tradition of *connaissance* with German idealism, and claims that the tradition reached its

[59] Slavoj Žižek, *The Sublime Object of Ideology* (London: Verso, 1989), p. 144.

[60] Žižek defines the symptom as 'a particular element which subverts its own universal foundation, a species subverting its own genus'. *The Sublime Object of Ideology*, p 16.

[61] Lacan, 'On the Subject Who is Finally in Question', in *Écrits*, pp. 189–196 (p. 194). See Chapter 4, pp. 200–204. Lacan gestures to this idea once again in the passage of the second lesson of *Seminar XVI*, when he describes surplus value as being, for Marx, 'the conflictual element which is the truth of the system' of capitalism. See *Seminar XVI*, p. 27.

'culmination' in Hegel.[62] In marking this tradition of *connaissance* as a 'fundamental dupery', he says, Marx introduced the dimension of what Lacan calls 'semblance' as a critical weapon.[63] In *Seminar XVIII*, Lacan uses the notion of the 'semblance' to refer to a false appearance in the realm of the imaginary that can be utilised to serve a particular discursive function. The key question of *Seminar XVIII* as a whole is to identify a discourse that, as referred to in its title, would not operate on the level of semblance. Marx's development of a logic of the symptom was a break that announced the semblamatic nature of *connaissance*. It was, as Lacan frames it, a result of Marx's attempt to sweep aside the distortions of the semblance as they are manifested in capitalism, primarily in the commodity fetish. After denouncing the reign of *connaissance*, Marx puts forward surplus value as an alternative support for truth, based on the logic of the symptom. Surplus value is, Lacan says, presented by Marx both as the object on which capitalism absolutely depends, and as that which undermines the semblance of capitalism's rational functioning.[64]

It is worth pointing out that Lacan does not actually use the word 'invented' in *Seminar XVIII* to refer to Marx and the symptom. Instead, he says that Marx is 'the one who is responsible [*celui qui en est responsable*]' for the dimension of the symptom.[65] The difference is subtle, but the activity of the word 'invented' puts more emphasis on Marx's position,

[62] Lacan, Lesson of 16 June 1971, 'X. On the Myth Freud Made', in *Seminar XVIII: On a Discourse that Might not Be a Semblance*, trans. Bruce Fink, ed. by Jacques-Alain Miller (London: Polity, 2024), pp. 143–156 (p. 144).

[63] Lacan, *Seminar XVIII*, pp. 144.

[64] Lacan, *Seminar XVIII*, pp. 144–5.

[65] 'Il est important de s'apercevoir que, historiquement, ce n'est pas là que réside la nouveauté de l'introduction à la psychanalyse réalisée par Freud. Je l'ai plusieurs fois indiqué, et il est très facile de le repérer à la lecture, la notion de symptôme, celui qui en est responsable, c'est Marx'. Lacan, *Le Séminaire, Livre XVIII, D'un discours qui ne serait pas du semblant (1971)*, ed. by Jacques-Alain Miller (Paris: Seuil, 2007), p. 164. The idea reaches what is essentially its final form in this seminar, but Lacan does return to it in some of the later seminars, giving it slightly different emphases. See Lesson of 19 January 1972, 'IV. From Necessity to Inexistence', in *Seminar XIX: … or Worse (1971–1972)*, ed. by Jacques-Alain Miller, trans. by A.R. Price (Cambridge: Polity, 2018), pp. 37–48; Lesson of 4 May 1972, 'XI. An Issue of Ones', in *Seminar XIX*, pp. 128–145; Lesson of 2 December 1971, in *Seminar XIXa: The Knowledge of the Analyst*, published as 'II. On Incomprehension and Other Themes', in *Talking to Brick Walls: A Series of Presentations in the Chapel at Sainte-Anne Hospital*, trans. by A.R. Price (Cambridge: Polity, 2017), pp. 35–70; and Lesson 4, 21 January 1975 and Lesson 6, 18 February 1975, in *Seminar XXII: R.S.I.*, unpublished.

compared to the relative passivity implied by his 'responsibility' for the symptom. The Žižekian 'inventor' Marx suggests an infernal tinkerer, dividing heaven and hell like Blake's Newton—Lacan's 'responsible' Marx is invoked as more of a bystander, almost as someone who stumbled on something by mistake, or who made a lapsus that would later prove fateful when fully registered by Freud. This imprecision is somewhat characteristic of Žižek's reading of Lacan, into which other approximations do slip. From the way Lacan features in Žižek's work, it is not clear exactly what psychoanalysis was left to achieve after Marx introduced the procedure of collapsing an imaginary order by pinpointing its symptom—or what Lacan was intending to articulate by intervening here, beyond a summary of how Marx and psychoanalysis lock together that would merely anticipate more cryptically Žižek and Tomšič's own.

It is generally omitted by Žižek, too, that despite the obvious impact that Marx's critique of political economy made on this episode of Lacan's work, in the years following *Seminar XVI*, Lacan's attitude towards Marx is distinctly critical. Lacan begins to outline this more censorious position on Marx in *Seminar XVII* (1969–70). The seminar builds on the groundwork for the theory of discourse he laid the previous year, by articulating four possible modalities of human social bonds, which Lacan formulates in diagrams as the 'four discourses'.[66]

Seminar XVII also continues the close discussion of Marx that Lacan began in *Seminar XVI*. In the opening lesson of *Seminar XVII*, Lacan repurposes the formula of the signifier—'the signifier represents the subject for another signifier'—as the first, and most fundamental, of the four discourses, the 'discourse of the master'. Lacan represents the formula of the signifier by the following matheme: $\frac{S_1}{\$} \longrightarrow S_2$ the signifier (S_1) represents the subject ($\$$) for another signifier (S_2)

Lacan forms the discourse of the master by giving this formula a minor alteration. He adds the object *a*, as its 'product':

[66] By four discourses, Lacan means the four fundamental forms of possible social bond. These are given by Lacan in *Seminar XVII* as the following formulas:

$$\frac{S_1}{\$} \longrightarrow \frac{S_2}{a} \qquad \frac{\$}{a} \longrightarrow \frac{S_1}{S_2} \qquad \frac{S_2}{S_1} \longrightarrow \frac{a}{\$} \qquad \frac{a}{S_2} \longrightarrow \frac{\$}{S_1}$$

master hysteric university analyst

$$\frac{S_1}{\$} \rightarrow \frac{S_2}{a}$$

The formula Lacan gives to the master's discourse—the type of social bond based on mastery—is also the basic formula that he uses for the subject's relation to the symbolic order. In terms of the symbols Lacan uses here, the master signifier, represented as S_1, is what 'the essence of the master relies on'.[67] What he is saying here is that the representative of a subject for another signifier is what gives the subject the position of the master. Mastery, he is saying, amounts to making an effect in the symbolic order. The other significant feature of the discourse of the master is that, as indicated by the broken arrow on the bottom level, the object *a*—the *plus-de-jouir* produced by the master's discourse—cannot, under this discourse, be returned to the subject.

Later, in the fifth lesson of the seminar, Lacan outlines a historical shift that, he says, replaced the discourse of the master by a new 'discourse of the university'. The transition he describes here is a refinement of the one he refers to in *Seminar XVI* as the inauguration of a 'market' of knowledge after the rise of modern science. Lacan describes the discourse of the university as representing a departure from the classic Hegelian movement of knowledge described in the *Phenomenology of Spirit*, in which it accumulates linearly until absolute knowledge is reached. Lacan identifies this knowledge with the imaginary form of *connaissance*.[68] Lacan associates the discourse of the university, on the other hand, with thermodynamics, and the mechanisms of industry—with factories, formalisation, and the counting of units: with what Lacan calls a 'reign of the signifier', which he pinpoints as having been instantiated after the field of thermodynamics was unified by the formulas of the conservation of energy.[69] The rise of the discourse of the university heralded, he says, a new world based on 'pure numerical truths' and on 'that which is countable', where primacy is given to everything at the beginning and at the end of a process, and where everything in between is neglected.

[67] Jacques Lacan, Lesson of 10 December 1969, 'I. Production of the four discourses', in *Seminar XVII: The Other Side of Psychoanalysis*, trans. by R. Grigg (London: Norton, 1991), pp. 11–28 (p. 21).

[68] See Lacan, Lesson of 11 February 1970, 'V. The Lacanian field', in *Seminar XVII*, pp. 69–86 (p. 79).

[69] Lacan, *Seminar XVII*, p. 79.

$$\frac{S_2}{S_1} \longrightarrow \frac{a}{\$}$$

the discourse of the university

In *Seminar XVI*, the relationship between *plus-de-jouir* and surplus value was presented by Lacan as a 'homology'. What disparities or differences that might exist between surplus value and *plus-de-jouir* are left vague by him. In *Seminar XVII*, Lacan establishes a clear difference between surplus value and *plus-de-jouir*, based on the discursive shift from the master to the university that the seminar articulates. Even *plus-de-jouir* was not immune, he envisages, to the drive towards quantification entailed in this shift. It instigated a movement, says Lacan, towards a point where '*plus-de-jouir* is no longer *plus-de-jouir* but is inscribed simply as a value to be inscribed in or deducted from the totality of whatever it is that is accumulating [...] from out of an essentially transformed nature'.[70] Within the discourse of the university, in other words, a means exists to take *plus-de-jouir*—the point of excess that is produced as a loss occasioned by the symbolic order—and to subject it to the process to which this discourse, according to Lacan, also subjects everything in nature. The discourse of the university is able to draw *plus-de-jouir* back onto the level of the symbolic order, as a value that is quantifiable, countable, and reducible to *savoir*.

In a passage from the twelfth lesson of *Seminar XVII*, Lacan gives a small, allusive historical sketch of the moment when the decisive shift first occurred to make the numeralisation of *plus-de-jouir* possible. This, he says in the passage below, happened at the same moment when it became possible to accumulate capital through the recuperation of surplus value:

> Something changed in the master's discourse at a certain point in history. We are not going to break our backs finding out if it was because of Luther, or Calvin, or some unknown traffic of ships around Genoa, or in the Mediterranean Sea, or anywhere else, for the important point is that on a certain day *plus-de-jouir* became calculable, could be counted, totalised. This is where what is called the accumulation of capital begins.[71]

[70] Lacan, *Seminar XVII*, pp. 80–81.

[71] Lacan, Lesson of 10 June 1970, 'XII. The impotence of truth', in *Seminar XVII*, pp. 164–179 (p. 177). Though he withdraws from attributing a historical moment to this shift, based on the

Plus-de-jouir was made countable, Lacan says here, at the same moment when surplus value appeared in history. The discourse of the university Lacan puts forward in *Seminar XVII* is a technology that appeared at a certain point in history, which is capable of turning *plus-de-jouir* into calculable, countable knowledge. It does so by transforming *plus-de-jouir* into a surplus-as-loss on another level, a level that *can* be metabolised by the symbolic: that of monetary value. Surplus value, Lacan is saying in *Seminar XVII*, is only 'a memorial to *plus-de-jouir*', an 'equivalent of *plus-de-jouir*'.[72] Surplus value is a replica of *plus-de-jouir* that can be accumulated to combine effortlessly with capital, because both surplus value and capital exist in the field of value. The discourse of the university produced surplus value, a perverse fossil of what had remained unassimilable *plus-de-jouir* under the discourse of the master.

This idea, that surplus value is only derived from *plus-de-jouir*, is at the core of what Lacan finds to have been omitted from Marx. Lacan, as a result, takes Marx's politics to be out of step with the logic of his critique of political economy. What, for Lacan, Marx criticises about surplus value on a political level, is the 'spoliation of *jouissance*'.[73] Lacan charges Marx, in other words, with having understood surplus value as the ruinous theft of the proletarian's *jouissance*. Surplus value, for Marx, is what capital steals of the proletarian's *jouissance*. The way Lacan is presenting Marx here is significant in light of the theoretical shift he carried out in *Seminar XVI* the previous year. Lacan frames Marx as a critic of what capitalism spoils or prohibits of the proletarian's *jouissance*. Lacan therefore situates Marx's politics within the logic of his own *earlier* theoretical framework—the one he departed from in *Seminar XVI*. This framework saw the signifier as prohibiting the subject's *jouissance*. For Marx, as Lacan is reading him in *Seminar XVII*, surplus value serves to prohibit *jouissance*, in the same way that Lacan used to understand the signifier to prohibit *jouissance*.

The 'homology' Lacan announced in *Seminar XVI* attains a far more complicated status in light of this criticism of Marx in *Seminar XVII*. In *Seminar XVI*, just one year earlier, Marx had taken centre stage as the one

references he gives in this passage, he clearly situates it in Early Modern Europe, around the sixteenth century.

[72] Lacan, *Seminar XVII*, p. 81.

[73] Lacan, *Seminar XVII*, p. 81.

whose logic, when brought to its limit, pressed Lacan to move *beyond* that earlier theoretical framework, by identifying *plus-de-jouir* as the surplus of *jouissance* produced by the signifier. Lacan is not usually seen as one of those Marxists discussed in Chap. 4, who were keen to discover the break in Marx between the mystified remnants of his youth, and the true concepts that we ought to take from him. But Lacan, in *Seminar XVII*, is marking a division of his own within Marx. He is dividing Marx's thought between a politics, on the one hand, that wrongly sees surplus value as the vampiric enemy threatening the proletarian's *jouissance*—and, on the other hand, a logic of discourse that does not allow such clear lines of distinction to be drawn.

The discourse theory exemplifies, and formalises, a rhetorical manoeuvre that is characteristic of Lacan's work, of turning upside-down an ordinarily assumed notion or perspective. This is a manoeuvre that he often performs by uniting two co-ordinates that would initially appear to be directly opposed. The most illustrative example of this is the argument of 'Kant with Sade' (1963), that the Kantian moral will is structurally identical to a sadistic will to *jouissance*, and that both are united in the Freudian superego.[74] Another impressive instance of this rhetorical manoeuvre is a reinterpretation of the Hegelian dialectic of master and slave that Lacan makes in *Seminar XVI*. What the discourse of psychoanalysis is able to identify, he says here, is the act of renunciation that is made on the part, not of the slave, but of the *master*. This, he says, makes 'the function of the *plus-de-jouir*' appear as constitutive of the master's, not the slave's, position. In the first lesson of *Seminar XVI*, Lacan claims—against Hegel—that labour 'is what constitutes the master', and not the slave, because the master makes labour 'the principle of his power', in the form of a silent renunciation.[75] The master, having exposed himself to death, and having made himself a subject of the signifier, has 'renounced everything, and *jouissance* first up'.[76] The slave, on the other hand, though deprived of the disposal of his body, still has his *jouissance*—he chose to keep it when he opted for his life over his prestige, as in the famous epi-

[74] Lacan, 'Kant with Sade', in *Écrits*, pp. 645–670.

[75] Lacan, *Seminar XVII*, p. 107.

[76] Lacan, *Seminar XVII*, p. 107.

sode of the *Phenomenology*. In the revision of Hegel that Lacan carries out here, the master is the one who had to make a fundamental renunciation of *jouissance*, in order to achieve victory in the struggle for pure prestige. The master had to choose prestige over his life in order to attain his position. The slave, however, ultimately chose to keep his *jouissance*, against the threat of its being extinguished by his death. At the same time, of course, although a loss of *jouissance* is involved in the master's fulfilment of his function, 'something of *jouissance*' is nonetheless rendered to him, in *plus-de-jouir*, the trace in discourse of the loss of *jouissance*. The slave, counterintuitively, is the one who is able to keep his *jouissance*, and this is why he 'owes' *plus-de-jouir* to the master.[77]

The logic of *plus-de-jouir* is an extension of the revised function of the signifier that Lacan outlines in *Seminar XVI* in reference to Marx's critique of political economy. Whilst it is not a Hegelian logic, its role in Lacan's revised dialectic of master and slave makes clear that it is the shadow of a Hegelian logic. It is a negative imprint of the Hegelian dialectic; a tracing out of its limits that, as Chap. 2 described, Lacan had been attempting to extract from Hegel since the 1950s. Lacan is also making clear, in *Seminar XVII*, that this is the logic that escapes Marx. In this seminar, there is one specific instance of Lacan's manoeuvre of reversal that is central to this period of his work: he reads Marx, here, as being no less than the 'founder' of capitalism. In the seventh lesson of *Seminar XVII*, in a section that Miller subtitles 'Genealogy of Surplus Value', Lacan describes the role he understands Marx to have played in the origin of the capitalist discourse:

> If, by means of this relentlessness to castrate himself that he had, he hadn't computed [*comptabilise*] this *plus-de-jouir*, if he hadn't converted it into surplus value, in other words if he hadn't founded capitalism, Marx would have realised that surplus value is *plus-de-jouir*. None of this, of course, prevents it being the case that capitalism is founded by him [*que par lui le capitalisme est fondé*], and that the function of surplus value is designated with complete pertinence in its devastating consequences.[78]

[77] Lacan, *Seminar XVII*, p. 107.

[78] Lacan, *Seminar XVII* pp. 107–108. For the original French passage, see Lacan, 'VII. Oedipe et Moïse et le père de la horde' in *La Séminaire, Livre XVII, L'envers de la psychanalyse*, ed. Jacques-

In this impious portrait, Lacan argues that Marx did not, as is usually and obviously thought, simply articulate the operation of capitalist economies when he formulated the position and the function of surplus value. In light of Lacan's theory of discourse, and of his discernment of *plus-de-jouir*, Lacan instead identifies Marx's critique of political economy as having participated on a fundamental level in the operation and establishment of capitalism. Lacan's theory of discourse, as he articulated it in *Seminar XVI*, identifies the appearances of scientific knowledge and capitalism as having had direct effects on the level of *jouissance*. In doing so, Lacan makes his theory of discourse an alternative either to a naïve positivism, which would understand science as drawing knowledge directly from the real, or to the version of this—which was not fully escaped by Althusser—where a shadowy real is made progressively brighter and brighter by the enlightening effect of scientific knowledge. The way Lacan articulates his observations in the passage above identifies Marx as the figure who 'computes' *plus-de-jouir*, in the same way that the university discourse computes all of nature. Marx's critique of political economy, Lacan is announcing, not only takes place in the university discourse, but it also represented the very moment when the numeralising thrust of the university discourse was extended to the limit of *plus-de-jouir*. For Lacan, the appearance of capitalism amounted to a radicalised distortion in the position of *plus-de-jouir*, in a way that furthered the quantifying shift begun by the discourse of the university, and that amounted to the elision and metabolisation of *plus-de-jouir*. Marx's precise foreclosure of *plus-de-jouir* is understood by Lacan to represent the completion of this elision, and the founding, therefore, of the discourse of capitalism.

If Marx, as Althusser reads him, achieved his epistemological break by formulating the existence of surplus value, this, for Lacan, simultaneously made him the founder of capitalism. Lacan's theory of discourse

---

Alain Miller (Paris: Seuil, 1998), pp. 117–135 (pp. 123–124): 'Si, par cet acharnement qui est le sien de se castrer, il n'avait pas comptabilisé ce plus-de-jouir, s'il n'en avait pas fait la plus-value, en d'autres termes s'il n'avait pas fondé le capitalisme, Marx se serait apercu que la plus-value, c'est le plus-de-jouir. Tout cela n'empeche pas, bien sur, que par lui le capitalisme est fondé, et que la fonction de la plus-value est tout a fait pertinemment designée dans ses consequences ravageantes. Neanmoins, pour en venir a bout, il faudrait peut-etre savoir quel est au moins le premier temps de son articulation. Ce n'est pas parce qu'on nationalise, au niveau du socialisme dans un seul pays, les moyens de production, qu'on en a fini pour autant avec la plus-value, si on ne sait pas ce que c'est'.

allows him, thanks to a logic that he took from Marx, to present the historical movement of science as never taking place without a cost, and a loss. The invention of capitalism—as it is fully metabolised by science, and therefore, Lacan argues, fully *invented*, only in Marx's critique of political economy—is the most privileged dénouement in the history of science. This is because something about the very nature of discourse is fully operationalised and deployed only at the point when Marx 'computed' *plus-de-jouir*. If Marx's critique of political economy represents the first full and accurate theory of capitalism, then it also, Lacan is saying, represents the first expression of capitalism *as* scientific knowledge. Marx invented the symptom, then, because he brought into science the unstable object that exists at the heart of capitalism, and named it surplus value. He brought, to put it another way, the market of commodities *onto* the market of knowledge.

There is a significant shift between the way Lacan presents Marx in 1966, in 'On the Subject Who Is Finally in Question', and the way that he reads Marx in 1970, in light of the discourse theory. In 1966, Marx could already be acknowledged by Lacan as the differentiator of the dimension of the symptom (or, as he restates in *Seminar XVIII*, the one 'responsible for' the symptom) because he introduced surplus value as an alternative basis for truth to the semblance epitomised by the commodity fetish.[79] Marx, from this approach, is positioned by Lacan as a turning point in the progress of the Enlightenment, who punctured through the illusory mystifications and dupery epitomised by Hegel's ruse of reason. Marx appears differently in *Seminar XVII*. In *Seminar XVIII*, the year after, Marx goes back to being the one who was 'responsible for' the symptom. In *Seminar XVII*, however, Marx appears not in this beatified role, but as no less than the *founder* of capitalism. Marx's position for Lacan is divided. For him, Marx deludedly criticises the spoliation of the proletarian's *jouissance*, but also provides the logic for the formulation of *plus-de-jouir*. Marx founds capitalism by computing *plus-de-jouir*, but also invents the symptom by disenchanting the veil of *connaissance*.

But then, as this book has been attempting to demonstrate throughout, Marx's position was complex for every one of his serious readers

[79] Lacan, 'On the Subject Who Is Finally in Question', p. 194.

contemporary to Lacan. Althusser's later work would approach Marx with similar ambivalence, presenting him as having not achieved the break from idealism that Althusser described in the 1960s. Althusser's article 'Marx in his Limits' (1978) argues that materialist and idealist concepts are terminably and inseparably interwoven throughout Marx's work. However, despite the critical ambivalence with which Lacan treats Marx, he also understands the historical position of psychoanalysis to be comprehensible only with respect to Marx's own. It is not, reading Lacan carefully, that capitalism 'reproduces' something in the unconscious, poisoning our minds with some alien form of *jouissance*. Capitalism, on the other hand, is presented by Lacan to have utilised and technologised something of the structure *of* the unconscious, by taking its discursive logic to a limit. Only when capitalism is understood in this way can the position within its history that Lacan gives to psychoanalysis, and the position he holds it to take with respect to Marx, be properly comprehended. As the best readers of Marx have always known, a much more strategic, and in many ways much more pessimistic, critique of capitalism is required in order to register these subtleties.

'Radiophonie' and the Freudian Break

Lacan's critique of Marx might, from one perspective, be understood as his identification of a dimension of hypocrisy, or a repressed double standard, within Marx's thinking. This is how Žižek understands Lacan's 'reproach' to Marx. For Žižek, Lacan identifies and criticises Marx's unwitting participation in the underlying fantasy of capitalism—that of capital's limitless capacity for generation. According to Lacan, says Žižek, Marx's mistake was to imagine 'capitalism's self-revolutionising perpetual motion exploding freely when its inherent obstacle is removed'.[80] Marx erroneously concludes, for Žižek, that:

[80] Žižek, *The Parallax View* (Cambridge, Massachusetts: MIT Press, 2006), p. 263. Marx, says Žižek, perceived 'how capitalism unleashed the breathtaking dynamic of self-enhancing productivity', a world in which, famously, "everything melts into air". On the other hand, he also perceived 'how this capitalist dynamic is propelled by its own inner obstacle or antagonism'; how 'the ultimate limit [...] of capitalist self-propelling productivity is Capital itself' and 'the mad dance of its

> a new, higher social order (Communism) is possible, an order that would not only maintain but even raise to a higher level, and effectively release the potential of, the self-increasing spiral of productivity which, in capitalism, on account of its inherent obstacle ("contradiction"), is again and again thwarted by socially destructive economic crises.

This image of a post-capitalist plenitude, both enjoying the productive capability of capital, yet also free from its contradictions, is an inherently capitalist fantasy that Marx himself—Žižek argues—still entertains. Žižek borrows Derridean terms to articulate how Marx overlooks that the "condition of impossibility" of the full deployment of capitalism's productive forces is simultaneously its "condition of possibility". Marx, says Žižek, overlooks that the obstacle to and potential for capitalism's productivity are one and the same, so that 'if we take away the obstacle, the very potential thwarted by this obstacle dissipates'.[81] Žižek identifies this as the 'ultimate *capitalist* fantasy', because it disavows that the form of capitalism—the appropriation of surplus value—is 'the necessary [...] formal frame/condition of the self-propelling productive movement'.[82] Žižek also, however, makes the further step of reading this critique as the 'fundamental reproach to Marx' enabled by Lacan's identification of 'the ambiguous overlapping between surplus value and *plus-de-jouir*'.[83] Though Žižek does not elaborate on this, *plus-de-jouir* presumably represents the 'obstacle' here, which motivates its own always-incomplete metabolisation into surplus value (the equivalence of an obstacle with a condition of possibility is the way Žižek generally reads and deploys the Lacanian object *a*). This chapter has been attempting to give an account of Lacan's reproach to Marx that shows it to be more subtle, and more fundamental, than this. As the previous section showed, it is not just an error on Marx's part that Lacan is identifying. Lacan is attempting to diagnose a fundamental proximity between Marx's theories and

unconditional spiral of productivity is ultimately nothing but a desperate flight forward to escape its own debilitating inherent contradiction'. *The Parallax View*, p. 266.

[81] Žižek, *The Parallax View*, p. 266.

[82] Žižek, *The Parallax View*, p. 263.

[83] Žižek, *The Parallax View*, p. 266.

capitalism itself, which appears in light of the theory of discourse: a correspondence, on a structural level, between their respective operations.

Žižek uses Lacan, broadly speaking, to crystallise or to rescue something from Marx that was misunderstood by Marx's earlier readers, on the level of form and its surprising, paradoxical limit-effects. As Žižek outlines several times at length, there is a prioritisation of form in Marx that is structurally identical to that made by Freud in *The Interpretation of Dreams*.[84] Žižek uses this observation to unite psychoanalysis and Marx on the grounds that both are interested, fundamentally, in the objects that resist form. By mapping out the logic of the remainder in *plus-de-jouir*, as Žižek's reading goes, Lacan was also therefore identifying the significance of this logic for understanding capitalism. As this chapter has been arguing, however, there is something missing from this perspective on the relationship between Marx and Lacan. The present section will extend this idea, to show that this absence is, in its own way, symptomatic of how Lacan positions himself with respect to the traditions of philosophy that Žižek writes about. The *deux ex machina* role that Lacan tends to play in Žižek's arguments—being brought in at just the right moment to reframe an impossible problem, but in a way that always disregards the possibility of Lacan's own prior entanglement in the coordinates of this problem—avoids elaborating Lacan's position with respect to the history of these traditions. The position Žižek gives to Lacan can indirectly be read as an indicator of where, from the perspective of the early twenty-first century, Lacan falls with respect to the traditions of thought Žižek is using him as a Swiss Army knife to fix up.

The second chapter of this book described the way in which the very conflicts between readings of Hegel that prioritised different points of his system—the dialectic of master and slave; the unhappy consciousness; the philosophy of nature—ultimately highlighted something fundamental about his work: that there is an entire problematic internal to it of how to locate 'Hegel' in any meaningful, stable way. This first chapter argued that it is not possible to assimilate Lacan to Hegel if, following Lacan, we appreciate, firstly, that Hegel has only ever been able to appear as a series of fractional misperceptions of his philosophy, and secondly, that this

[84] Žižek, *The Parallax View*, p. 50.

spectral nature of Hegel is at the core of Hegelian philosophy—that Hegel determined this aspect of how his philosophical system would be interpreted. Žižek is correct, in other words, to connect up Lacan's idea of the 'non-All' with Hegel; to find a seed of this logical operator in Hegel, and to understand it as a key to unlock the status of what Hegel uncovered. Reading Hegel as non-All, however, has more serious implications than Žižek is prepared to acknowledge. Where Žižek is wrong is in eliding the passage that led from Hegel to Lacan, and that therefore led to the very emergence of the idea of the non-All out of the Hegelian fall-out. The position of Lacan as an inheritor of a destabilising element within German idealism that first raised its head in Hegel—and which we find again in Marx's 'symptomatic' thinking—is censored by Žižek's presentation of this position as a frozen set of final co-ordinates, when it is this passage itself, and only this passage, that reveals the true nature of the shift produced by Lacan.

An attempt can be identified in the philosophers of the Ljubljana School, to make Lacan into the missing piece completing the traditions of German idealism and dialectical materialism that concern the majority of their writings.[85] However, something is unregistered here with regards to what Lacan is articulating about the nature of structure in his theory of discourses. Žižek makes the comparisons he does as if the terms he refers to are fixed, stable, and lacking a history. Psychoanalysis, however, as Lacan puts it in *Seminar XVI*, 'appeared as a symptom because of a turning point of knowledge in history'.[86] Lacan's claim that psychoanalysis is the symptom of this 'turning point' cannot be accurately comprehended if the attempt is made to contain psychoanalysis within the limits of what came before.[87]

In June 1970, a radio interview with Lacan was recorded and broadcast over a series of instalments, a slightly edited version of which was

[85] See, for example, the position Zupančič gives Lacan within the history of philosophy in her book *Ethics of the Real* (London: Verso, 1995, p. 17); or the passage in Žižek's *The Metastases of Enjoyment* (London: Verso, 1994) in which he argues that the phallus, or 'the phallic element as the signifier of "castration"' is 'the fundamental category of dialectical materialism' (p. 130).

[86] Lacan, *Seminar XVI*, p. 33. Translation modified.

[87] There is even something of the discourse of capitalism in the work of the Ljubljana School, precisely in their attempt (possibly the only successful attempt as of yet) to bring the object *a* as a trans-logical, trans-structural operator back into line with the discourse of the university.

later published in *Scilicet 2/3* as 'Radiophonie'—the title under which it would also be printed in the *Autres écrits* (2001).[88] The interview develops several themes introduced in *Seminar XVII*, which Lacan had been teaching in the same year.[89] Lacan responds—with a healthy dose of subversion—to seven questions addressed to him by the interviewer Robert Georgin, which attempt to pin Lacan down on what had clearly by this point become one version of the received understanding of his work—a version that centres on psychoanalysis' relationship with linguistics, and its implications for revolutionary politics.[90] This gives Lacan the opportunity to specify with precision where he falls with regards to these co-ordinates. Out of this emerges a text that is as lucidly direct as it is obscure and enigmatic at times. One of its central themes—and the one that the remainder of this chapter will focus on—is the question of the position of psychoanalysis with respect to scientific knowledge, and its status as a

[88] Lacan, 'Radiophonie', *Scilicet 2/3* (September 1970), 55–99. Republished in *Autres écrits* (Paris: Seuil, 2001), pp. 403–447. Subsequent references to 'Radiophonie' will be to the republished version in the *Autres écrits*, in my translation. Two unofficial English translations, by Anthony Chadwick and Jack W. Stone, are available online. For pdfs containing both translations of each individual question of the interview, see <www.freud2lacan.com/lacan/>

[89] Lacan read out the text of some of his replies in lessons of *Seminar XVII*. He read the first three replies in the Lesson of 9 April 1970; see 'VIII. From Myth to Structure', in *Seminar XVII*, pp. 118–132 (pp. 130–132). He then read the sixth reply in the Lesson of 17 June 1970; see 'XIII. The Power of the Impossibles', in *Seminar XVII*, pp. 180–192 (pp. 184–187).

[90] The seven interview questions were:

'1. In the *Écrits*, you affirm that Freud anticipates, without being aware of it, the researches of Saussure and the Prague circle. Can you explain yourself on this point?

2. Linguistics, psychoanalysis and ethnology have in common the notion of structure; beginning with this notion, can one not imagine the statement [*énoncé*] of a common field that will one day reunite psychoanalysis, ethnology, and linguistics?

3. Would not one of the possible articulations between psychoanalysis and linguistics be the privilege awarded to metaphor and metonymy, by Jakobson on the linguistic plane, and by you on the psychoanalytic plane?

4. You say that the discovery of the unconscious led to a second Copernican revolution. How is the unconscious a key notion that subverts every theory of *connaissance*?

5. What are its consequences on the plane of: (a) science, (b) philosophy, (c) more particularly, of Marxism, even of Communism?

6. How are *savoir* and truth incompatible?

7. To govern, to educate, to psychoanalyse are three wagers impossible to make. However, the psychoanalyst must indeed hook onto this perpetual contestation of all discourse, and notably his own. He hooks onto a *savoir*—analytic *savoir*—the one which by definition he contests. How do you resolve—or not—this contradiction? Status of the impossible? The impossible is the Real?'

disruptive element within the history of this scientific knowledge that Lacan describes.

'Radiophonie' is a particularly important text for the argument of this book as a whole, that Lacan's position with respect to Marx appears significantly different in light of the details of some particular co-ordinates in the history of Marxism. The interview foregrounds some central notions that readers of Marx had been moving towards and circling around for decades by the late 1960s. The fact that the themes of 'Radiophonie' are introduced by an interlocutor demonstrates not just that these were, at the time, co-ordinates within which Lacan was commonly being viewed, or that it was these that characterised the position psychoanalysis was understood to hold more broadly in France, but also that this very position was in question in significant ways. There was clearly a space, and a demand, for psychoanalysis to intervene in this set of co-ordinates, and the interview represents Lacan's clarification, and de-centring, of exactly where it was located in this respect. Georgin's questions are symptomatic of what psychoanalysis seemed, to many, to be able to achieve: the bridging together of linguistics, ethnology, philosophy, and politics in a uniquely disruptive, enigmatic way. On each account, Lacan argues that to rely on psychoanalysis as such a bridge is to misrecognise its status with respect to what knowledge fundamentally is.[91]

The first three questions of the interview prompt a return by Lacan to the calibration of the unconscious with structural linguistics that he first articulated in the 1950s. Lacan clarifies here, in 1970, with particular vividity, his view of language as independent of, and as acting on and through, subjectivity.[92] On one level, this amounts to a slightly more lyri-

---

[91] Georgin went on to study at Paris VIII, and later published books about Lacan, psychoanalysis, and linguistics. See Robert Georgin, *Le temps freudien du verbe* (Lausanne: L'Âge d'Homme, coll. "Spinx", 1975); *Lacan* (Lausanne: L'Âge d'Homme, 1977); and *L'inceste et ses tabous: Essai sur le mythe de la déesse* (Paris: Cistre, 1993).

[92] Lacan illustrates this through the image of the poet, who 'produces himself by being [...] eaten by worms/lines [*vers*], which find amongst themselves their arrangement without bothering, it's clear, whether the poet knows anything about them or not' ('Radiophonie', in *Autres écrits*, p. 405). The poet evoked here is seemingly modelled on the surrealist automatic writer, with echoes, too, of Rimbaud's 'Je est un autre'—though this also has its precedents in a much longer history of poetic inspiration, by a muse other than the unconscious. This poet is Lacan's archetypal figure of the 'subject [who] is not the one who knows what he is saying, when indeed something is said by the word which is lacking, but also in the oddness of a behaviour that he believes his own'; whose

cal rendition of the theory of the materiality of the signifier developed in 'The Instance of the Letter in the Unconscious' (1957). Chapter 4 explored some of the silent assumptions that existed behind Lacan's dovetailing of Saussure and Freud, and discussed Lacan's deployment, in making this connection, of an implicit historical argument. As François Dosse sees it, Lacan's projection of metaphor and metonymy back onto the Freudian mechanisms of condensation and displacement, in 'The Instance of the Letter', has the effect of making Freud look like the inventor of structuralism.[93] In 'Radiophonie', Lacan develops explicitly these historical implications of his return to Freud. Georgin's first question asks Lacan to explain his supposed 'affirm[ation] that Freud anticipates, without being aware of it, the researches of Saussure and the Prague circle'.[94] Lacan responds by emphasising that he is steadfastly opposed to the idea that Freud "influenced" Saussure. He instead makes a far more radical argument: that Freud's work amounted to an opening of the unconscious that made Saussurean linguistics possible.

Lacan's return to Freud is not, he makes clear, pointing out how 'Freud anticipates linguistics'.[95] Instead, he says, it traces out 'the formula I now liberate: the unconscious is the condition of linguistics'.[96] The 'eruption of the unconscious' enabled by Freud is, as Lacan presents it, what allowed linguistics 'to emerge from the doubtful light by which the University, by the name of human sciences, still eclipses science'.[97] Lacan is rejecting the idea of a historical progression, that would see some kind of flame of genius having been passed from Freud to Saussure. Instead, he says, something radical was opened up by Freud on the level of discourse, or

speech, in other words, is overdetermined by unconscious knowledge. In this independence of language with respect to the subject—its ability to speak through the subject, without the subject having any knowledge of this speech—is 'the order of facts that Freud calls the unconscious' (pp. 405–6).

[93] Dosse, *History of Structuralism*, p. 106.

[94] Lacan, 'Radiophonie', p. 406.

[95] Lacan, 'Radiophonie', p. 406.

[96] Lacan, 'Radiophonie', p. 406. '[L]a formule que je libère maintenant: l'inconscient est la condition de la linguistique'.

[97] Lacan, 'Radiophonie', p. 406. 'Sans l'éruption de l'inconscient, pas moyen que la linguistique sorte du jour douteux dont l'Université, du nom des sciences humaines, fait encore eclipse à la science'.

social bond. As he puts it here, Freud made the unconscious, in the sense of an independent language that speaks through subjects, the object of a science. The effect, on the level of discourse, of inaugurating this status for language is, he says, what made Saussurean linguistics possible. In response, then, to Georgin's first question, which asked Lacan to clarify how Freud 'anticipated' Saussure and the Prague circle of linguistics, Lacan instead outlines how the opening of the unconscious was the event that made their work possible. This was a historical event, for Lacan, in which Freud was involved. As we know from Lacan's comments on Marx, however, he sees this as an event that took place in a way that makes Freud only one player in its occurrence. Psychoanalysis, as Lacan declares in *Seminar XVI*, is the symptom of 'a turning point of knowledge in history'.[98] What this opening section of 'Radiophonie' also implies is that psychoanalysis amounts to a turning point in knowledge *of* history. Lacan is suggesting that, with psychoanalysis, history—and certainly the history of science—can be approached in a different way to that which is implied by Georgin.

Lacan's response to this first question of the interview begins with his reiteration of his theory of the materiality of the signifier. It then makes a continuous movement through to his reappraisal of the historical position of the unconscious with respect to science. One of Lacan's concerns in 'Radiophonie' is to elaborate how these dimensions—the signifier, the history of science, and the position *of* psychoanalysis in history—are locked together by his theory of discourses. In another equally important way, however, Lacan is resisting the kind of unification that Georgin proposes. He is resisting an integration of psychoanalysis with other fields of science. Georgin's following two questions to Lacan press him, firstly, on the possibility of a 'common field that will one day reunite psychoanalysis, ethnology, and linguistics' based on the 'notion of structure' that these disciplines share. After this, he asks whether Lacan's identification of metonymy and metaphor, as principles of the function of the unconscious, could serve as a fulcrum between the fields of psychoanalysis and linguistics. Lacan responds by describing where psychoanalysis exceeds either of these two other fields. On the one hand, linguistics, he says,

[98] Lacan, *Seminar XVI*, p. 33. Translation modified.

omits the position of the object *a* in the gap between the body of the symbolic and the individual human body, which is made by the organic body being 'incorporated' into the symbolic.[99] On the other hand, structuralist ethnology violates the principle of there being no metalanguage, because it treats mythemes as if they are untranslatable, and therefore outside of language.[100]

Lacan's response to this question also contains a reemphasis of the idea that the unique status of psychoanalysis boils down to the distinction between *connaissance*—the imaginary knowledge that takes things as wholes—and *savoir*—knowledge on the level of the symbolic. It is *savoir* alone, he says, that facilitates the logical calculus able to circumscribe the real. Lacan's distinction between *connaissance* and *savoir* provides the main co-ordinates for his new account of the history of science. Lacan describes this later in the interview, building on the shifts mapped out in *Seminar XVI* and *Seminar XVII*. Georgin's fourth question presses Lacan on his claim that 'the discovery of the unconscious led to a second Copernican revolution', by asking how the unconscious serves, in Georgin's words, as 'a key notion that subverts every theory of *connaissance*'.[101] In a typically contrarian response, Lacan gives a penetrating analysis of this notion of the Copernican break and its consequences. He begins with a revised account of the history of astronomy, which frames this history as a romance of *connaissance* and *savoir*. For Lacan, amending Freud's famous formulation, Copernicus does not offer the archetypal image of revolution, nor does the unconscious necessarily amount to the liquefier of *connaissance*.[102] Lacan begins his answer to this fourth question by addressing the way that it evokes, in its reference to

[99] Lacan, 'Radiophonie', pp. 409–10. As a result, he adds, the body amounts to an 'empty set' in the mathematical sense.

[100] Lacan, 'Radiophonie', p. 411.

[101] Lacan, 'Radiophonie', p. 420.

[102] See Sigmund Freud, 'Lecture XVII. Fixation to Traumas—The Unconscious', in *The Standard Edition of the Complete Psychological Works of Sigmund Freud, Vol. XVI (1916–1917): Introductory Lectures to Psycho-Analysis (Part III)*, trans. by James Strachey (London: The Hogarth Press, 1963), pp. 271–285 (pp. 284–285). The idea is rephrased in 'A Difficulty in the Path of Psycho-Analysis', *SE, Vol. XVII*, pp. 135–144 (pp. 140–141), and it is described as a cosmological blow, a biological blow, and a psychological blow in 'The Resistances to Psycho-Analysis', *SE, Vol. XIX*, pp. 211–224 (p. 221).

the scientific 'revolution' brought about by Copernicus, both the political sense of revolution, and also the very astral movement that Copernicus described in making the world revolve around the sun.[103] Lacan deflates the notion of the Copernican 'revolution', by pitching it merely as an act that made the sun the image of the master signifier. The sun in the Copernican model remains centralised, motionless, and unchanged in the centre of the world, just as the S_1 is the fixed point around which other signifiers are made to work, and around which transfer of knowledge is made to occur, in Lacan's theory of discourse. In Freud's famous allegorical allusion to Copernicus, to which Georgin is referring in his question, Freud was comparing the Copernican revolution to the displacement of psychic unity that was achieved by psychoanalysis.[104] But Freud's appeal to Copernicus actually amounts, says Lacan, to a devaluation, on a more fundamental, structural level, of any 'monocentrism'.[105] What Lacan elaborates from this in the interview is a topological principle, of how psychoanalysis presses towards an alternative to a world that would be envisaged as monocentric in any respect—towards a world that would be opposed to the topology of a sphere. What psychoanalysis achieves, then, is not the displacement of a centre, so much as the abdication of any idea of geometrical completeness, or sphericality, which monocentric assumptions carry with them.

In order to develop this idea of the anti-monocentrism of the Freudian turn, Lacan spends the remainder of his response to Georgin's fourth question presenting an abridged history of science. This culminates in his account of the specific way that Marx and Freud facilitated a departure from the reign of *connaissance*. Lacan's history of science amounts to a sweeping and heavily abridged roster of the central figures in Enlightenment thought, positioning them in such a way that they converge onto the point of crisis that Lacan understands the unconscious to crystallise with respect to knowledge. A true revolutionary break did not, for Lacan, occur with Copernicus, because he still imagined the universe

[103] Lacan, 'Radiophonie', p. 420–21.

[104] Hence in both cases Lacan's use of language. He takes advantage of puns and wordplay to demonstrate these as the true material of language, behind which no overarching structure exists.

[105] Lacan, 'Radiophonie', p. 421.

in a way that preserves a spherical topology. There *was* a 'Copernican' break—but it was carried out later, he says, by Kepler, in his theory of the elliptical solar orbit. This step, as Lacan sees it, performed a departure from an imaginary universe governed by abstract symmetries, towards a symbolic one understood in terms of mathematical calculation. Lacan describes this shift, with reference to Alexandre Koyré, as a *connaissance* that has—in a departure from the veneer of imaginary wholeness—begun to fold back onto itself:

> That around which turns, but that's precisely the word to avoid, around which gravitates the effort of a *connaissance* on the way to finding itself as imaginary, it is clearly, as one reads it by making with Koyré the chronicle of Kepler's approach, by ridding oneself of the idea that the movement of rotation, because it engenders the circle (that is: the perfect form), can alone be appropriate for the affection of the heavenly body that is the planet.[106]

As Lacan traces out here, the introduction of an elliptical trajectory for heavenly bodies opened the way for the Galilean assertion that the planets turn according to a movement that is dependent on their masses.

This Galilean model required complex mathematical calculation, and an awareness of the wealth of variables involved in this planetary motion. Lacan positions Newton as a continuation along the historical path of this movement of knowledge. Newton's formulas, he says, fully isolated the independence of structure from the imaginary—their 'assembly with the real', as Lacan puts it.[107] At the same time, Newton's theories retained, says Lacan, the 'scandal' of proposing that elements of mass attract one another without having any medium to transmit this force; his theories therefore preserved the occult idea of matter being able, in effect, to communicate with itself.[108] As discussed in Chap. 2, in *Seminar XII: Crucial Problems for Psychoanalysis* (1964–65), Lacan uses this same critique of

[106] Lacan, 'Radiophonie', p. 421–422.

[107] Lacan, 'Radiophonie', p. 423.

[108] This was the criticism that had originally been made of Newton by Leibniz, as discussed in detail by Koyré in *Newtonian Studies* (1965), and as referred to by Lacan in *Seminar XII* (1964–65). See Koyré, *Newtonian Studies* (London: Chapman & Hall, 1965), p. 139; Lacan, Lesson 18, of 12 May 1965, in *Seminar XII: Crucial Problems for Psychoanalysis* (1964–1965), unpublished. For an unofficial translation, see Gallagher, <http://www.lacaninireland.com/web/wp-content/uploads/2010/06/12-Crucial-problems-for-psychoanalysis.pdf>, p. 239; and Chapter 2, pp. 70–72.

Newton to demonstrate the function of the 'subject supposed to know' that silently underpins Newton's theories. It is also a good example of the assumption of knowledge in the real. For Newton, as Lacan—following Leibniz—criticises him here, elements of mass are assumed to 'know' how far away they are from each other, and what force to exert on one another as a result. Newton's *hypotheses non fingo*—his refusal to explain this phenomenon—amounted, says Lacan in 1970, to the 'charter for structure', which decisively located structure in the real. The 'true reach' of the Newtonian innovation, however, was 'stifled' by this obscurantism. Newton therefore does not, says Lacan, reach the point of being able to isolate and identify the paradoxical element that is inherent to structure.

This is the background onto which Marx's discovery of surplus value is placed by Lacan. Surplus value represents, for Lacan, the point of ultimate structural flux, and the inscribed co-ordinate of its breakdown. In making surplus value both the point that is foreclosed by the capitalist discourse, and that which 'motivates' the discourse, Marx, says Lacan, made a break with respect to *savoir* that was not possible before him. Lacan presents this break as an adjournment of the liberal revolution, which was characterised, as Lacan illustrates it, by the spherical subjectivity of the master's discourse. Marx, he says, interrupted this 'from the unconscious and the symptom'.[109] Lacan takes Freud to have made an extension of this odyssey of structure that took it to its limit. Freud, as Lacan points it out here, discovered a *savoir* that operates independently of consciousness, that is structured, as Lacan identified it, like a language, and that is articulated only from a point of lack.[110] Lacan makes a new definition of the unconscious on this basis:

[109] Lacan, 'Radiophonie', p. 424. The full passage reads as follows: 'Il en serait ainsi si Marx ne l'avait replacée de la structure qu'il en formule dans un discours du capitaliste, mais de ce qu'elle ait forclos la plus-value dont il motive ce discours. Autrement dit c'est de l'inconscient et du symptôme qu'il prétend proroger la grande Révolution: c'est de la plus-value découverte qu'il précipite la conscience dite de classe.' Lacan denounces the Leninist revolution, on the other hand, as amounting merely to a '*passage a l'acte*'. As the remainder of this fourth section of 'Radiophonie' argues, the October Revolution betrayed the sense of revolution that Lacan is attempting to articulate.

[110] Lacan, 'Radiophonie', p. 424–5.

> The unconscious, one sees, is only a metaphoric term to designate the *savoir* that only sustains itself in presenting itself as impossible, so that from that it is confirmed as being real (to be understood: real discourse). The unconscious disqualifies nothing worthwhile in that *connaissance* of nature, which is a point of myth, or even inconsistency, to be demonstrated by the unconscious.[111]

The Freudian discovery, as this definition casts it, amounted to the writing of a metaphor. As Lacan articulates in this passage, the unconscious represents the impossible gap within *savoir*, onto which Marx's theories first converged. At the same time, Lacan subverts here Georgin's assumption that the Freudian revolution overthrows all theories based in *connaissance*. These are instead appreciated by Lacan to be of great value. The central example he gives of this is the psychoanalytic idea of the sexual 'non-rapport'. This is the name Lacan gives for what psychoanalysis demonstrates about sexuality: that the original myth of sexual union is a semblance. The idea of a sexual non-rapport is dependent, he says, *on* the very original myth of sexual union or symmetry. As Chap. 4 pointed out, for Lacan, Marx invented the symptom not because he managed to escape the *conaissance* of Hegel's ruses of reason, but because he managed to formulate the truth of them. In the same way, the sexual non-rapport is not the alternative to the myth of sexual rapport, but it is the truth of it; a truth that is dependent on this original error.

Lacan is clear, however, as discussed above, that this stance towards *connaissance* was ultimately missing from Marx's work. This meant that he unintentionally preserved it, even whilst seeking to pierce through it. Lacan makes a series of stabs throughout 'Radiophonie' at contemporary communists on the basis of their failure to comprehend this. Communists in general have, Lacan adds, failed to receive the way that his theories demand a swerve away 'from imaginary impotence', and onto an 'impossible that establishes itself as being the real in only founding itself on logic'.[112] This is Lacan's description of the point where he locates the

[111] Lacan, 'Radiophonie', p. 425. 'L'inconscient, on le voit, n'est que terme métaphorique à designer le savoir qui ne se soutient qu'à se presenter comme impossible, pour que de ça il se confirme d'être réel (entendez discours réel)'.

[112] Lacan, 'Radiophonie', p. 438.

unconscious. It comes into play, as he puts it in passing here, through the impossibility by which sex, as a non-rapport, is inscribed in it.[113]

Lacan offers his idea of 'logical time' as an underlying motor for the historical movement of knowledge that he is describing in 'Radiophonie'. He first introduced the idea of 'logical time' in the 1945 article 'Logical Time and the Assertion of Anticipated Certainty', where he deduces the temporal dimension that he identifies as existing to any logical deduction. The 'moment of concluding' [*moment de conclure*] is the name he gives in the article to an act that redeems a previous error, and transforms

---

[113] Communists, as Lacan claims here, have failed to comprehend the need for a turn away from *connaissance*. He makes a pointed comparison between followers of 'master Marx', and the psychoanalysts who entertain the essentialist idea of 'genital maturity'. These psychoanalysts, in their obscurantism, 'want to know nothing of politics'; but this reproach against them, says Lacan, comes from Marxists who themselves 'make an obligation of the insignias of conjugal normalisation' (p. 438). The unconscious, he adds, by contrast, 'will not subvert our science in making honourable amends with any form of *connaissance*'. He explains this with the idea that communists only 'end up counterfeiting' everything that the bourgeois order makes honourable—including work, family, and country (p. 440).

Lacan's criticisms of Marx continue in the following years of his Seminar. He continues to position psychoanalysis antagonistically with respect to Marx in *Seminar XIX: Or Worse...*, where he adds: 'The promotion of what I am putting forward precisely discolours [...] and finishes off the effect of Marx's discourse. I should like to underscore something in this discourse that constitutes its limit.' Lesson of 8 March 1972, 'VIII. What is Involved in the Other', in *Seminar XIX: Or Worse... (1971–1972)*, ed. by Jacques-Alain Miller, trans. by A. R. Price (Cambridge: Polity, 2018), pp. 95–104 (pp. 101–102).

He returns to this idea again in *Seminar XIXa: The Knowledge of the Analyst*: 'A symptom is not cured in the same way in Marxist dialectic and in psychoanalysis. In psychoanalysis, it has to do with something that is the translation of its truth value into speech. That this should give rise to what is felt by the analyst to be a Being of refusal on no account allows it to be seeded as to whether this feeling deserves to be retained in any way, because equally, in other registers, precisely in the register I mentioned earlier, the symptom has to yield to altogether different procedures.

I'm not according preference to any one of these procedures, and even less so given that I want to enable you to hear that there is another dialectic besides the one that is imputed to history.' Lesson of 2 December 1971, 'II. On Incomprehension and Other Themes', in *Talking to Brick Walls: A Series of Presentations in the Chapel at Sainte-Anne Hospital*, trans. by A.R. Price (Cambridge: Polity, 2017), pp. 35–70 (pp. 45–46).

In another lesson of this seminar, he gives a clearer indictment of Marx as having perpetuated the discourse of the master: 'Again, history has shown that this discourse was alive and kicking for centuries in a way that was profitable for everyone up until a particular inflection, whereupon, by virtue of a fractional slippage that went unnoticed by the very people concerned by it, it turned into the discourse of the capitalist, of which we wouldn't have had the faintest idea had Marx not set himself to completing it, to giving it its subject, the proletariat. Thanks to this, the discourse of capitalism has flourished in every nation-state that has taken a Marxist form'. Lesson of 6 January 1971, 'III. I've Been Talking to Brick Walls', in *Talking to Brick Walls*, pp. 71–104 (p. 90).

it into truth.[114] Projecting this process onto the historical path of science, Lacan frames Newton's theory of gravity as the 'moment of concluding' of the movement that was first inaugurated by Copernicus. In the following passage of 'Radiophonie', Lacan describes poetically how he promotes this principle to one operating on the level of history:

> My proof does not touch being except by making it be born from the fault that the being produces by saying itself.
>
> Whence the author is to be reduced to making himself a means for a desire which is beyond him.
>
> But there is an intermediary other than what Socrates said in act.
>
> He knew like us that for the being, it takes time to get used to being.
>
> This "*faut le temps*" [it takes/needs time] is the being that solicits from the unconscious to return to it each time that it will have to take, yes, *faudra le temps*.[115]

In general, Lacan is presenting the history of science here as a gradual emergence from a world governed by the spherical totality of *connaissance*. This, for him, was enabled not by the mere appearance of *savoir*, but because this new form of knowledge eventually made discernible the fault in structure that Freud identified as the unconscious. Two implications of the above passage are, firstly, that the truth that emerges from science as a result is not tethered to the particular figure who attempted to enunciate it, and secondly, that this truth is never fully realised by

---

[114] Lacan, 'Logical Time and the Assertion of Anticipated Certainty' (1945), in *Écrits*, pp. 161–175 (pp. 171–172). For an extended summary of this article's logic, and a discussion of its uptake of theories of W.H. Bion, see Max Maher, 'Post-World War II Group Psychology and the Limits of Leadership: Bion, Lacan and the Leaderless Group', in *Psychoanalysis and History*, 22, no. 3 (2020), 317–339.

[115] Lacan, 'Radiophonie', p. 426:

> Mon épreuve ne touche à l'être qu'à le faire naître de la faille que produit l'étant de se dire.
>
> D'où l'auteur est à reléguer à se faire moyen pour un désir qui le dépasse.
>
> Mais il y a entremise autre qu'a dir Socrate en acte.
>
> Il savait comme nous qu'à l'étant, faut le temps de se faire à être.
>
> Ce "faut le temps", c'est l'être qui sollicite de l'inconscient pour y faire retour chaque fois que lui faudra, oui faudra le temps.

these attempted enunciations. At the same time, it is not located in some ideal plane waiting to be channelled by a sufficiently intuitive oracle. The psychoanalytic break amounts to an indexing of the history of science onto the 'fault in being' produced by language, which can only be realised, as Lacan makes clear here, by its contextualisation in a sequence of events that precipitated this fault. The axis of history is crucial, therefore, to his understanding of what science is. Truth, for him, only appears from structure in partial flashes, through the passage of time.

It is through this projection of logical time onto history that Lacan, motivated by a general frustration with what he sees as the impoverished idea of revolution still harboured by his contemporary Marxists, gives a brief prescription, in his response to the sixth question of the interview, of the political function of the psychoanalyst. In 'Radiophonie', he has been outlining a reading of the Freudian symptom as a failure within *savoir*, from which truth—in the transient and partial way that Lacan conceives of it—can appear. It emerges, he says, through the movement of logical time, in an appearance that he says comes as a surprise, in what he calls an act of 'Freudian grace [*la grâce freudienne*]'. It is, says Lacan, 'at this joint in the real that is found the political incidence where the psychoanalyst would have his place if he were capable of it':

> There would be the act that puts into play the *savoir* to make a law of. [A] Revolution that happens because a *Savoir* is reduced to making a symptom, seen from the very gaze that it [*Savoir*] has produced.[116]

This reconditely articulated passage frames the political function of the analyst as a circling-back onto the flaw in *savoir* that Lacan, in 'Radiophonie', is equating to the symptom. This dimension of the symptom would then, he says, have a privileged position in the realm of politics.[117] In the ambiguous style of this text as a whole, Lacan is formulating

[116] Lacan, 'Radiophonie', p. 443, from Lacan's answer to the sixth question. 'Là serait l'acte qui met en jeu de quel savoir faire la loi. Révolution qui arrive de ce qu'un Savoir de réduise à faire symptôme, vu du regard même qu'il a produit.' Lacan's answer to this question is also translated by Russell Grigg in 'VIII. From Myth to Structure', in *Seminar XVII*, pp. 130–132.

[117] For a reading of this aspect of 'Radiophonie', see Éric Laurent, 'La société du symptôme', *Quarto*, 79 (June 2003), 3–9.

the political 'incidence', or position, that he thinks the psychoanalyst is able to take in civilisation. There is, however, nothing like a political programme given by Lacan here—or even a politics at all. He has been describing in 'Radiophonie' the way in which he thinks modern science historically deployed *savoir* as knowledge in the real. Because Lacan understands the psychoanalyst as the product of a turning point in knowledge, they would, by this account, be able to look *back* at knowledge in a way that was not possible before, and to appreciate the *effects* of knowledge in a new way as a result. Lacan is not invoking any envisaged future of society. He is, however, establishing that psychoanalysis—and psychoanalysts, understood as subjects of the shift in knowledge that he has been tracing—can have a political effect, or 'incidence', based on the privileged position that he gives to them in the text.

The Symptom: 'A Turning Point of Knowledge in History'

In 'Radiophonie', Lacan is indexing the entire history of science onto the emergence of the unconscious in Freud's work, to the extent that the Freudian unconscious becomes the decisive event, and the most important turning point or crisis, in this history. Lacan presents the origin of psychoanalysis as a moment when knowledge, after a process of revolution beginning with modern science, fully turned back onto itself, to achieve a registering of its own necessary internal division. This is not, however, a moment of unification, consolidation, or becoming, but a decisive shift from what came before. As a direct consequence of this, psychoanalysis also makes possible, for Lacan, a transformed understanding of this historical process itself, which Lacan presents in the reframed history of science that he describes in 'Radiophonie'.

Freud, Lacan says, responded to a transformation on a radical level; what Lacan refers to as a 'turning point of *savoir* in history'. This, as he clarifies in *Seminar XVI*, is not the same thing as a turning point 'in the history of *savoir*'.[118] For Lacan, the Freudian unconscious is not just one

[118] Lacan, *Seminar XVI*, p. 33. Translation modified.

more meander in the river that would amount to the history of knowledge. It is not a shift that could be registered as having taken place, in a history that could, at least in principle, be mapped out. Instead, he thinks of knowledge—*savoir*—as itself having gone through a major transformation, which resulted in the appearance of psychoanalysis. This makes a view of the 'history of *savoir*' redundant. This view would in itself preserve a belief in knowledge in the real, by assuming that *savoir* has a history, in the sense of an inert historical trajectory, rather than being the very discursive material out of which *jouissance* is produced, and through which *objets a* metastasise human reality. Lacan thinks of knowledge as something that changes through history, in a way that psychoanalysis can make visible and determinable, because the psychoanalyst, as he says in *Seminar XVI*, occupies a position from which they are able to point out the gaps in the structure to which any history would amount.[119] Knowledge, in short, is fundamentally different after Freud.

One of the aims of this book as a whole has been to trace a significant but neglected arc of the interaction between Marxist thought, German idealism, and psychoanalysis in twentieth-century France. The book has sought to give an account of Lacan's position in these traditions. Lacan, it argues, attempted to make his work into a focal point for a set of questions that were generated at this moment around readings of Marx. In 'Radiophonie', Lacan uses the Freudian unconscious to produce a levelling effect on the co-ordinates that generated these questions. This is why he keeps deflating or subverting assumptions that lay behind the questions of Robert Georgin to which he responds in the text. These questions repeatedly assume that psychoanalysis can act as a suturing point for a set of disciplines, that would deliver the knowledge generated by those disciplines into a real, coherent politics. In this, these questions anticipate the position into which Lacan is pressed by the Ljubljana School: in Žižek's rescuing of Hegel and Althusser through Lacan; in Tomšič's stitching together of Lacan and Marx; or in Zupančič's enlistment of Lacan as a missing piece to unite Kant, Marx, and Freud, nowhere is it considered that these might not be achievable tasks; that they might be self-defeating on some level—or that psychoanalysis might itself manifest

[119] See Lacan, *Seminar XVI*, p. 15.

the very point representing the limit of such a consolidation.[120] This, however, is what Lacan is saying by positioning psychoanalysis as the symptom—the object *a*—of knowledge in history. For Lacan, psychoanalysis does not fit back together pieces of knowledge that have been broken apart by modernity. It situates itself as a co-ordinate outside of them, which is able therefore to approach this knowledge in a new way. In doing so, psychoanalysis can have a levelling effect on existing knowledge, one that these philosophers exploit to make possible a cascade of connections, equations, and parallels. These flow so effortlessly only because Lacan has, in removing all friction opposed to them, already fundamentally undermined and subverted their significance.

Another aim of this thesis, and of this chapter in particular, has been to make clear where Lacan stands with respect to Marx, because of the degree to which their conjunction has been cathected by contemporary theoretical attention. Lacan did, with reference to Althusser, make a reading of *Capital* in the late 1960s and early 1970s, that had a decisive role in his theories. As this chapter has attempted to show, however, this reading did not just amount to a shift in the narrative of Lacan's theories, but also attempted to produce a radically altered portrayal of Marx. From Lacan, we receive a version of Marx whose critique of political economy represented the inauguration of capitalist discourse. This dual impact of Marx is the central example of the rupture in knowledge that, as has been a theme in this and prior chapters, Lacan demonstrates to be what is identified by a true materialism. Hence that centrality of unintended consequences to Lacan's theories, and the proximities he registers between points that are structurally opposed. What the reality of the unconscious brings to light on an ethical level is that, after psychoanalysis, knowledge, banished from the real where it was once believed to have secreted itself away, cannot be taken for granted to function on its own—as the naïve Marxists whom Lacan pillories in 'Radiophonie' as the 'babysitters of history' assume.[121] Instead, it requires attention, ingenuity, and constant work to keep it from slipping into the death-driven circuit on whose edge

[120] See Zupančič, *Ethics of the Real* (London: Verso, 1995), p. 17, as summarised in n.88, above.
[121] Lacan, 'Radiophonie', p. 415.

it sits.[122] Lacan attributes joint discoveries to Marx: the invention of the symptom, on the one hand, and the founding of capitalism, on the other. The key thing uncovered by Lacan is that you cannot have one without the other. The symptomatic point manifested by *plus-de-jouir* could only be discovered once a discourse appeared that attempted to metabolise it in surplus value, and psychoanalysis and Marx are, as a result, both implicated on the deepest of levels with capitalism. The idea that the unconscious is capitalist should therefore be understood not as a positioning of psychoanalysis as the antidote to capitalism, but as the moment of psychoanalysis's Oedipal dénouement: when it first sees itself for what it truly always has been. For Lacan, psychoanalysis does not open up a means to exit capitalism, but a means to realise something new, and more extensive, about the deadlock to which capitalism ultimately amounts.

It is possible, as many increasingly do, to read the Lacanian algebra developed throughout his work, and epitomised by the four discourses, as a semiotics of all philosophy—as the switchboard connecting the loose ends of the history of knowledge, or a nuclear scan lighting up its points of symptomatic conflict, so that they can be polished off by the philosophers at the end of history. Lacan's true intention, though, was to bring to a head a crisis in what he understands knowledge fundamentally to be after Freud, by demonstrating the subterranean faultlines that exist in the nature of knowledge itself, which, in his portrayal of them, continue to

---

[122] Lacan elaborates the connection between capitalism and the death drive in *Seminar XIXa: The Knowledge of the Analyst* (1971–1972): 'What differentiates the discourse of capitalism is *Verwerfung*, the fact of rejecting, outside all the fields of the symbolic. This brings with it the consequence I have already said it has. What does it reject? Well, castration. Any order, any discourse that aligns itself with capitalism, sweeps to one side what we may simply call, my fine friends, matters of love. You see, it's a mere nothing' (*Talking to Brick Walls*, pp. 90–91).

In the 'Milan Discourse' of 1972, Lacan represents the discourse of capitalism as a figure of eight, formed by an inversion of the discourse of the master, and describes it as follows: 'After all, it is the cleverest discourse that we have made. It is no less headed for a blowout. This is because it is untenable. It is untenable… in a thing that I could explain to you… because capitalist discourse is here, you see… a little inversion simply between the S_1 and the S… which is the subject… it suffices so that that goes on casters [*ça marche comme sur des roulettes*], indeed that cannot go better, but that goes too fast, that consumes itself, that consumes itself so that is consumed [*ça se consomme, ça se consomme si bien que ça se consume*]' (Discourse of 12 May 1972, University of Milan, in *Lacan in Italia-Lacan en Italy 1953–1978* (Milan: La Salmandra, 1978), pp. 32–55 (p. 46)). For an unofficial translation, see Jack W. Stone, <https://freud2lacan.b-cdn.net/DISCOURSE_OF_CAPITALISM-bilingual.pdf>.

animate a haunted civilisation. Lacan does not, for this reason, represent a missing piece of a puzzle made up of German idealism and dialectical materialism. The unconscious cannot be placed on the side of what came before it, or bracketed in with an earlier paradigm. It has a history, and part of that history is what this book has been articulating. According to Lacan, however, it manifests a turning point in that history that penetrates through it and transforms it. It is possible to read the Ljubljana philosophers as demonstrating a key awareness of this—but only if the history this book has started to articulate is comprehended. Without this, these philosophers look less like products of the Lacanian shift, and more like reactionary attempts to overlook what it achieved. To borrow Žižek's own description of Hegel in *Less Than Nothing*, these philosophers themselves are significant because of their not-All quality—because something does not quite fully emerge in them of the Lacanian discovery. There is a parallax gap inherent within their work: it represents a registering of the crux of Lacan's thought, but at the same time an avoidance of it; a failure to register what it claims to have transformed.

6

Conclusion: 'A Lot of Fireworks'

This book has been attempting to present a fuller, more subtle account of the relationship between the work of Lacan and Marx than those that currently exist, by positioning Lacan in the context of the history of Marxism. It has described how developments in milieux of thought within and associated with Marxism contemporary to Lacan pressed towards dramatic shifts in how Marx was being perceived and understood in the early-twentieth century. These, it has argued, formed the background for Lacan's own ambivalent and critical interpretation of Marx, which reads *Capital* as the site, not only of a decisive shift in the history of science, but also as the introduction of a problematic deadlock into this history. It is inadequate, therefore, to read Lacan as either an ally or an enemy of Marx. Lacan's work was so dependent on the set of paradoxes and problems that concerned Marxists contemporary to him that, in order to articulate what he found to be most important about Marx, he was led to dissolve some of the fundamental co-ordinates of Marx's thought. It took Lacan time to develop this position. Abstracting Lacan from either this context, or this process of his own development, obscures the position of his work with respect to Marx.

M. Maher, *Symptom Invented*, The Palgrave Lacan Series,
https://doi.org/10.1007/978-3-032-12267-4_6

The four chapters of this book have described how a stark revision of the relationship between Marx and Hegel, and that of materialism and idealism more broadly, can be identified in Lacan's work. This was made possible, for one, as a result of the way Lacan read Hegel. The functions of knowledge that Lacan learns and distils from Hegel are not ones that, for him, would disappear if capitalism no longer existed. The imaginary element of knowledge that Lacan, in *Seminar XVIII* (1971), names the semblance is, it is important to emphasise, in no way simply the enemy for him. From his perspective, the lure of the semblance has to be regarded as an inevitable component of knowledge, and as something that knowledge depends on. Chapter 2 summarised how this was deduced by Lacan in the early years of his Seminar in ways that directly adapted the work of the French Hegelians in the 1920s and 1930s, and their questions, regarding the Hegelian notion of absolute knowledge and the consequences posed to it by Kierkegaard's critique. Lacan presents the semblance as being mobilised in the subject supposed to know, the receptacle of transference which is operative as the skeletal core of all knowledge. This is one reason why Marx is given two faces by Lacan in *Seminar XVII* (1969–70). One basis for Lacan's reproaches of Marx is that he is not able to take the dimension of the semblance seriously enough, but attempts simply to pierce through it, by dismissing the Hegelian dialectic as an ideological mirage. This is a classical reading of Marx that was being put under great pressure in France at the time—most clearly, in concerns about the Hegelianism of his early work—in a way that Lacan is taking to a limit. Althusser had articulated something similar, in his own terms, by emphasising the significance of ideology, and of the superstructural components of society, which this more classical Marxism had regarded as mere apparitions produced by an economic base. Althusser did so not as a criticism of Marx, but in order to complete Marx's theory of production by including in it the function of ideology. Lacan, however, argues that the function of the semblance is operative in *all* knowledge—a notion that he took from a reading of Hegel in the 1950s—and that this undermines Marx's own project without him realising it. As Kojève identified, despite Marx's disregard for the Hegelian dialectic, he did not jettison absolute knowledge, but reinstated it in the form of the Communist State at the End of History. Marx remains, therefore, in this way especially, under the sway of the semblance, whilst being unable to identify the function of the semblance theoretically. The old, classic question of Marx's 'inversion' of Hegel is thereby given a new articulation by Lacan. For him, there is something in Hegel's limits, as recognised by the French Hegelians, that continues to determine the materialist dialectic.

What this led to, in Lacan's critical view, was the rebirth within materialism of a new, spiritualistic idealism. Lacan's idea that knowledge depends on the artifice of the semblance is redeployed in his claim that modern science assumes that there is 'knowledge in the real'. This, as Chap. 3 discussed, was the core of Lacan's critique of Pavlovian reflexology: that it is based on the spiritualistic belief that knowledge exists inscribed within material reality. This assumption, for Lacan, denies the dimension of artifice that he locates at the transferential core of all knowledge. It forecloses the dimension that had troubled readers of Hegel, from Kierkegaard onwards, in the form of 'subjectivity' or 'existence'—the dimension psychoanalysis had always understood as that of libido, or love—and the one on which, for Lacan, all knowledge in fact depends. The error of assuming knowledge in the real is one that Lacan ascribes to materialism more generally. He identifies it especially, however, in the attempt to give psychology a materialist revival. In this context, Wallon holds much more significance for Lacan's work than that of a defeated master or repressed influence. He represents an anchoring point for Lacan's position in a history of thinking about dialectical materialism, and in a history of the problems posed to dialectical materialism by psychology; a science of subjectivity marked, from its name onwards, by remnants of spiritualistic idealism. Hence why, as Chap. 3 described, Lacan repeats amended forms of the theoretical steps made by Vygotsky and Politzer when they attempted to use Freud to address these problems. For Lacan, Freud is the one who made a turning point in this hubris of science, and its assumption of knowledge in the real, because it was he who first theorised the operation of transference in human experience. Lacan thereby makes Freud the bearer of a new way to approach the problem of subjective existence, which had been such a dominant theme, and such a stumbling-block, in French Marxist thought.

This is in no way, however, Lacan's pitting of Freud against Marx. Lacan's means of theorising the nature of history makes it clear that he is putting forward an entirely different conception of their relationship. It was Althusser who made Marx a turning point in the history of science, by arguing that one particular epistemological object that had been previously invisible to science—surplus value—was the lynchpin of the structure of all of human experience. Freud, for Althusser, then inaugurated a science capable of uniting biology with sociology, a fusion that he takes Lacan to have completed. Althusser implies that Marx, Freud, and Lacan (and, it would follow, also Althusser himself) were accomplishing a gradual triangulation onto a complete field of science. Lacan deliberately undermines this approach to studying history, because he extends his own critique of the assumption of knowledge in the real also to the study of history itself. Both this tendency to destined completion that is latent in Althusser's theory of history, and his reliance on the force of 'necessity' in the life of the individual, then appear as the remnants of a belief in knowledge in the real—this time, in the real of history.

In Lacan's hands, psychoanalysis becomes the science whose object is that which is lost from modern science, because of modern science's belief in knowledge in the real. Lacan identifies this object of psychoanalysis as the metabolised form of *jouissance* that science produced by triggering the subsumption of all human life by the logic of capitalist industry. This is what Lacan names *plus-de-jouir*, or the object *a*, in 1968. For Lacan, as Chap. 5 described, Marx made the definitive turning point in the history of enabling this subsumption, because his critique of political economy completed the hubristic metabolisation of *plus-de-jouir* effected by modern scientific knowledge. In this way, Lacan agrees with Althusser—but only by pointing out the unintended consequences of Marx's act. Marx replaced all of the mystified bases for human social bonds with surplus value. In doing so, he invented the symptom, but he also, Lacan argues, founded capitalism. Lacan obviously is not suggesting, by saying this, that factory owners, entrepreneurs, and stockbrokers read *Capital* as an economic handbook. Nor, of course, is he suggesting any allegiance of Freud with Marx. But Lacan is arguing that, when the deceitful farce that had been undertaken for about a century before Marx was fully unveiled by him, for the first time, for what it truly was, it made just as profound an effect on human life as the articulation of the formulas of thermodynamics deployed in the industrial revolution had. This is an argument made possible by Lacan's conception of discourse as an unconscious logic underpinning all social bonds, all subjectivity, and all *jouissance*. Lacan is arguing that Marx's invention of the symptom—and with it, the founding of capitalism, the misrecognition of *plus-de-jouir*, and the conjuring of the mirage of the Communist revolution—had to take place in order to make the field of psychoanalysis possible.

Lacan makes psychoanalysis inherit what is, by his strategic estimation, most fundamental about Marx. Even so, he is clearly still pitting psychoanalysis against Marx in significant ways. So what does he think psychoanalysis can do that Marxism can't? What is certain is that Lacan prescribes nothing politically to replace what he denounces in Marx. In a passage discussed in Chap. 5, from towards the end of the sixth section of 'Radiophonie', he invokes the 'political incidence' that the psychoanalyst is capable of occupying, as a vantage-point on the history of knowledge he describes in the interview. This replacement of Marxist politics, and of the promise of Communism, with the pretence of positioning the psychoanalyst in what sounds like a historical panopticon, is not popular with Marxists. In response to the first question of 'Radiophonie', Lacan recounts how a young Marxist attacked him following his presentation on 'The Subversion of the Subject and the Dialectic of Desire in Psychoanalysis' in 1960. 'Do you think, he said to me, that it is enough that you have produced something, written letters on a blackboard, in order to expect a result from them?'.[1] This preceded the very similar reproach voiced by the would-be revolutionaries of May 1968, in the anti-structuralist slogan "structures don't march in the streets". The response Lacan gives in 'Radiophonie' to this criticism is that the letters and formulas he writes on the blackboard do not communicate something, but produce the 'displacement of discourse'. Without the effect of this displacement, he says, 'the convulsions of history remain an enigma'.[2] Both the attempted revolution of May '68, and Lenin's October Revolution, were mere actings-out, says Lacan in 'Radiophonie', because each was performed by subjects who identified with a logic in the real of

[1] Lacan, 'Radiophonie', in *Autres écrits* (Paris: Seuil, 2001), pp. 403–447 (p. 407).

[2] Lacan, 'Radiophonie', p. 407.

history.[3] They made a 'mockery' of this dialectic, he says, because they made themselves its 'slaves'.[4]

Lacan is criticised by these Marxists, for regressing into a naïve, liberal conservatism.[5] His denouncement of Marx is accused of replacing political action and organisation with arrogant, cerebral intellectual games, and with a clinic that is staunchly and proudly apolitical. His reading of Marx, from this perspective, achieved a blunting aestheticisation of Marx's politics; his reticence and complexity, this argument goes, avoids politics, and draws revolutionary Marxism back into obscure scholasticism. The melodrama of continuous dissolution triggered by Lacan in French psychoanalysis, and the failure of the pass as an attempt to solve this problem, can then be read conveniently as a correlate of this political failure. As Miller puts it, ventriloquising a fictional critic of Lacan in his introduction to *Television* (1990), '[h]e brags, repeats himself, makes erroneous claims and disappears into the shadows, while shooting off a lot of fireworks'.[6]

Something this book has been highlighting is that this complication and deferral of politics in any clear sense was already an uncomfortable presence in Marxist thought contemporary to Lacan. What was the *politics* of the materialist psychologists, who attempted to form a new subject for Communism, but who discovered only theoretical impasses? What would it mean *politically* to have a *Capital*, not of political economy, but of psychology? How was Communist politics to break from Hegelian liberalism if Marx really *was* still somehow conditioned by the Hegelian dialectic? How far did capitalism extend as a frame for a subject's reality, and could this frame be escaped, or even perceived? In each case, these were questions that many were realising could not be answered by Marx. Lacan is arguing that something could not be seen by his contemporaries. He is saying that there is something about what capitalism *is* that was

[3] Lacan, 'Radiophonie', p. 424.

[4] Lacan, 'Radiophonie', p. 407.

[5] See Lacan, 'Analyticon', in *Seminar XVII: The Other Side of Psychoanalysis* (1969–70), trans. by Russell Grigg (London: Norton, 2007), pp. 197–208 (pp. 207–8).

[6] Miller, 'Microscopia: An Introduction to the Reading of *Television*' (1990), in *Television* (1974), trans. by Denis Hollier, Rosalind Kruss, and Annette Michelson, ed. by Joan Copjec (London: Norton, 1990), pp. xxi–xxxi (p. ixx).

going unregistered by them—and not because there was a missing object from the epistemological field of Marxism that was waiting to emerge. For him, this is why psychoanalysis is so important. Lacan's position in the history of Marxism is difficult to register, because Lacan is part of the history of the *failure* of Marxism; a failure that is, as many of Lacan's contemporaries were becoming aware, integral to what Marxism is.

This is why there is not something in Lacan that can be allied to an existing political project. Lacan deliberately struck to the very foundations of something about his historical moment, and left them in disarray. What it would mean to extract a politics from this is not established by Lacan, except for the provisional, potential position he gives to the psychoanalyst. Lacan was attempting to articulate the underlying structures of civilisation at a particular moment in history. He is in no way suggesting that these structures will not change, that he gives a complete articulation of them, or that psychoanalysis marks some kind of ending or completion of knowledge in history. What he is saying is that psychoanalysis makes it possible to be aware of these changes in a new way. Hence the importance of understanding what he thinks is missing in Marx, and of not conflating his position to Marx's.

There is a tendency in existing literature to absorb Lacan back into other co-ordinates, and particularly to Hegel and Marx. This, however, is not the way Lacan himself reads his interlocutors. Lacan's own approach to history, particularly the history of philosophy, is not one of completion, competition, or succession. As he articulates in his readings of Marx's and of Kierkegaard's critiques of Hegel, what he instead prioritises, and implicitly aspires to, is the realisation of 'the truth' of a given, pre-existing formula.[7] As he says in 1946, 'neither Socrates nor Descartes, nor Marx, nor Freud, can be "gone beyond", insofar as they carried out their research with the passion to unveil that has an object: truth'.[8] The

[7] Kierkegaard, says Lacan, is 'the one who imparts the truth of the Hegelian formula'. See Lacan, Lesson of 21 November 1962, 'Chapter II: Anxiety, Sign of Desire', in *Seminar X: Anxiety* (1962–63), ed. by Jacques-Alain Miller, trans. by A.R. Price (Cambridge: Polity, 2014), pp. 16–28 (p. 25); and Chap. 2, pp. 73–75. As Chap. 4 argued, Lacan takes Marx to make a similar articulation of the truth of Hegel. See p. 204 above.

[8] Lacan', 'Presentation on Psychical Causality', in *Écrits* (London: Norton, 2006), pp. 123–160 (p. 157).

reason he says that psychoanalysis responds to a turning point of knowledge in history is not because he thinks that it goes 'beyond' Marx, but because, for him, psychoanalysis allows something to be understood about the unstoppable, death-driven movement to which science and capitalism amount—and also about Marx's own part in that movement. Without psychoanalysis, any politics derived from Marx therefore defeats itself. With psychoanalysis, something else becomes possible. This would be a realisation of the truth of Lacan's own formulas, something that can only be achieved by understanding his own position in history.

Bibliography

Alquié, Ferdinand, *The Philosophy of Surrealism*, trans. by Bernard Waldrop (University of Michigan Press, 1965)

Althusser, Louis, 'Contradiction and Overdetermination' (1962), in *For Marx*, trans. by Ben Brewster (London: Verso, 2005a), pp. 87–128

———, 'Freud and Lacan' (1964), in *Writings on Psychoanalysis*, ed. by Olivier Corpet and Françoise Matheron, trans. by Jeffrey Mehlman (Columbia University Press, 1999a) pp. 7–32

———, 'From *Capital* to Marx's Philosophy' (1965), in *Reading Capital*, trans. by Ben Brewster and David Fernbach (London: Verso, 2016a), pp. 11–70

———, 'Ideology and Ideological State Apparatuses' (1970), in *On the Reproduction of Capitalism: Ideology and Ideological State Apparatuses*, trans. by G.M. Goshgarian (London: Verso, 2014), pp. 232–272

———, 'On the Materialist Dialectic' (1962), in *For Marx*, trans. by Ben Brewster (Verso, 2005b), pp. 161–218

———, 'On the Young Marx' (1961), *For Marx*, trans. by Ben Brewster (London: Verso, 2005c), pp. 49–86

———, 'The Place of Psychoanalysis in the Human Sciences' (1963–4), in *Psychoanalysis and the Human Sciences*, trans. by Steven Rendall (New York: Columbia University Press, 2016b), pp. 1–44

M. Maher, *Symptom Invented*, The Palgrave Lacan Series,
https://doi.org/10.1007/978-3-032-12267-4

———, 'Psychoanalysis and Psychology' (1963–4), in *Psychoanalysis and the Human Sciences*, trans. by Steven Rendall (New York: Columbia University Press, 2016c), pp. 45–88

———, *Lire le Capital* (Paris: Maspero, 1965)

———, *Reading Capital*, trans. by Ben Brewster and David Fernbach (London: Verso, 2016d)

———, *Essays in Self-Criticism*, trans. by Grahame Lock (London: New Left Books, 1976)

———, 'Correspondence with Jacques Lacan', in *Writings on Psychoanalysis*, ed. by Olivier Corpet and Françoise Matheron, trans. by Jeffrey Mehlman (Columbia University Press, 1999b), pp. 145–174

———, 'On Lévi-Strauss' (1966), in *The Humanist Controversy*, ed. by Françoise Matheron, trans. by G.M. Goshgarian (London: Verso, 2003), pp. 19–32

Anan'yev, B. G., ed., *Psychological Science in the USSR, Vol. 1* (1959), trans. by US Joint Publications Research Service (1961)

Anderson, Kevin, 'The "Unknown" Marx's *Capital*, Volume I: The French Edition of 1872–75, 100 Years Later', *Review of Radical Political Economics*, 15, no. 4 (1983), 71–80

Aron, Raymond, *Mémoires: Cinquante Ans de réflexion politique* (Paris: Julliard, 1938)

Hollier, Denis ed., *The College of Sociology, 1937–39* (University of Minnesota Press, 1988)

Askofaré, Sidi, 'Le symptôme sociale' (1989), in *Marx et Lénine, Freud et Lacan, Actes de 2e Colloque de La Découverte Freudienne*, ed. by André Soueix (Toulouse, Mirail, 1992)

Asratyan, E.A., 'Switching in Conditioned Reflex Activity as a Basic Form of its Changeability', *Voprosy Psikhologii*, 1 (1955), 49–57

Bachelard, Gaston, *La formation de l'esprit scientifique: Contribution à une psychanalyse de la connaissance objective* (Paris: Vrin, 1938)

Bandyopadhyay, Pradeep, 'The Many Faces of French Marxism', *Science & Society*, 36, no. 2 (Summer, 1972) 129–157

Barrett, Michèle, 'Althusser's Marx, Althusser's Lacan', in *The Althusserian Legacy*, ed. E. Ann Kaplan and Michael Sprinkler (London: Verso, 1993), pp. 169–182

Baugh, Bruce, *French Hegel: From Surrealism to Postmodernism* (London: Routledge, 2003)

Bekhterev, *Obshchie osnory rejleksologii cheloveka* (Moscow–Petersburg, 1923)

Bekhterev, Vladimir, *Kollektivnaja refleksologija* (Petersburg, 1921)

Benton, Ted, *The Rise and Fall of Structural Marxism: Althusser and His Influence* (London: Macmillan, 1984)

Bianchi, Pietro, 'The Discourse and the Capitalist. Lacan, Marx, and the Question of the Surplus', *Filosofski vestnik*, 31, no. 2 (2010), 123–137

Billig, Michael, 'Lacan's Misuse of Psychology: Evidence, Rhetoric and the Mirror Stage', *Theory, Culture & Society*, 23, no. 4, 1–26

Breton, André, 'Surrealist Situation of the Object' (1935), in *Manifestoes of Surrealism*, trans. by Richard Seaver and Helen R. Lane (University of Michigan Press, 1969a), pp. 255–278

———, 'What is Surrealism?' (1934), in *What is Surrealism? Selected Writings*, ed. by Franklin Rosemont (New York: Monad, 1978), pp. 151–187

———, 'Manifesto of Surrealism' (1924), in *Manifestoes of Surrealism*, trans. by Richard Seaver and Helen R. Lane (University of Michigan Press, 1969b), pp. 1–48

Bruner, Jermone, 'Prologue to the English Edition', in *The Collected Works of L.S. Vygotsky, Vol. 1: Problems of General Psychology*, ed. by Robert W. Rieber and Aaron S. Carton, trans. by Norris Minick (London: Plenum Press, 1987), pp. 1–16

Brunschvicg, Léon, *Le progrès de la conscience dans la philosophie occidentale* (Paris: Alcan, 1927)

Bykhovsky, Bernard, 'O Metodologicheskih Osnovaniyah Psikhoanaliticheskogo Ucheniya Freuda', *Pod Znamenem Marxizma*, 11–12 (1923)

Caillois, Roger, 'Introduction' (1938), in *The College of Sociology*, ed. by Hollier (University of Minnesota Press, 1988a), pp. 9–11

Caillois, Roger, et. al., 'Note on the Foundation of a College of Sociology' (1937), in *The College of Sociology*, ed. by Hollier (University of Minnesota Press, 1988b), pp. 3–5

Canguilhem, Georges, *La connaissance de la vie* (Paris: Vrin, 1952)

———, *La formation du concept de réflexe aux XVIIe et XVIII siècles* (Paris: Vrin, 1955)

Cardoso, Mauricio, and Vinicius Darriba, 'A Referência a Marx no Ensino de Lacan', *Psicologia; Teoria e Pesquisa*, 32, no. 1 (January–March 2016)

Cléro, Jean-Pierre, 'Hyppolite et Lacan', *La Cause freudienne*, 70, no. 3 (2008), 122–128

Colletti, Lucio, *Il Marxismo e Hegel* (Laterza, 1969)

Coombs, Nathan, *History and Event: From Marxism to Contemporary French Theory* (Edinburgh: Edinburgh University Press, 2015)

Cornu, Auguste, *Karl Marx, l'homme et l'œvure: De l'hégélianisme au matérialisme historique (1818–1845)* (Paris: Librairie Félix Alcan, 1934)
Corpet, Oliver, and Francois Matheron, 'Introduction to "Freud and Lacan"', in *Writings on Psychoanalysis*, ed. by Olivier Corpet and Françoise Matheron, (Columbia University Press, 1999), pp. 7–12
Crevel, Renée, 'Notes en vue d'une psychodialectique', *Le Surréalisme au service de la révolution* 5 (May 1933). Reprinted in *Le Surréalisme au service de la revolution: Collection complète*, ed. André Breton (Paris, 1976), pp. 48–52
Dalí, Salvador, 'Paranoiac-Critical Interpretations of the Obsessive Image of Millet's "Angelus", in *The Tragic Myth of Millet's Angelus,* trans. and ed. by Albert Reynolds Morse (The Salvador Dalí Museum, 1986), pp. 215–16
Dews, Peter, 'Structuralism and the French Epistemological Tradition', in *Althusser: A Critical Reader*, ed. by Gregory Elliott (Wiley-Blackwell, 1994), pp. 104–141
Dolar, Mladen, and Slavoj Žižek, *Opera's Second Death* (London: Routledge, 2001)
Dolto, Françoise, 'Notes de Françoise Dolto à la S.P.P. le 16 juin 1936', in Gérard Guillerault, *Le miroir et la psyché. Dolto, Lacan et le stade du miroir* (Paris: Gallimard, 2003), pp. 267–272
Dosse, François, *History of Structuralism* (University of Minnesota Press, 1998)
Éluard, Paul, *Poésie involontaire et poésie intentionnelle* (Villeneuve-les-Avignon: Seghers, 1942)
Engels, Friedrich, *Dialektik der Natur* (1925) (Berlin: Dietz Verlag, 1978)
——, 'The Part Played by Labour in the Transition from Ape to Man', *Die Neue Zeit*, 14, 545–556.
——, *The Dialectics of Nature* (London: Lawrence and Wishart, 1955)
Etkind, Alexander, *Eros of the Impossible* (London; Routledge, 1997)
Ford, Russell, 'Introduction to "Hegel and Kierkegaard"', in *Transcendence and the Concrete*, pp. 90–92
Foucault, Michel, 'Discourse on Language', in *The Archaeology of Knowledge and the Discourse on Language*, trans. by Alan Mark Sheridan Smith (New York: Pantheon, 1972), pp. 215–237
Freud, Sigmund, 'Project for a Scientific Psychology' (1950 [1895]), in *The Standard Edition of the Complete Psychological Works of Sigmund Freud, Vol. 1 (1866–1899): Pre-Psycho-Analytic Publications and Unpublished Drafts*, trans. by James Strachey (London: The Hogarth Press, 1966), pp. 281–391
———, 'Formulations on the Two Principles of Mental Functioning' (1911), in *The Standard Edition of the Complete Psychological Works of Sigmund Freud,*

Vol. XII (1911–1913), trans. by James Strachey (London: The Hogarth Press, 1957a), pp. 213–226

———, 'Repression' (1915), in *The Standard Edition of the Complete Psychological Works of Sigmund Freud, Vol. XIV (1914–1916): On the History of the Psycho-Analytic Movement, Papers on Metapsychology and Other Works*, trans. by James Strachey (London: The Hogarth Press, 1957b), pp. 146–158

———, 'The Resistances to Psycho-Analysis' (1925 [1924]), *The Standard Edition of the Complete Psychological Works of Sigmund Freud, Vol. XIX (1923–1925): The Ego and the Id and Other Works*, trans. by James Strachey (London: The Hogarth Press, 1961), pp. 211–224

———, 'Lecture XVII. Fixation to Traumas—The Unconscious' (1917 [1916–17]), in *The Standard Edition of the Complete Psychological Works of Sigmund Freud, Vol. XVI (1916–1917): Introductory Lectures to Psycho-Analysis (Part III)*, trans. by James Strachey (London: The Hogarth Press, 1963), pp. 271–285

———, Sigmund 'A Difficulty in the Path of Psycho-Analysis' (1925), *The Standard Edition of the Complete Psychological Works of Sigmund Freud, Vol. XVII: An Infantile Neurosis and Other Works*, trans. by James Strachey (London: The Hogarth Press, 1955), pp. 135–144

———, 'Lecture XXXV: The Question of a *Weltanschauung*' (1933), in *The Standard Edition of the Complete Psychological Works of Sigmund Freud, Vol. XXII (1932–1936): New Introductory Lectures on Psycho-Analysis and Other Works*, trans. by James Strachey (London: The Hogarth Press, 1964), pp. 158–184

Fridman, B.D., 'Osnovnye psikhologicheskie vozrenija Frejda i teorija istoricheskogo materializma' (1925), In *Pstkhologija i marksizm*, ed. by K. N. Kornilov, pp. 113–159

Georgin, Robert, *Le temps freudien du verbe* (Lausanne: L'Âge d'Homme, coll. "Spinx", 1975)

———, *Lacan* (Lausanne: L'Âge d'Homme, 1977)

———, *L'inceste et ses tabous: Essai sur le mythe de la déesse* (Paris: Cistre, 1993)

Godelier, Maurice, *Rationalité et Irrationalité en Economie* (Paris: Éd. Maspéro, 1966)

van Haute, Phillippe, 'Psychanalyse et existentialisme: A propos de la theorie lacanienne de la subjectivitie' *Man and World: An International Philosophical Review* (October 1990), 453–472

Heckman, John, 'Introduction', in Jean Hyppolite (1946), *Genesis and Structure of Hegel's Phenomenology of Spirit*, trans. Samuel Cherniak and John Heckman (Illinois, Northwestern University Press, 1974), pp. xv–xli

Hegel, Georg Wilhelm Friedrich, *Early Theological Writings*, trans. by Thomas Malcolm Knox (Chicago: University of Chicago Press, 1948)

———, *The Phenomenology of Mind*, trans. by James Black Baillie (London: George Allen and Unwin, 1964)

Hirch, Arthur, *The French New Left: An Intellectual History from Sartre to Gorz* (Boston: South End Press, 1981)

Hudgins, Clarence Virginius, 'Conditioning and the Voluntary Control of the Pupillary Light Reflex', *Journal of General Psychology*, 8, no. 3 (1933), 3–51

Hyppolite, Jean, 'Les Travaux de Jeunesse de Hegel d'après des ouvrages récents', *Revue de Métaphysique et de Morale*, 3 (July 1935), 399–426

———, 'Vie et prise de conscience de la vie dans la philosophie Hégélienne d'Iéna', *Revue de Métaphysique et de Morale*, 1 (January 1938), 45–61

———, *La Phénomenologie de l'esprit* (Paris: Aubier, 1939)

———, 'L'existence dans la phénoménologie de Hegel', *Etudes germaniques* 1 (1946), pp. 131–141

———, 'The Concept of Existence in the Hegelian Phenomenology' (1946), in *Studies on Marx and Hegel*, trans. by John O'Neill (New York: Harper, 1969), pp. 22–34

———, *Introduction to Hegel's Philosophy of History* (1948), trans. by Bond Harris and Jacqueline Bouchard Spurlock (Gainesville: University Press of Florida, 1996)

———, *Logic and Existence: An Essay on Hegel's Logic* (1953), trans. by Leonard Lawler and Amit Sen (New York: State of New York Press, 1997)

Jalley, Émile, 'Introduction a la lecture de *La Vie Mentale*', in Wallon, *La Vie Mentale* (Paris: Lacan, *De la psychose paranoïaque dans ses rapports avec la personalité, suivi de Premiere écrits sur la paranoia*, (1932) (Paris: de Seuil, 1975) pp. 149–215

Jay, Martin, *Marxism and Totality: The Adventures of a Concept from Lukáks to Habermas* (Berkeley: University of California Press, 1984)

Jones, Irwin, and Helena Motoh, 'From Structuralism to Lacan—Interview with Mladen Dolar', in *Zizek and his Contemporaries: On the Emergence of the Slovenian Lacan* (2014, Bloomsbury), pp. 93–111

Joravsky, David, *Russian Psychology: A Critical History* (Oxford: Basil Blackwell, 1989)

Judt, Tony, *Marxism and the French Left: Studies on Labour and Politics in France, 1830–1981* (Oxford: Oxford University Press, 1985)

Kelly, Michael, *Modern French Marxism* (London: Wiley-Blackwell, 1982)

Kierkegaard, Søren, *Concluding Unscientific Postscript* (1846), trans. by David Ferdinand Swenson (Princeton: Princeton University Press, 1944)

Knudsen, Daniel C., Jillian M. Rickly, and Elizabeth S. Vidon, 'The Fantasy of Authenticity: Touring with Lacan', *Annals of Tourism Research*, 58 (May 2016), 33–45

Kojève, Alexandre, 'Résumé du cours 1934–1935 (Extrait de l'Annuaire de 1935–1936 de l'Ecole Pratique des Hautes Études, section des Sciences religieuses)', in *Introduction à la lecture de Hegel: Leçons sur la "Phénoménologie de l'Esprit professes de 1933 à 1939 à l'École des Hautes Études*, ed. by Raymond Queneau (Paris: Gallimard, 1947), pp. 74–76

———, 'A Note on Eternity, Time, and the Concept: Complete Text of the Sixth through Eight Lectures of the Academic Year 1938–1939', in *Introduction to the Reading of Hegel: Lectures on the "Phenomenology of Spirit"*, ed. by Allan Bloom, trans. by James H. Nichols, Jr. (London: Cornell University Press, 1969a), pp. 100-149

———, 'Philosophy and Wisdom: Complete Text of the First Two Lectures of the Academic Year 1938–1939', in *Introduction to the Reading of Hegel: Lectures on the "Phenomenology of Spirit"*, ed. by Allan Bloom, trans. by James H. Nichols, Jr. (London: Cornell University Press, 1969b), pp. 75–99

———, 'In Place of an Introduction' (1939), in *Introduction to the Reading of Hegel: Lectures on the "Phenomenology of Spirit"*, ed. by Allan Bloom, trans. by James H. Nichols, Jr. (London: Cornell University Press, 1969c), pp. 3–30

Koyré, Alexandre, (1930), 'Rapport sur l'état des études hégéliennes en France', in *Études d'histoire de la pensée philosophique* (Paris: A. Colin, 1961), pp. 205–230

———, 'Review of *Le malheur de la conscience dans la philosophie de Hegel* by Jean Wahl', *Revue Philosophique de la France et de l'Étranger* (July-December 1930), 136–143

———, *From the Closed World to the Infinite Universe* (Baltimore: John Hopkins Press, 1957)

———, *Newtonian Studies* (London: Chapman & Hall, 1965)

Kozulin, Alex, *Psychology in Utopia: Toward a Social History of Soviet Psychology* (Massachusetts: MIT Press, 1984)

Krementsov, Nikolai, *Stalinist Science* (Princeton: Princeton University Press, 1997),

Kubie, Lawrence, 'Pavlov, Freud and Soviet Psychiatry', *Behavioural Science*, 4 (1959), 29–34

Kurzweil, Edith *The Age of Structuralism* (London: Transaction Publishers, 1996)

Lacan, Jacques, J. Lévy-Valensi and Pierre Migault, 'Écrits « inspirés » : schizographie', *Les Annales Médico-Psychologiques*, 2 (1931), 508–522

——, 'Motifs du crime paranoïaque: le crime des sœurs Papin' (1933), *Le Minotaure* 3/4: 100–103

——, Jacques, 'La Famille' (1938), in *Encyclopedie Française, Vol. 8: La Vie mentale*, ed. by Henri Wallon (Paris: Société de gestion de l'Encyclopédie Française, 1938)

——, 'Logical Time and the Assertion of Anticipated Certainty' (1945), in *Écrits*, trans. by Bruce Fink (London: Norton, 2006a), pp. 161–175

——, Jacques, 'Presentation on Psychical Causality' (1946), in *Écrits*, trans. by Bruce Fink (London: Norton, 2006b), pp. 123–160

——, Jacques, 'Aggressiveness in Psychoanalysis', (1948) in *Écrits* (London: Norton, 2006c), pp. 82–101

——, 'The Mirror Stage as Formative of the *I* Function as Revealed in Psychoanalytic Experience', in *Écrits* (London: Norton, 2006d), pp. 75–81

——, 'Presentation on Transference' (1951), in *Écrits*, trans. by Bruce Fink (London: Verso, 2006e), pp. 176–188

——, 'The Symbolic, the Imaginary, and the Real' (1953), in *On the Names-of-the-Father*, trans. by Bruce. Fink (London: Polity, 2015a), pp. 1–52

——, 'The Function and Field of Speech and Language in Psychoanalysis' (1953), in *Écrits*, trans. by Bruce Fink (London: Norton, 2006f), pp. 197–268

——, 'Seminar on "The Purloined Letter"' (1955), in *Écrits*, trans. by Bruce Fink (London: Verso, 2006g), pp. 6–48

——, *Seminar I: Freud's Papers on Technique (1953–1954)*, ed. by Jacques-Alain Miller, trans. by John Forrester (London: Norton, 1991a)

——, *Seminar II: The Ego in Freud's Theory and in the Technique of Psychoanalysis (1954–1955)*, ed. by Jacques-Alain Miller, trans. by Sylvana Tomaselli (London: Norton, 1991b)

——, *Seminar III: The Psychoses (1955–1956)*, ed. by Jacques-Alain Miller, trans. by Russell Grigg (London: Norton, 1997)

——, *The Seminar of Jacques Lacan, Book V: Formations of the Unconscious*, ed. by Jacques-Alain Miller, trans. by Russell Grigg (London: Polity, 2017a)

——, *Seminar VIII: Transference* (1960–61), ed. by Jacques-Alain Miller, trans. by Bruce Fink (Cambridge: Polity, 2015b)

——, 'The Subversion of the Subject and the Dialectic of Desire in the Freudian Unconscious' (1960), in *Écrits*, trans. by Bruce Fink (London: Norton, 2006h), pp. 671–702

——, *Seminar IX: Identification* (1961–1962), unpublished

——, *Seminar IX: Identification* (1961–1962), trans. by Cormac Gallagher, <http://www.lacaninireland.com/web/wp-content/uploads/2010/06/Seminar-IX-Amended-Iby-MCL-7.NOV_.20111.pdf>, [accessed 26 March 2022]

——, *Seminar X: Anxiety* (1962–63), ed. by Jacques-Alain Miller, trans. by A.R. Price (Cambridge: Polity, 2014)

——, *Seminar XI: The Four Fundamental Concepts of Psychoanalysis* (1964–1965), ed. by Jacques-Alain Miller, trans. by Alan Sheridan (London: Norton, 1998a)

——, *Seminar XII: Crucial Problems for Psychoanalysis* (1964–1965), unpublished

——, *Seminar XII: Crucial Problems for Psychoanalysis* (1964–1965a), trans. by Cormac Gallagher, <http://www.lacaninireland.com/web/wp-content/uploads/2010/06/12-Crucial-problems-for-psychoanalysis.pdf>, [accessed 26 March 2022]

——, *Seminar XIII: The Object of Psychoanalysis* (1965–1966), unpublished

——, *Seminar XIII: The Object of Psychoanalysis* (1965b–1966), trans. by Cormac Gallagher, <http://www.lacaninireland.com/web/wp-content/uploads/2010/06/13-The-Object-of-Psychoanalysis1.pdf>, [accessed 26 March 2022]

——, 'On the Subject Who Is Finally In Question' (1966), in *Écrits*, trans. by Bruce Fink (London: Verso, 2006i), pp. 189–196

——, *Écrits* (1966), trans. B. Fink (London: Norton, 2006j)

——, *Seminar XIV: The Logic of Phantasy* (1966–1967a), unpublished

——, *Seminar XIV: The Logic of Phantasy* (1966–1967), trans. by Cormac Gallagher, <http://www.lacaninireland.com/web/wp-content/uploads/2010/06/14-Logic-of-Phantasy-Complete.pdf>, [accessed 26 March 2022]

——, *Seminar XV: The Psychoanalytic Act* (1967–1968), unpublished

——, *Seminar XV: The Psychoanalytic Act* (1967b–1968), trans. by Cormac Gallagher, <http://www.lacaninireland.com/web/wp-content/uploads/2010/06/Book-15-The-Psychoanalytical-Act.pdf>, [accessed 26 March 2022]

——, *Le Séminaire de Jacques Lacan, Livre XVI: D'un Autre à l'autre (1968–1969)*, ed. by Jacques-Alain Miller (Paris: Éditions de Seuil, 2006k)

——, *Seminar XVI: From an Other to the other* (1968–69), ed. by Jacques-Alain Miller, trans. by Bruce Fink (London: Polity, 2024a)

——, *La Séminaire, Livre XVII, L'envers de la psychanalyse (1969–1970)*, ed. by Jacques-Alain Miller (Paris: Seuil, 1998b)
——, *Seminar XVII: The Other Side of Psychoanalysis* (1969–1970), trans. by Russell Grigg (London: Norton, 1991c)
——, 'Radiophonie', *Scilicet 2/3* (September 1970), 55–99
——, 'Radiophonie', in *Autres écrits* (Paris: Seuil, 2001), pp. 403–447
——, *Le Séminaire, Livre XVIII, D'un discours qui ne serait pas du semblant (1971)*, ed. by Jacques-Alain Miller (Paris: Seuil, 2007)
——, *Seminar XVIII: On a Discourse that Might not Be a Semblance* (1971), ed. by Jacques-Alain Miller, trans. by Bruce Fink (London: Polity, 2024b)
——, *Le Séminaire, Livre XIX, … ou pire (1971–1972)*, ed. by Jacques-Alain Miller (Paris: Éditions du Seuil, 2011)
——, *Seminar XIX: Or Worse… (1971–1972)*, ed. by Jacques-Alain Miller, trans. by Adrian R. Price (Cambridge: Polity, 2018)
——, *Talking to Brick Walls: A Series of Presentations in the Chapel at Sainte-Anne Hospital*, trans. by Adrian R. Price (Cambridge: Polity, 2017b)
Langford, Peter E., *Vygotsky's Developmental and Educational Psychology* (Hove: Psychology Press, 2005)
Laurent, Éric, 'La société du symptôme', *Quarto*, 79 (June 2003), 3–9
Lefebvre, Henri, *Les temps des méprises* (Paris: Stock 1975)
Lefebvre, Henri, and Norbert Guterman, *La Conscience mystifiée* (Paris: Gallimard, 1936)
Lenin, Vladimir, *Materialism and Empirio-Criticism* (1908) (Peking: Foreign Languages Press, 1972)
Leont'ev, Alexei Nikolaevich, 'On Vygotsky's Creative Development', in *The Collected Works of L.S. Vygotsky, Vol. 3: Problems of the Theory and History of Psychology*, trans. by René van der Veer (New York: Springer, 1997), pp. 9–32
Lévi-Strauss, Claude, *Triste Tropiques* (1955) (Penguin Classics, 2011)
Levitin, Karl, 'A Criminal Investigation', *Journal of Russian and Eastern European Psychology*, 36, no. 5 (1998), 46–75
Lewis, William S., *Louis Althusser and the Traditions of French Marxism* (Lanham: Lexington Books, 2005)
Lucchelli, Juan Pablo, and Todd McGowan, 'The Early Lacan: Five Unpublished Letters from Jacques Lacan to Alexandre Kojève', *American Imago*, 73, No. 3 (Fall 2016): 325–341
Luria, Alexander, 'Psikhoanaliz, kak sistema monistieheskoj psikhologii' (1925), in *Psikhologija i rnarksizm*, ed. by Konstantin Nikolaevich Kornilov (Leningrad: Gosudarstvennoe Izdatel'stvo), pp. 47–80

Macey, David, 'Althusser and Lacan', in *Althusser: A Critical Reader*, ed. Gregory Elliott (Oxford: Blackwell, 1994), pp. 142–158

———, *Lacan in Contexts* (London: Verso, 1988),

Marx, Karl, and Friedrich Engels, 'Theses on Feuerbach' (1845), in *The German Ideology*, trans. by Christopher John Arthur (New York: International Publishers, 1973), pp. 121–123

Marx, Karl, *Capital: A Critique of Political Economy, Volume 1* (1867), trans. by Ben Fowkes (London: Penguin, 1976)

———, 'Afterword to the Second German Edition' (1873), in *Capital: A Critique of Political Economy*, trans. by Samuel Moore and Edward Aveling (London: Lawrence and Wishart, 1974), pp. 12–22

Masserman, Jules Homan, 'Language, Behaviour and Dynamic Psychiatry', *International Journal of Psychoanalysis* (1944), 1–7

Maublanc, René, 'Hegel et Marx', in *A la lumière de Marxisme* (Paris: Editions Sociales Internationales, 1935), pp. 189–232

McGarr, Paul, Alex Callinicos, and John Rees, *Marxism and the Great French Revolution* (London: International Socialism, 1989)

Miller, Jacques-Alain, 'Microscopia: An Introduction to the Reading of *Television*' (1990), in *Television* (1974), trans. by Denis Hollier, Rosalind Kruss, and Annette Michelson, ed. by Joan Copjec (London: Norton, 1990)

———, 'A Reading of the Seminar *From an Other to the other*, Part I', trans. by Barbara P. Fulks, *lacanian ink*, 29 (2007), 8–61

Miller, Martin A., *Freud and the Bolsheviks: Psychoanalysis in Imperial Russia and the Soviet Union* (New York: Yale University Press, 1998)

Montag, Warren, 'Spinoza and Althusser Against Hermeneutics: Interpretation or Invention?', in *The Althusserian Legacy* ed. by E. Ann Kaplan and Michael Sprinkler (London: Verso, 1993), pp. 51–58

Özselçuk, Ceren, and Yahya M. Madra, 'Enjoyment as an Economic Factor: Reading Marx with Lacan', *Subjectivity*, 3 (2010), 323–347

Pavón-Cuéllar, David, *Lacan, lecteur de Marx* (Rouen: Universite de Rouen, 2013)

———, 'Lacanianizing Marxism: The Effects of Lacan in Readings of Marx and Marxist Thinkers', *Critique*, 6, no. 1 (May 2019), 262–289

Politzer, Georges, *Critique of the Foundations of Psychology: The Psychology of Psychoanalysis* (1928), trans. by Maurice Apprey (Pittsburgh: Duquesne University Press, 1994)

———, *Principes élémentaire de philosophie* (1935–1936) (Paris: Éditions sociales, 1970)

———, [under the pseudonym Th. W. Morris], 'Le fin de la psychanalyse', *La Pensée* 3 (October–December 1939), 13–23

———, *La Crise de la Psychologie Contemporaine* (Paris: Éditions Sociales, 1947)

———, *Écrits II: Les Fondements de la Psychologie*, ed. by J. Debouzy (Paris: Editions Sociales, 1969)

Poster, Mark, *Existential Marxism in Postwar France: From Sartre to Althusser* (Princeton: Princeton University Press, 1975)

Proctor, Hannah, '"A Country Beyond the Pleasure Principle": Alexander Luria, Death Drive and Dialectic in Soviet Russia, 1917–1930', *Psychoanalysis and History*, 18, no. 2 (2016), 155–182

Regnault, François, 'Le Marx de Lacan', *La Lettre Mensuelle de l'ECF*, 242 (2005), 4–6

Ricoeur, Paul 'Althusser's Theory of Ideology', in *Althusser: A Critical Reader*, ed. by Gregory Elliot (Wiley-Blackwell, 1994), pp. 44–72

Rieber Robert W., and Jeffrey Wollock, 'Prologue: Vygotsky's "Crisis" and Its Meaning Today', in *The Collected Works of L.S. Vygotsky, Vol. 3: Problems of the Theory and History of Psychology*, trans. by René van der Veer (New York: Springer, 1997), pp. vii–xii

Roth, Michael Scott, *Knowing and History: Appropriations of Hegel in Twentieth-Century France* (Cornell University Press, 1988)

Roudinesco, Elisabeth, *Jacques Lacan & Co.: A History of Psychoanalysis in France, 1925–1985* (1986), trans. by Jeffrey Mehlman (Chicago: University of Chicago Press, 1990)

———, *Jacques Lacan: An Outline of a Life and History of a System of Thought* (1993), trans. Barbara Bray (New York: Columbia University Press, 1997)

———, 'The Mirror Stage: An Obliterated Archive', in *The Cambridge Companion to Lacan* (Cambridge: Cambridge University Press, 2010), 25–34

Salerno, Roger A., 'Imagining Marx Imagining Lacan', *Critical Sociology*, 44, no. 2 (2018), 259–266

Sass, Louis A., 'Lacan: The Mind of the Modernist', *Continental Philosophy Review*, 48, no. 4 (December 2015), 409–443.

Simone de Beauvoir, *Memoirs of a Dutiful Daughter* (1958), trans. by James Kirkup (New York: Harper, 1959)

Stalin, Joseph, 'Dialectical and Historical Materialism', in *Leninism: Selected Writings* (New York, 1942) pp. 406–433.

Stavrakakis, Yannis, 'Wallon, Lacan and the Lacanians: Citation Practices and Repression', in *Theory, Culture and Society*, 24, no. 4 (2007), 131–138

Sturrock, John, *Structuralism and Since* (Oxford: Oxford Paperbacks, 1980)

Tomšič, Samo, 'Homology: Marx and Lacan', in *Journal of the Jan van Eyck Circle for Lacanian Ideology Critique*, 5 (2012), 98–112

———, *The Capitalist Unconscious* (London: Verso, 2013)
Trần Đức Thảo, 'Le "noyau rationnel" dans la dialectique hégélienne', in *La Pensée* (January–February 1965), 4–5
———, *Investigations into the Origin of Language and Consciousness*, trans. Daniel J. Herman and Robert L. Armstrong (Boston: Reidel, 1984)
Valente, Joe, 'Lacan's Marxism, Marxism's Lacan (from Žižek to Althusser)', in *The Cambridge Companion to Lacan*, ed. Jean-Michel Rabaté (Cambridge: Cambridge University Press, 2010), 153–172
van der Veer, René, 'Henri Wallon's Theory of Early Child Development: The Role of Emotions', *Developmental Review*, 16 (1996), 364–390
Véra, Augusto, *La Philosophie de l'esprit* (Paris: Germer Baillière, 1867)
Vighi, Fabio, 'Capitalist Bulimia: Lacan on Marx and Crisis', *Crisis and Critique*, 3 (2016), 414–432
Vladimir Petrovich Zinchenko, 'Thought and Word: The Approaches of L.S. Vygotsky and G.G. Shpet', in *The Cambridge Companion to Vygotsky*, ed. by Harry Daniels, Michael Cole and James V. Wertsch (Cambridge: Cambridge University Press, 2007), pp. 212–245
Vygotsky, Lev Semyonovich, 'Consciousness as a Problem for the Psychology of Behaviour' (1925), in *The Collected Works of L.S. Vygotsky, Vol. 3: Problems of the Theory and History of Psychology*, trans. by René van der Veer (New York: Springer, 1997a), pp. 63–80
———, and Alexander Luria, 'Introduction to the Russian translation of Freud's *Beyond the Pleasure Principle*' (1925), in *The Vygotsky Reader*, ed. by René van der Veer and Jaan Valsiner (Oxford: Blackwell, 1994), pp. 10–18
———, 'The Methods of Reflexological and Psychological Investigation' (1926), in *The Collected Works of L.S. Vygotsky, Vol. 3: Problems of the Theory and History of Psychology*, trans. by René van der Veer (New York: Springer, 1997b), pp. 35–50
———, 'Mind, Consciousness, the Unconscious' (1930), in *The Collected Works of L.S. Vygotsky, Vol. 3: Problems of the Theory and History of Psychology*, trans. by René van der Veer (New York: Springer, 1997c), pp. 109–122
———, 'The Instrumental Method in Psychology' (1930), in *The Concept of Activity in Soviet Psychology*, ed. by James V. Wertsch (New York: Armonk, 1981), pp. 134–143
———, 'The Meaning of the Historical Crisis in Psychology', in *The Collected Works of L.S. Vygotsky, Vol. 3: Problems of the Theory and History of Psychology*, trans. by René van der Veer (New York: Springer, 1997d), pp. 233–244

———, *Thinking and Speech* (1934), in *The Collected Works of L.S. Vygotsky, Vol. 1: Problems of General Psychology*, ed. by Robert W. Rieber and Aaron S. Carton, trans. by Norris Minick (London: Plenum Press, 1987), pp. 39–288

Wahl, Jean 'Commentaire d'un passage de la "*Phénoménologie de l'Esprit*"', *Revue de Métaphysique et de Morale*, 34 (1927), 441–71

——— 'Commentaire d'un passage de la "*Phénoménologie de l'Esprit*"', *Revue de Métaphysique et de Morale*, 34, 'Note sur les démarches de la pensée de Hegel', *Revue Philosophique de la France et de l'Étranger* (January–June 1926), 281–289

——— 'Commentaire d'un passage de la "*Phénoménologie de l'Esprit*"', *Revue de Métaphysique et de Morale*, 34, 'Note sur les démarches de la pensée de Hegel', *Revue Philosophique de la France et de l'Étranger* (January–June, 'Commentary on a Passage from Hegel's *Phenomenology of Spirit*' (1929), in *Transcendence and the Concrete: Selected Writings*, ed. by Alan D. Schrift and Ian Alexander Moore, trans. by Bruce Baugh (New York: Fordham University Press, 2017), pp. 54–89

——, *Le Malheur de la conscience dans la philosophie de Hegel* (Paris: Les Editions Rieder, 1929)

Wallon, Henri, 'La conscience et la vie subconsciente' (1920), in Emile Jalley, *Wallon, lecteur de Freud et de Piaget* (Paris: Éditions sociales, 1981)

———, 'De l'image au réel, dans la pensée de l'enfant', *Revue philosophique de la France et de l'Étranger* (January–June 1930), 446–458

———, 'Comment se développe chez l'enfant la notion du corps propre' (1931), *Enfance*, 16, nos. 1–2 (1963), 121–150

———, 'Sur la septième conference internationale de psychotechnique' (1932), *Revue de Psychologie Appliquée de l'Est* (September 1931), 3–12

———, Henri, *La Vie Mentale* (1938) (Paris: Editions Sociales, 1982)

Westphal, Merold, 'Kierkegaard and Hegel', in *The Cambridge Companion to Kierkegaard*, ed. by Hannay, Alastair, and Gordon D. Marino (Cambridge: Cambridge University Press, 1998), pp. 101–124

Williams, Caroline, 'Philosophy and Psychoanalysis: Lacan, Kojève and Hyppolite on the Concept of the Subject', *Parallax*, 3, No. 1 (1997), 41–53

Zaretsky, Eli, *Secrets of the Soul: A Social and Cultural History of Psychoanalysis* (London: Three Rivers Press, 2005)

Žižek, Slavoj, *The Sublime Object of Ideology* (1989) (London: Verso, 2009)

———, *The Parallax View* (Cambridge, Massachusetts: MIT Press, 2006a)

———, *Lacan: The Silent Partners* (London: Verso, 2006b)

———, *Less Than Nothing: Hegel and the Shadow of Dialectical Materialism* (London: Verso, 2013)
———, *The Most Sublime Hysteric: Hegel with Lacan* (London: Polity, 2014)
Zupančič, Alenka, *What is Sex?* (London: MIT Press, 2017)
———, *Ethics of the Real* (London: Verso, 1995)
———, *Why Psychoanalysis? Three Interventions* (Aarhus University Press, 2008)

Index[1]

[1] Note: Page numbers followed by 'n' refer to notes.

M. Maher, *Symptom Invented*, The Palgrave Lacan Series,
https://doi.org/10.1007/978-3-032-12267-4

FSC
www.fsc.org
MIX
Papier | Fördert gute Waldnutzung
FSC® C083411

Kolibri 360 GmbH
Ferdinand-Jühlke-Straße 7
99095 Erfurt, Deutschland
produktsicherheit@kolibri360.de